Comprehensive Textbook of
APPLIED MICROBIOLOGY FOR NURSES

Comprehensive Textbook of
APPLIED MICROBIOLOGY FOR NURSES

As per the Revised Nursing Syllabus

Upasana Bhumbla MBBS MD CIC (Microbiology)
Associate Professor
Member Secretary and Infection Control Officer
In-Charge, Central Laboratory
Adesh Institute of Medical Sciences
Bathinda, Punjab, India

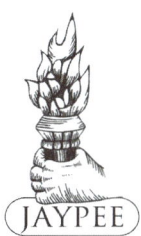

JAYPEE BROTHERS MEDICAL PUBLISHERS
The Health Sciences Publisher

New Delhi | London | Panama

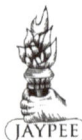

Jaypee Brothers Medical Publishers (P) Ltd.

Headquarters
Jaypee Brothers Medical Publishers (P) Ltd.
EMCA House
23/23-B, Ansari Road, Daryaganj
New Delhi - 110 002, India
Landline: +91-11-23272143, +91-11-23272703
+91-11-23282021, +91-11-23245672
Email: jaypee@jaypeebrothers.com

Corporate Office
Jaypee Brothers Medical Publishers (P) Ltd
4838/24, Ansari Road, Daryaganj
New Delhi 110 002, India
Phone: +91-11-43574357
Fax: +91-11-43574314
Email: jaypee@jaypeebrothers.com

Overseas Office
J.P. Medical Ltd.
83 Victoria Street, London
SW1H 0HW (UK)
Phone: +44 20 3170 8910
Fax: +44 (0)20 3008 6180
Email: info@jpmedpub.com

Website: www.jaypeebrothers.com
Website: www.jaypeedigital.com

© 2024, Jaypee Brothers Medical Publishers (P) Ltd.

The views and opinions expressed in this book are solely those of the original contributor(s)/author(s) and do not necessarily represent those of editor(s) and publisher of the book.

All rights reserved. No part of this publication may be reproduced, stored or transmitted in any form or by any means, electronic, mechanical, photocopying, recording or otherwise, without the prior permission in writing of the publishers.

All brand names and product names used in this book are trade names, service marks, trademarks or registered trademarks of their respective owners. The publisher is not associated with any product or vendor mentioned in this book.

Medical knowledge and practice change constantly. This book is designed to provide accurate, authoritative information about the subject matter in question. However, readers are advised to check the most current information available on procedures included and check information from the manufacturer of each product to be administered, to verify the recommended dose, formula, method and duration of administration, adverse effects and contraindications. It is the responsibility of the practitioner to take all appropriate safety precautions. Neither the publisher nor the author(s)/editor(s) assume any liability for any injury and/or damage to persons or property arising from or related to use of material in this book.

This book is sold on the understanding that the publisher is not engaged in providing professional medical services. If such advice or services are required, the services of a competent medical professional should be sought.

Every effort has been made where necessary to contact holders of copyright to obtain permission to reproduce copyright material. If any have been inadvertently overlooked, the publisher will be pleased to make the necessary arrangements at the first opportunity.

Inquiries for bulk sales may be solicited at: jaypee@jaypeebrothers.com

Comprehensive Textbook of Applied Microbiology for Nurses

First Edition: **2024**

ISBN: 978-93-5696-111-1

Printed at: Sterling Graphics Pvt. Ltd. India

Dedicated to

My Guruji
Grandparents
Parents and my beloved Sisters
whose blessings and encouragement have always
been with me throughout my endeavor

Preface

It gives me immense pleasure to announce the release of much awaited, First Edition of my book *Comprehensive Textbook of Applied Microbiology for Nurses,* designed as per newer nursing curriculum and covering detailed explanation of various aspects of hospital infection and patient safety. Compilation of this book was actually "Need of the hour" for nursing students. The revised curriculum embraces competency-based and outcome-based approach throughout the program, integrating and mastery learning and self-directed learning. The undergraduate nursing program is broad-based education within an academic curricular framework specifically directed to the development of critical thinking skills, competencies, appropriate to human and professional values.

Section I: Applied Microbiology

This book has been compiled and designed as per the latest curriculum so that the students can acquire understanding of fundamentals of microbiology, compare and contrast different microbes and comprehend the means of transmission and control of spread by various microorganisms. Section A comprises of four chapters focusing on General Introduction to Microbiology, General Characteristics of Microbes, Various Pathogenic Organisms and Immunity.

Section II: Infection Control and Safety

It will help students to acquire knowledge and develop competencies required for fundamental patient safety and infection control in delivering quality patient care. It also focuses on identifying patient safety indicators, preventing and managing hospital acquired infections and also in following universal precautions. This book will provide opportunities to students for practicing infection control measures in hospital and community settings. Section B comprises of eleven chapters focusing on Hospital Acquired Infections, Isolation Precautions and Use of Personal Protective Equipment, Hand Hygiene, Disinfection and Sterilization, Specimen Collection, Biomedical Waste Management, Antibiotic Stewardship, Patient Safety Indicators, International Patient Safety Goals, Safety Protocols and Employee Safety Indicators.

I hope the readers will find this book more informative and up-to-date. If any reader wishes to share any feedback, suggestions, updates, please feel free to write to us. Suggestions and new ideas for further improvement of this book shall always be appreciated.

Upasana Bhumbla

Acknowledgments

I wish to express my gratitude to my mentors, teachers for being a constant support during this venture. I am indebted to my teachers, Dr AS Dalal, Ex-Professor and Head, Department of Microbiology, RNT Medical College, Udaipur, Dr Gyaneshwari, Dr Dinesh Raj Mathur, Dr Balramji Omar, Professor, Department of Microbiology, All India Institute of Medical Sciences and Research, Rishikesh, for their valuable guidance and encouragement while writing this book.

My sincere thanks to my seniors in Microbiology, Dr Sunite A Ganju, Professor and Head, Department of Microbiology, SLB Government Medical College and Hospital, Mandi, Himachal Pradesh, Dr Bella Mahajan, Professor and Head, Department of Microbiology, ASSCOM, Jammu, Dr Sarabjit Sharma, Professor and Head, Department of Microbiology, SGRD, Amritsar, Dr Veenu Gupta, Professor and Head, Department of Microbiology, DMC, Ludhiana, Dr Ramgopal Saini, Registrar, Adesh University, Bathinda, for encouraging me to this endeavor and constantly inspiring me.

I am grateful to my team Ms Mandeep Kaur, for helping me to tackle the computer related issues and in compiling the manuscript. I am thankful to Mr Ansar for helping me in compiling few of the write-ups for a section. I am thankful to Dr Sabah Yaseen Shah, Assistant Professor, Department of Anatomy, Hamdard Institute of Medical Sciences and Research, New Delhi, Dr Pratibha Dhiman, Senior Consultant, Department of Haemato Oncology and BMT, Medanta Medicity, Gurugram who inspired me to accomplish the writing of this manuscript.

I also like to thank faculty and staff of my institute, whose support and help at various stages of preparation of this edition have been valuable.

I am very thankful to my nieces Sanya, Raisa and my nephew Ranraj for always being my support.

I am also thankful to M/s Jaypee Brothers Medical Publishers (P) Ltd, New Delhi, India, who helped and guided me, especially Shri Jitendar P Vij (Group Chairman), Mr Ankit Vij (Managing Director), Mr MS Mani (Group President), Dr Madhu Choudhary (Director–Educational Publishing), Ms Pooja Bhandari [Director–Production (Books and Journals)], Ms Sunita Katla (Executive Assistant to Group Chairman and Publishing Manager), Mr Ajay Kumar Sharma (Deputy General Manager), Ms Samina Khan (Executive Assistant to Director–Educational Publishing), Ms Jitika Royal (Content Strategist), Mr Rajesh Sharma (Production Coordinator), Ms Seema Dogra (Cover Visualizer), Mr Laxmidhar Padhiary (Proofreader), Mr Jagvir Singh Tomar (Typesetter), Mr Radhe Shyam Singh (Graphic Designer), and their team for helping me in making this book compiled.

Upasana Bhumbla

Contents

SECTION I: APPLIED MICROBIOLOGY

Chapter 1: Introduction 3–7
- Importance and Relevance to Nursing 3–4
- Historical Perspective 4–5
- Concepts and Terminology 6–7
- Principles of Microbiology 7

Chapter 2: General Characteristics of Microbes ... 8–37
- Structure and Classification of Microbes 8–9
- Morphological Types 10–11
- Size and Form of Bacteria 12–14
- Motility 15–16
- Colonization 17
- Growth and Nutrition of Microbes 18–19
- Temperature 20
- Moisture 20
- Laboratory Methods for Identification of Microorganisms 21–27
- Types of Staining: Simple, Differential Gram's, AFB, Special Capsular Staining, Negative Staining, Spore, LPCB, KOH Mount 28–31
- Culture and Media Preparation—Solid and Liquid; Types of Media—Semi-synthetic, Synthetic, Enriched, Enrichment, Selective and Differential Media. Pure Culture Techniques—Tube Dilution, Pour, Spread, Streak Plate, Anaerobic Cultivation of Bacteria 32–37

Chapter 3: Pathogenic Organisms.......................... 38–93
- Micro-organisms: Cocci—Gram Positive and Gram Negative; Bacilli—Gram Positive and Gram Negative 38–72
- Viruses 73–80
- Fungi: Superficial and Deep Mycosis 81–84
- Parasites 85–93

Chapter 4: Immunity 94–108
- Immunity: Types, Classification 94–97
- Immunoglobulins: Structure, Types and Properties 97–99
- Antigen and Antibody Reactions 99–100
- Serological Test 100–105
- Vaccines: Types and Classification, Storage and Handling, Cold Chain, Immunization for Various Diseases 106
- Immunization Schedule 107–108

SECTION II: INFECTION CONTROL AND SAFETY

Chapter 5: Hospital Acquired Infections 111–126
- Hospital Acquired Infections 111–113
- Bundle Approach:
  – Prevention of Central Line Associated Infections CLABSI 113–114
  – Prevention of Urinary Tract Infections (UTI) 114–116
  – Prevention of Surgical Site Infections (SSI) 116–119
  – Prevention of Ventilator Associated Events (VAE) 119–122
- Surveillance of HAI—Infection Control Team and Infection Control Committee 123–126

Chapter 6: Isolation Precautions and Use of Personal Protective Equipments 127–136
- Types of Isolation System, Standard Precaution and Transmission Based Precautions, Direct Contact, Droplet, Indirect 126–128
- Epidemiology and Infection Prevention—CDC Guidelines 128
- Effective Use of PPE 129–136

Chapter 7: Hand Hygiene....................................137–141
- Types of Hand Hygiene 137–138
- Hand Washing and Use of Alcohol Rub 139
- Moments of Hand Hygiene 139–140
- WHO Hand Hygiene Promotion 141

Chapter 8: Disinfection and Sterilization 142–146
- Definitions 142
- Types of Disinfection and Sterilization 143–144
- Environment Cleaning 144–145
- Equipment Cleaning 145
- Guides on Usage of Disinfectants 146
- Spaulding's Principle 146

Chapter 9: Specimen Collection 147–156
- Principles of Specimen Collection 147
- Type of Specimens 147–149
- Appropriate Vacutainers 149
- Collection Techniques and Special Considerations 150–156

Chapter 10: Biomedical Waste Management ..157–163
- Laundry Management Process and Infection Control and Prevention *157–159*
- Waste Management Process and Infection Prevention *160–161*
- Country Ordinance and BMW; National Guidelines 2017: Segregation of Wastes, Color Coded Waste Containers, Waste Collection and Storage, Packaging and Labeling; Transportation *162–163*

Chapter 11: Antibiotic Stewardship 164–166
- Importance of Stewardship *164*
- Antimicrobial Resistance *164–165*
- Prevention of MRSA, MDRO in Healthcare Setting *165–166*

Chapter 12: Patient Safety Indicators 167–189
- Care of Vulnerable Patients *167–169*
- Prevention of Iatrogenic Injury *170*
- Care of Lines, Drains and Tubings *170–171*
- Restrain Policy and Care—Physical and Chemical *171–173*
- Blood and Blood Transfusion Policy *173–175*
- Prevention of IV Complication *176–177*
- Prevention of Fall *177–178*
- Prevention of DVT *178–179*
- Shifting and Transporting of Patients *179–181*
- Surgical Safety *181*
- Prevention of Communication Errors *182–183*
- Documentation *184–185*
- Prevention of HAI *185–187*

Incidents and Adverse Events
- Capturing of Incidents *188*
- Root Cause Analysis (RCA) *188*
- Corrective and Preventive Action (CAPA) *189*

Chapter 13: International Patient Safety Goals 190–195
- Identify Patient Correctly *190–191*
- Improve Effective Communication *191–192*
- Improve Safety of High Alert Medication *193*
- Ensure Safe Surgery *193*
- Reduce the Risk of Healthcare Associated Infections *194*
- Reduce the Risk of Patient Harm Resulting from Falls *195*

Chapter 14: Safety Protocol 196–211
- 5'S (Sort, Set in Order, Shine, Standardize, Sustain) *196–197*
- Radiation Safety *198*
- Laser Safety *198–199*
- Fire Safety: Types and Classification of Fire; Fire Alarms; Firefighting Equipment *199–204*
- Hazardous Materials (HAZMAT) *205*
  - Types of Spill and Spillage Management *205–207*
  - Material Safety Data Sheet (MSDS) *208*
- Environmental Safety *208*
  - Risk Assessment *208–209*
  - Aspect Impact Analysis *209–210*
- Emergency Codes *210*
- Role of Nurse in Disaster *211*

Chapter 15: Employee Safety Indicators 212–218
- Vaccination—Needle Stick Injuries (NSI) Prevention *212–213*
- Annual Health Check Up *214*

Healthcare Worker Immunization Program and Management of Occupational Exposures
- Occupational Health Ordinance *215*
- Vaccination Program for Healthcare Staff *215*
- Needle Stick Injuries and Prevention and Postexposure Prophylaxis *215–218*

Index — *219*

Syllabus

SECTION I: APPLIED MICROBIOLOGY

PLACEMENT: III Semester

THEORY: 2 Credits (40 Hours)

PRACTICAL: 1 Credit (40 Hours) (Laboratory/Experiential Learning—L/E)

DESCRIPTION: This course is designed to enable students to acquire understanding of fundamentals of microbiology, compare and contrast different microbes and comprehend the means of transmission and control of spread by various microorganisms. It also provides opportunities for practicing infection control measures in hospital and community settings.

COMPETENCIES: On completion of the course, the students will be able to:
1. Identify the ubiquity and diversity of microorganisms in the human body and the environment
2. Classify and explain the morphology and growth of microbes
3. Identify various types of microorganisms
4. Explore mechanisms by which microorganisms cause disease
5. Develop understanding of how the human immune system counteracts infection by specific and non-specific mechanisms
6. Apply the principles of preparation and use of vaccines in immunization
7. Identify the contribution of the microbiologist and the microbiology laboratory to the diagnosis of infection

Unit	Time (hours) T	P	Learning outcomes	Contents	Teaching/learning activities	Assessment methods
I.	3		Explain concepts and principles of microbiology and its importance of nursing	**Introduction** • Importance and relevance to nursing • Historical perspective • Concepts and terminology • Principles of microbiology	• Lecture cum discussion	• Short answer • Objective type
II.	10	10 (L/E)	Describe structure, classification morphology and growth of bacteria	**General Characteristics of Microbes** • Structure and classification of microbes • Morphological types • Size and form of bacteria • Motility • Colonization • Growth and nutrition of microbes • Temperature • Moisture • Blood and body fluids • Laboratory methods for identification of Microorganisms • Types of staining—simple, differential (Gram's, AFB), special capsular staining (negative), spore, LPCB, KOH mount • Culture and media preparation solid and liquid. Types of media semisynthetic, synthetic, enriched enrichment selective and differential media. Pure culture techniques tube dilution, pour spread, streak plate. Anaerobic cultivation of bacteria	• Lecture cum discussion • Demonstration • Experiential learning through visual	• Short answer • Objective type

Unit	Time (hours) T	P	Learning outcomes	Contents	Teaching/learning activities	Assessment methods

III.	4	6 (L/E)	Describe the different disease producing organisms	**Pathogenic Organisms**
				• **Microorganisms:**
				  – Cocci—gram-positive and gram-negative
				  – Bacilli—gram-positive and gram-negative
				• Viruses
				• **Fungi:** Superficial and deep mycoses
				• Parasites
				• **Rodents and vectors:** Characteristics, source, portal of entry transmission of infection, identification of disease producing microorganisms
					• Lecture cum discussion
					• Demonstration
					• Experiential Learning through visual
						• Short answer
						• Objective type

IV.	3	4(L/E)	Explain the concepts of immunity, hypersensitivity and immunization	**Immunity** • **Immunity:** Types, classification • Antigen and antibody reaction • Hypersensitivity reaction • Serological tests • Immunoglobulins structure, types and properties • **Vaccines:** Types and classification, storage and handling, cold chain, Immunization for various diseases • Immunization schedule	• Lecture cum discussion • Demonstration • Visit to observe vaccine storage • Clinical practice	• Short answer • Objective type • Visit report

SECTION II: INFECTION CONTROL AND SAFETY

THEORY: 20 Hours

PRACTICAL/LABORATORY: 20 hours (Laboratory/Experiential Learning—L/E)

DESCRIPTION: This course is designed to help students to acquire knowledge and develop competencies required for fundamental patient safety and infection control in delivering patient care. It also focuses on identifying patient safety indicators, preventing and managing hospital acquired infections, and in following universal precautions.

COMPETENCIES: The students will be able to:
1. Develop knowledge and understanding of hospital acquired Infections (HAI) and effective practices for prevention.
2. Integrate the knowledge of isolation (barrier and reverse barrier) techniques in implementing various precautions.
3. Demonstrate and practice steps in hand washing and appropriate use of different types of PPE.
4. Illustrate various disinfection and sterilization methods and techniques.
5. Demonstrate knowledge and skill in specimen collection, handling and transport to optimize the diagnosis for treatment.
6. Incorporate the principles and guidelines of biomedical waste management.
7. Apply the principles of antibiotic stewardship in performing the nurses' role.
8. Identify patient safety indicators and perform the role of nurse in the patient safety audit process.
9. Apply the knowledge of International Patient Safety Goals (IPSG) in the patient care settings. Identify employee safety indicators and risk of occupational hazards.
10. Develop understanding of the various safety protocols and adhere to those protocols.

COURSE OUTLINE
T—Theory, L/E—Laboratory/Experiential Learning

Unit	Time (hours) T	Time (hours) P	Learning outcomes	Contents	Teaching/learning activities	Assessment methods

I.	2	2 (E)	Summarize the evidence based and effective patient care practices for the prevention of common healthcare associated infections in the healthcare setting	**Hospital-acquired Infection (HAI)**
				• Hospital-acquired infection
				• Bundle approach
				  – Prevention of urinary tract infection (UTI)
				  – Prevention of surgical site infection (SSI)
				  – Prevention of ventilator associated events (VAE)
				  – Prevention of central line associated bloodstream infection (CLABSI)
				• Surveillance of HAI—infection control team and infection control committee
					• Lecture cum discussion
					• Experiential learning
						• Knowledge assessment
						• MCQ
						• Short answer

II.	3	4 (L)	Demonstrate appropriate use of different types of PPEs and the critical use of risk assessment	**Isolation Precautions and use of Personal Protective Equipment (PPE)** • Types of isolation system, standard precaution and transmission-based precautions (direct contact, droplet, indirect) • Epidemiology and infection prevention CDC guidelines • Effective use of PPE	• Lecture • Demonstration and re-demonstration	• Performance assessment • OSCE
III.	1	2 (L)	Demonstrate the hand hygiene practice and its effectiveness on infection control	**Hand Hygiene** • Types of hand hygiene • Hand washing and use of alcohol hand rub • Moments of hand hygiene • WHO hand hygiene promotion	• Lecture • Demonstration and re-demonstration	• Performance assessment

Unit	Time (hours) T	Time (hours) P	Learning outcomes	Contents	Teaching/learning activities	Assessment methods
IV.	1	2 (E)	Illustrates disinfection and sterilization in the healthcare setting	**Disinfection and Sterilization** • Definitions • Types of disinfection and sterilization • Environment cleaning • Equipment cleaning • Guides on use of disinfectants • Spaulding's principle	• Lecture • Discussion • Experiential learning through visit	• Short answer • Objective type
V.	1	2 (E)	Illustrate on what, when, how, why specimens are collected to optimize the diagnosis for treatment and management	**Specimen Collection (Review)** • Principle of specimen collection • Types of specimens • Collection techniques and special considerations • Appropriate containers • Transportation of the sample • Staff precautions in handling specimens	• Discussion	• Knowledge assessment • MCQ • Performance assessment • Checklist
VI.	2	2 (E)	Explain on biomedical waste management and laundry management	**Biomedical Waste Management (BMW)** Laundry management process and infection control and prevention • Waste management process and infection prevention • Staff precautions • Laundry management • Country ordinance and BMW National Guidelines 2017: Segregation of waste, color coded waste containers, waste collection and storage, packaging and labeling, transportation	• Discussion • Demonstration • Experiential learning through visit	• Knowledge assessment by short answers, objective type • Performance assessment
VII.	2		Explain in detail about antibiotic stewardship, AMR Describe MRSA/MDRO and its prevention	• Antibiotic stewardship • Importance of antibiotic stewardship • Antimicrobial resistance • Prevention of MRSA, MDRO in healthcare setting	• Lecture • Discussion • Written assignment–recent AMR (antimicrobial resistance guidelines)	• Short answer • Objective type • Assessment of assignment
VIII.	3	5 (L/E)	Enlist the patient safety indicators followed in a healthcare organization and the role of nurse in the patient safety audit process	**Patient Safety Indicators** • Care of vulnerable patients • Prevention of iatrogenic injury • Care of lines, drains and tubing's • Restrain policy and care—physical and chemical • Blood and blood transfusion policy • Prevention of IV complication • Prevention of fall • Prevention of DVT • Shifting and transporting of patients • Surgical safety • Care coordination event related to medication reconciliation and administration • Prevention of communication errors • Prevention of HAI • Documentation	• Lecture • Demonstration • Experiential learning	• Knowledge assessment • Performance assessment • Checklist/OSCE
			Captures and analyzes incidents and events for quality improvement	**Incidents and Adverse Events** • Capturing of incidents • Root cause analysis (RCA) • Corrective and preventive action (CAPA) • Report writing	• Lecture • Role play • Inquiry based learning	• Knowledge assessment • Short answer • Objective type

Unit	Time (hours) T	Time (hours) P	Learning outcomes	Contents	Teaching/learning activities	Assessment methods
IX.			Enumerate IPSG and application of the goals in the patients care settings	**International Patient Safety Goals (IPSG)** • Identify patient correctly • Improve effective communication • Improve safety of high alert medication • Ensure safe surgery • Reduce the risk of healthcare associated infection • Reduce the risk of patient harm resulting from falls • Reduce the harm associated with clinical alarm system	• Lecture • Role play	• Objective type

X.	2	3 (L/E)	Enumerate the various safety protocol and its applications	**Safety Protocol**
				• 5S (Son Set in order, Shine, Standardize, Sustain)
				• Radiation safety
				• Laser safety
				• Fire safety:
				  – Types and classification of fire
				  – Fire alarms
				  – Firefighting equipments
				• HAZMAT (Hazardous Materials) safety:
				  – Types of spill
				  – Spillage management
				  – Material safety data sheets (MSDS)
				• Environmental safety:
				  – Risk assessment
				  – Aspect impact analysis
				  – Maintenance of temperature and humidity
				  – Audits
				  – Emergency codes
				  – Role of nurse in times of disaster
					• Lecture
					• Demonstration
					• Experiential learning
						• Mock drills
						• Post tests
						• Checklist

XI.	2		Explain importance of employee safety indicator Identify risk of occupational hazards, prevention and post exposure prophylaxis	**Employee Safety Indicators** • Vaccination • Needle stick injuries (NSI) prevention • Fall prevention • Radiation safety • Annual heath check **Healthcare Worker Immunization Program and Management of Occupational Exposure** • Occupational health ordinance • Vaccination program for healthcare staff • Needle stick injuries and prevention and postexposure prophylaxis	• Lecture • Discussion • Lecture method • Journal review	• Knowledge assessment by short answers, objective type • Short answer

Experiential learning: Experiential learning is the process by which knowledge is created through the process of experience in the clinical field. Knowledge results from the combination of grasping transforming experience (Kolb, 1984). The experiential learning cycle begins with an experience that the student has had, followed by an opportunity to reflect on that experience. Then students may conceptualize and draw conclusions about what they experienced and observed, leading to future actions in which the students experiment with different behaviors. This begins the new cycle as the students have new experiences based on their experimentation. These steps may occur in nearly and order as the learning progresses. As the need of the learner, the concrete components and conceptual components can be in different order as they may require a variety of cognitive and affective behaviors

Plate 1

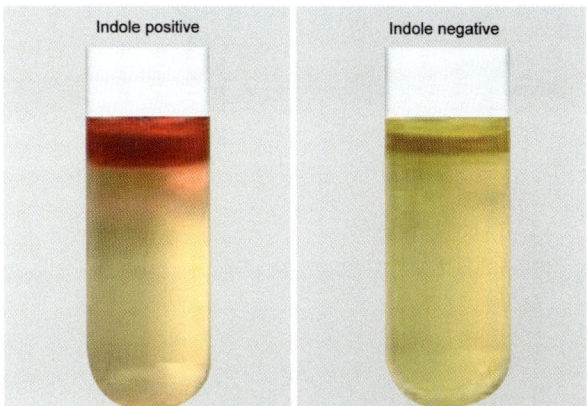

Fig. 2.11: Indole test.

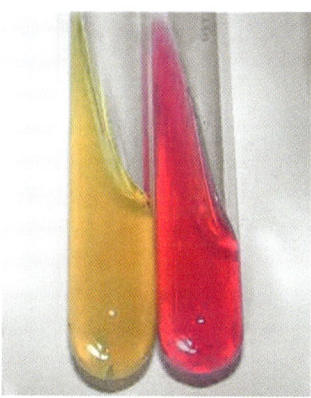

Fig. 2.12: Urease test.

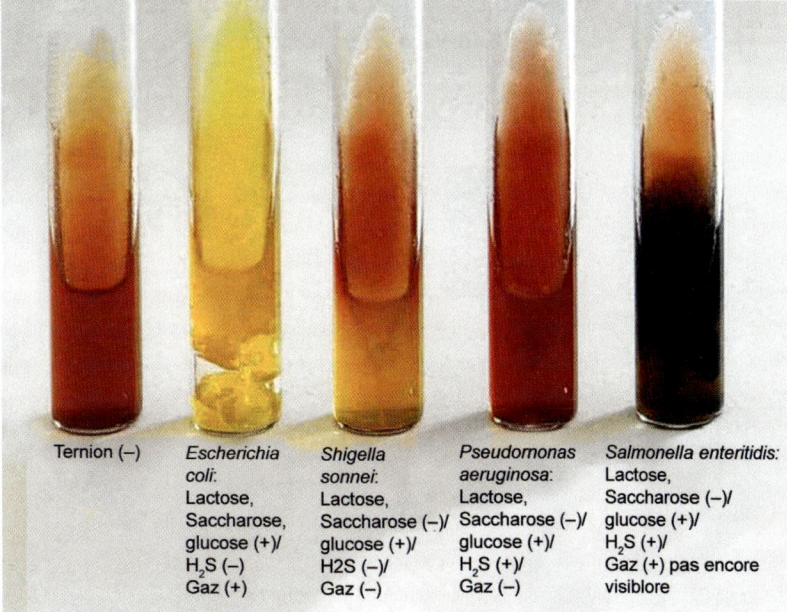

Fig. 2.13: Triple sugar iron agar test.

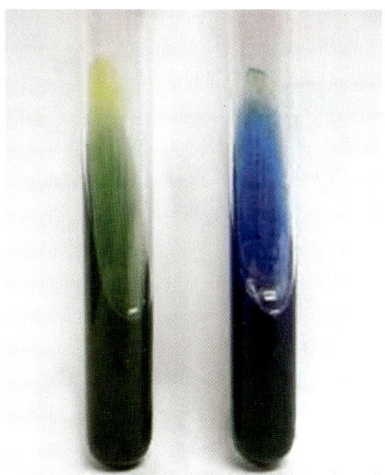

Fig. 2.14: Citrate utilization test.

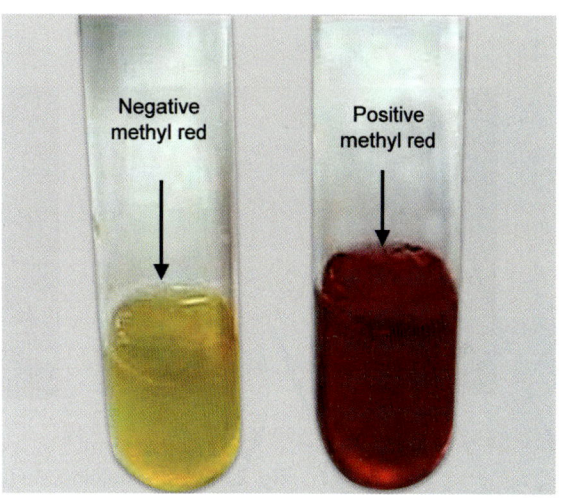

Fig. 2.15: Methyl red test.

Plate 2

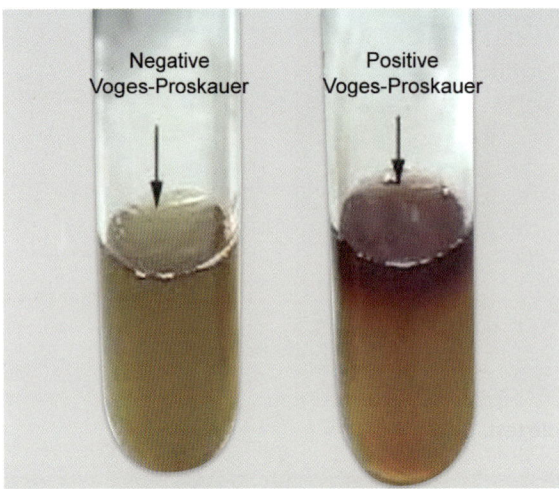

Fig. 2.16: Voges-Proskauer test.

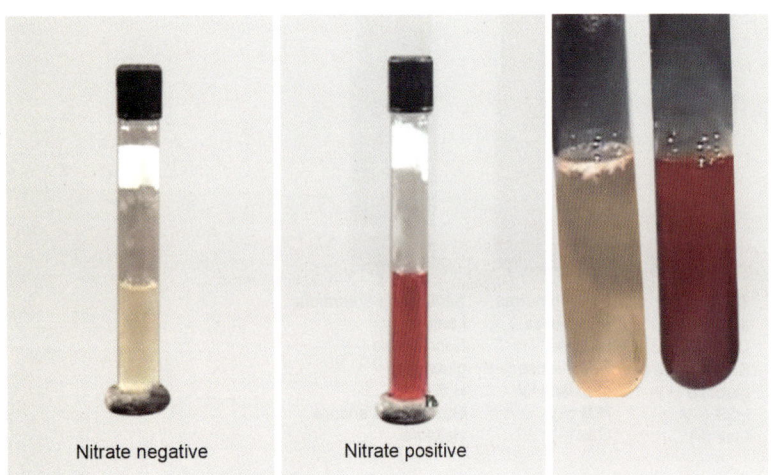

Fig. 2.17: Nitrate reduction test.

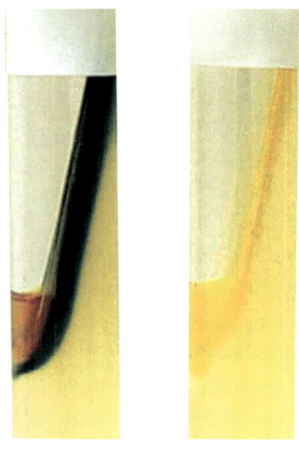

Fig. 2.18: Phenylalanine deaminase test.

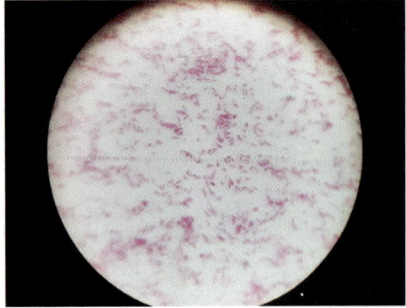

Gram-negative bacilli.

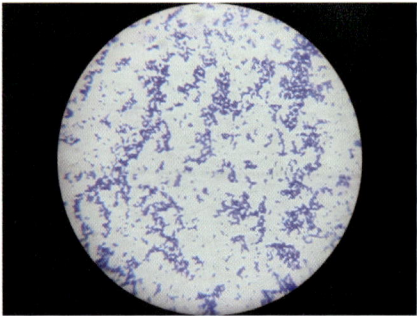

Gram-positive cocci.

Fig. 2.19: Gram staining (negative and positive).

Plate 3

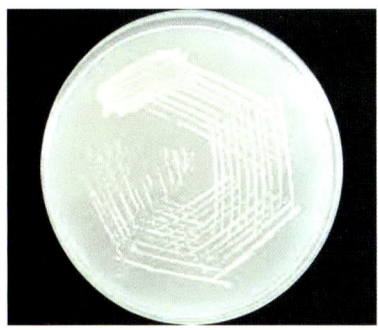
Nutrient agar.

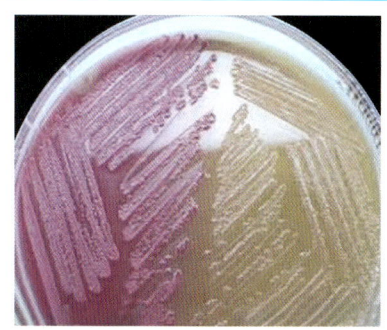
MacConkey's agar.

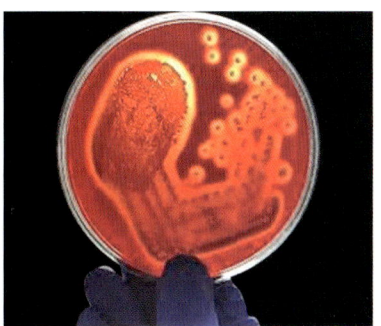
Blood agar.

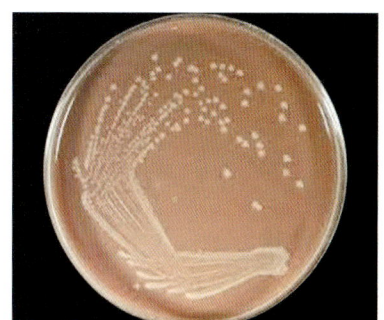
Chocolate agar.

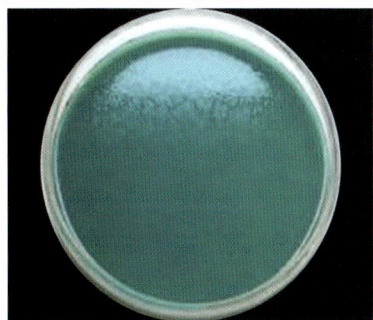
Wilson and Blair medium.

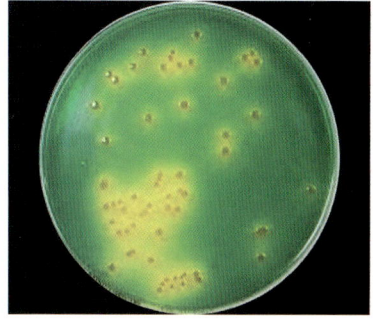
TCBS medium.

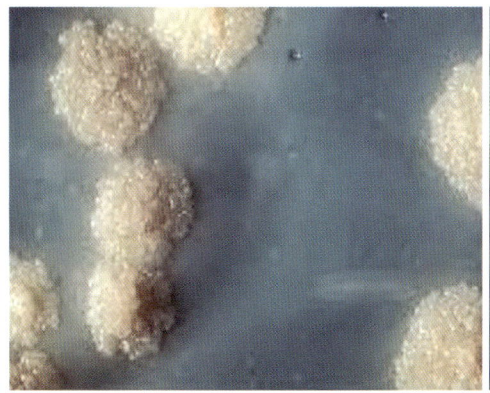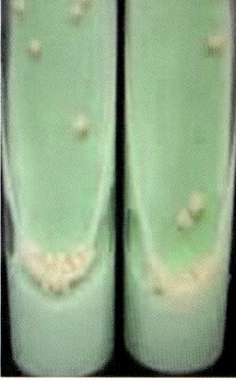
Lowenstein-Jensen medium.

Plate 4

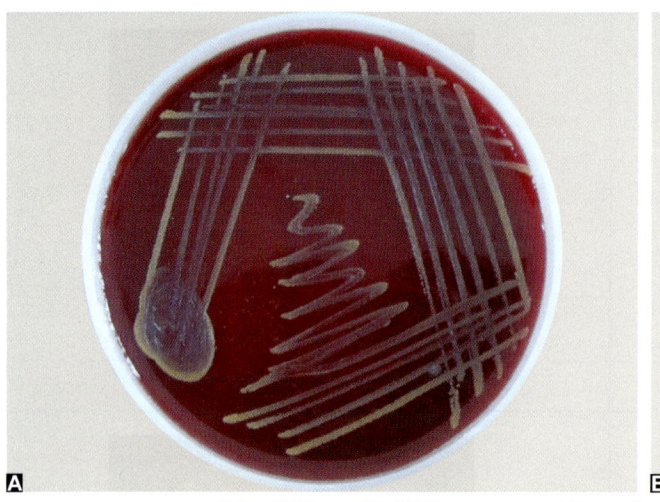 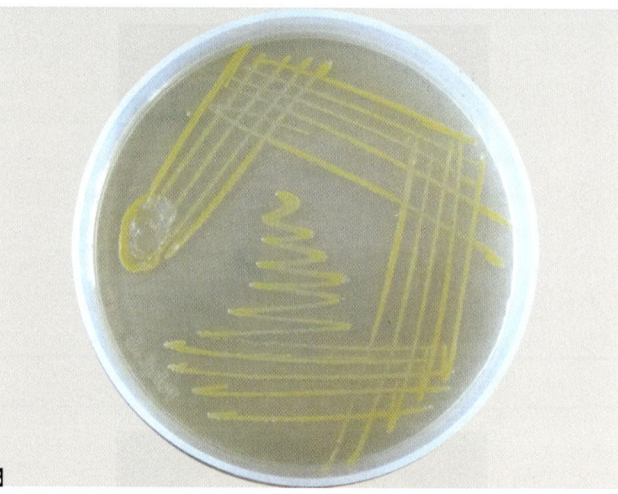

Figs. 3.2A and B: (A) *S. aureus*—golden yellow colonies on nutrient agar; (B) Blood agar.

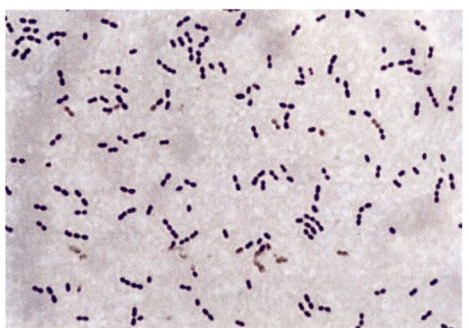 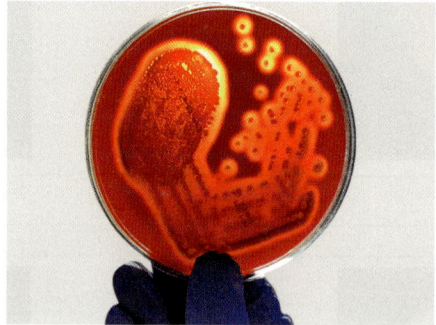 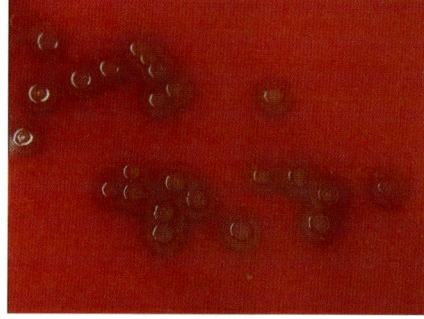

Fig. 3.3: *Streptococcus pyogenes* arranged in long chains.

Fig. 3.4: *Streptococcus pyogenes* on blood agar.

Fig. 3.5: *Pneumococcus* colonies on blood agar.

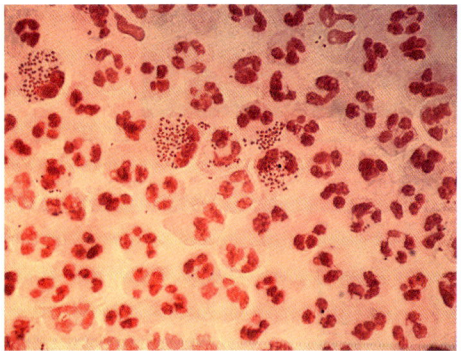 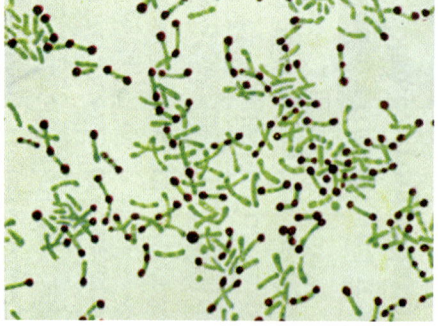 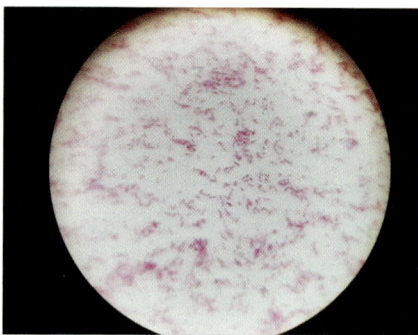

Fig. 3.7: *N. gonorrhoeae*—gram-negative cocci in pairs.

Fig. 3.8: *C. diphtheriae*—Chinese letter or cuneiform arrangement.

Fig. 3.13: Gram staining—gram-negative bacilli.

Plate 5

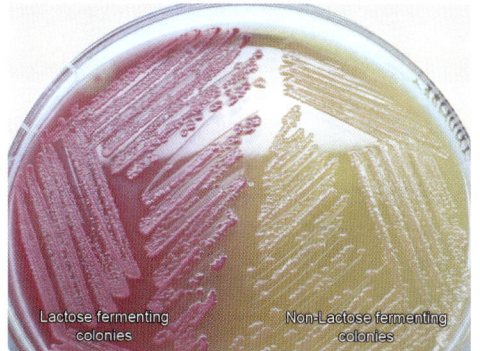

Fig. 3.14: MacConkey's agar—pink colored lactose fermenting colonies.

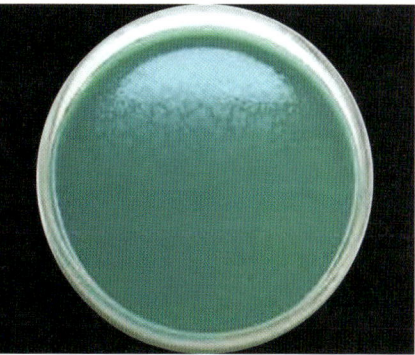

Fig. 3.16: Wilson and Blair medium.

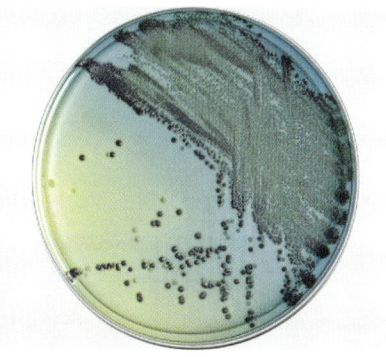

Fig. 3.17: Wilson and Blair medium—Jet black colonies of *Salmonella typhi*.

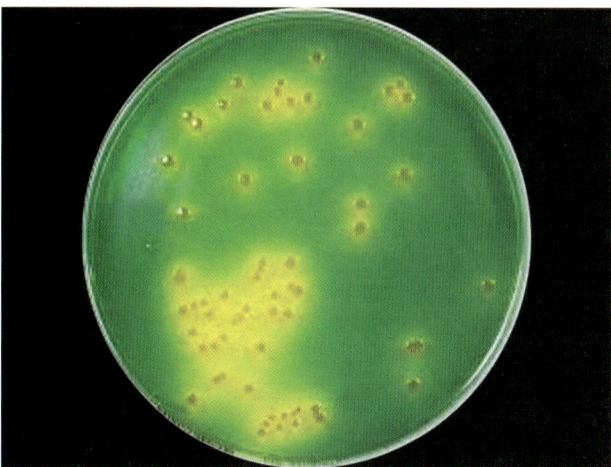

Fig. 3.19: On TCBS agar—yellow color colonies of *V. cholerae*.

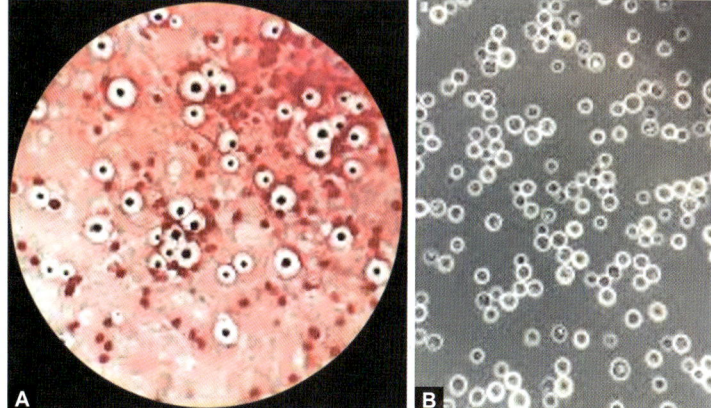

Figs. 3.21A and B: (A) Round yeast cells India ink; (B) Capsule of *Cryptococcus*.

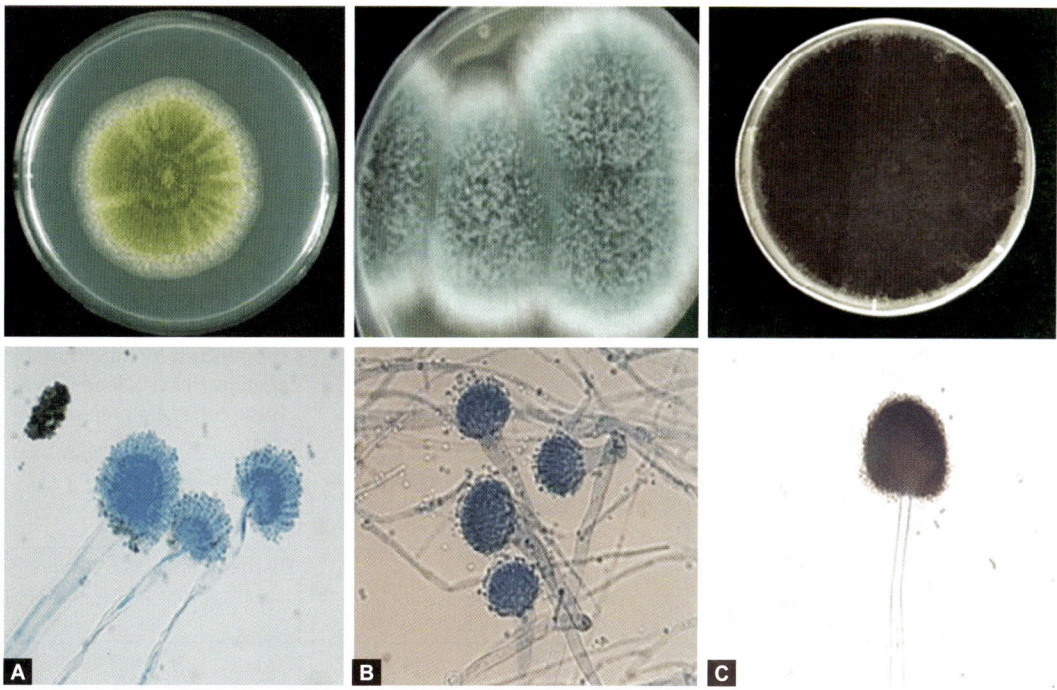

Figs. 3.22A to C: (A) *A. flavus*; (B) *A. fumigatus*; (C) *A. niger*.

Plate 6

Stages \ Species	P. falciparum	P. vivax	P. malariae	P. ovale
Ring stage				
Trophozoite				
Schizont				
Gametocyte				

Fig. 3.25: Draw malarial smear.

TABLE 9.1: Tubes commonly used in blood collection and their specifications.

Tube	Color	Name	Additive	Test used for
	Blood culture bottle	Culture bottle	Sodium polyanethol sulfonate (anticoagulant) and growth media for microorganisms	Two bottles are typically collected, in one blood draw; one for aerobic organisms and one for anaerobic organisms
	Light blue	Sodium citrate	3.2% sodium citrate (anticoagulant)	Coagulation tests
	Red	Red or plain	No additive No anticoagulant	Immunology, serological examination
	Gold	Serum separating tube	Serum separating gel and clot activator	All biochemistry test
	Light green	Heparin tube	Sodium heparin or lithium heparin (anticoagulant)	Prevent clotting chromosome testing HLA typing ammonia, lactate
	Purple/lavender	EDTA	Ethylene diamine tetra acetic acid (EDTA) (Anticoagulant)	Hematological examination like complete hemogram
	Pink		Ethylene diamine tetra acetic acid (EDTA) (Anticoagulant) Used only for whole blood sample being send to transfusion lab	Blood typing and cross-matching direct coombs test for autoimmune haemolytic anemia, HIV viral load (G & S) These tubes are preferred for blood bank tests
	Grey	Sodium fluoride	Sodium fluoride (glycolysis inhibitor) Potassium oxalate (anticoagulant)	Glucose, lactate testing
	Yellow	Acid-citrate-dextrose (anticoagulant)		Tissue typing, DNA studies, HIV cultures

Plate 7

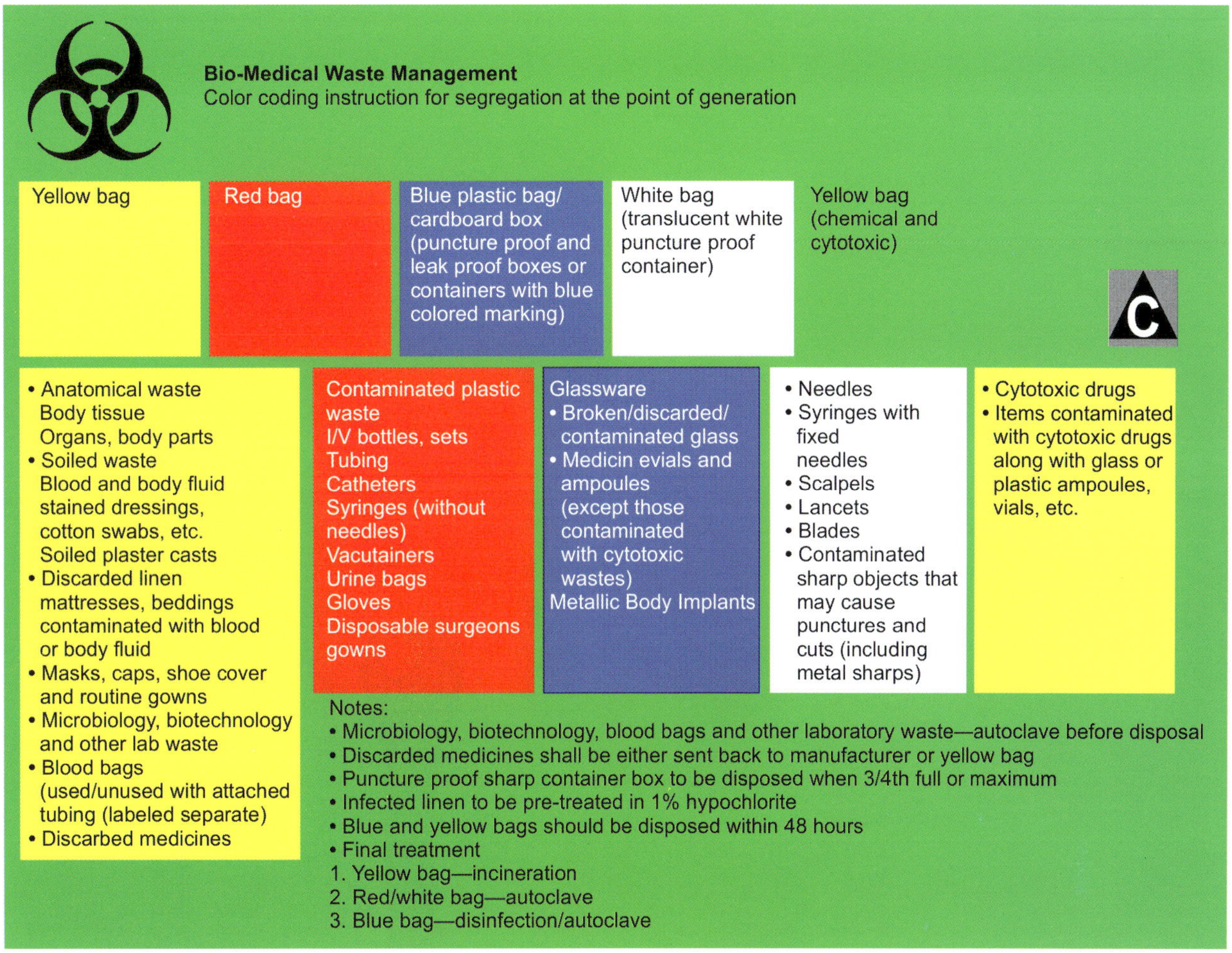

Bio-Medical Waste Management
Color coding instruction for segregation at the point of generation

Yellow bag	Red bag	Blue plastic bag/ cardboard box (puncture proof and leak proof boxes or containers with blue colored marking)	White bag (translucent white puncture proof container)	Yellow bag (chemical and cytotoxic)

• Anatomical waste
  Body tissue
  Organs, body parts
• Soiled waste
  Blood and body fluid stained dressings, cotton swabs, etc.
  Soiled plaster casts
• Discarded linen mattresses, beddings contaminated with blood or body fluid
• Masks, caps, shoe cover and routine gowns
• Microbiology, biotechnology and other lab waste
• Blood bags (used/unused with attached tubing (labeled separate)
• Discarbed medicines
	Contaminated plastic waste
	I/V bottles, sets
	Tubing
	Catheters
	Syringes (without needles)
	Vacutainers
	Urine bags
	Gloves
	Disposable surgeons gowns
		Glassware
		• Broken/discarded/ contaminated glass
		• Medicin evials and ampoules (except those contaminated with cytotoxic wastes)
		Metallic Body Implants
			• Needles
			• Syringes with fixed needles
			• Scalpels
			• Lancets
			• Blades
			• Contaminated sharp objects that may cause punctures and cuts (including metal sharps)
				• Cytotoxic drugs
				• Items contaminated with cytotoxic drugs along with glass or plastic ampoules, vials, etc.

Notes:
• Microbiology, biotechnology, blood bags and other laboratory waste—autoclave before disposal
• Discarded medicines shall be either sent back to manufacturer or yellow bag
• Puncture proof sharp container box to be disposed when 3/4th full or maximum
• Infected linen to be pre-treated in 1% hypochlorite
• Blue and yellow bags should be disposed within 48 hours
• Final treatment
1. Yellow bag—incineration
2. Red/white bag—autoclave
3. Blue bag—disinfection/autoclave

Fig. 10.1: Biomedical waste management.

SECTION I

Applied Microbiology

Chapter 1: Introduction to Microbiology
Chapter 2: General Characteristics of Microbes
Chapter 3: Pathogenic Organisms
Chapter 4: Immunity

CHAPTER 1

Introduction to Microbiology

Chapter Outline

- Microbiology
- Importance of Microbiology
- History of Microbiology
- Terminology in Microbiology
- Scope of Microbiology

LEARNING OBJECTIVE: EXPLAIN CONCEPTS AND PRINCIPLES OF MICROBIOLOGY AND ITS IMPORTANCE IN NURSING

Microbiology (Micro = small, Logy = study) means the study of microorganisms, such as bacteria, viruses, fungi, etc. Medical microbiology is the part of medical sciences in which microorganisms and their role in human health and disease is studied.

Clinical Microbiology

This is the branch of medical sciences that deals with the diagnosis, treatment and prevention of infectious disease. The various branches of this field are in **Table 1.1**.

TABLE 1.1: Branches of applied microbiology.

Branch/field	Definition
General microbiology	Study of general properties of microorganisms, such as morphology, classification, pathogenesis, laboratory diagnosis, sterilization and disinfection, etc.
Immunology	Study of immune system (body's defense mechanisms against disease)
Bacteriology	Study of bacteria, e.g., *E. coli, Mycobacterium tuberculosis*
Virology	Study of viruses, e.g., COVID-19, Ebola virus
Mycology	Study of fungi, e.g., *Candida, Aspergillus*
Parasitology	Study of parasites, e.g., malaria, filaria
Protozoology	Branch of parasitology that deals with the study of protozoa (unicellular parasites), e.g., amoeba, etc.
Helminthology	Branch of parasitology that deals with the study of helminths (multicellular parasites), e.g., tapeworm
Medical entomology	Branch of parasitology that deals with the study of medically important arthropods, e.g., sandfly, soft ticks, etc.

THE IMPORTANCE OF MICROBIOLOGY IN NURSING

Nursing students as well as staff should have sufficient education and knowledge in microbiology to perform many roles within clinical nursing practice (e.g., administering antibiotics, collecting specimens, preparing specimens for transport and delivery, educating patients and families, communicating results to the healthcare team, and developing healthcare plans based on results of microbiology studies and patient immunological status). Learning microbiology for nurses is helpful in the diagnosis, treatment and prevention of diseases. Importance of microbiology in nursing is for:

- Learning infection control by understanding the basic mechanism of infection spread, i.e., how an infection is spread.
- Collection and transport of specimens for diagnosis
- Immunization
- In prevention of healthcare-associated infections (HAIs). Burn patients in burn ward are more prone for infections. Thus having good knowledge of microbiology to a nurse can lower the infection in burn patients.
- Central sterilization sterile department (CSSD) in a hospital must work efficiently so that proper sterile conditions are maintained in a healthcare setting. A nurse must have sound knowledge about the sterilization methods and controls of sterilization so that good quality can be maintained while nursing care.
- They also help in proper disposal of biomedical waste generated in healthcare settings.
- Proper knowledge of medical microbiology also helps to understand the causative organism of disease and patient's normal flora because some of them may turn pathogenic under specific conditions and can cause disease.
- Nurses are eminent part of Hospital Infection Control Committee (HICC) where the knowledge of microbiology and microorganisms is important.

HISTORY OF MICROBIOLOGY

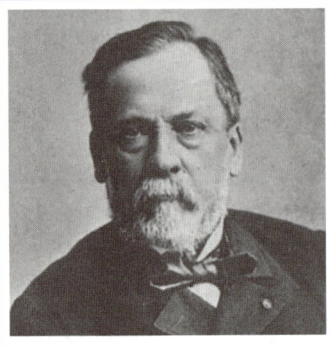

Louis Pasteur
(Father of Microbiology)

Important Contributions

Louis Pasture known as 'Father of Microbiology' (1822–1895).

- He was a Professor of Chemistry in France. His studies on fermentation led him to take interest to work in Microbiology
- He had proposed the principles of fermentation for preservation of food
- Introduced sterilization techniques and developed steam sterilizer, hot air oven and autoclave
- Described method of pasteurization of milk
- Contributed for vaccine development against several diseases, such as anthrax, cholera and rabies
- Postulated "germ theory of disease".
- Introduced liquid media concept
- Founder of Pasteur Institute, Paris

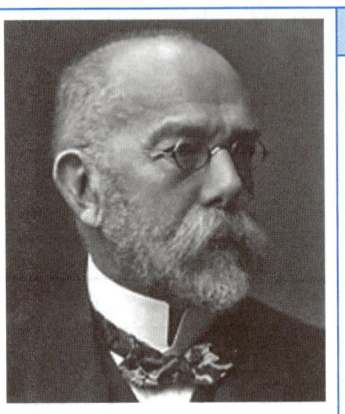

Robert Koch
(Father of Bacteriology)

Important Contributions

Robert Koch known as 'Father of Bacteriology' (1843–1901).

- He got Nobel Prize in year 1905 for the discovery of tubercle bacilli
- Introduced solid media for culture of bacteria and use of agar
- Methods of isolation of bacteria in pure culture
- Described hanging drop method for motility of organism
- Discovered bacteria, such as anthrax, cholera and tubercle bacilli
- Introduced staining techniques by using aniline dyes
- Koch's postulates and Koch's phenomenon was given by him

Koch's Postulates

- The microorganism should be constantly associated with the lesion.
- It should be possible to isolate the organism in pure culture from the lesion of the disease.
- The same disease must result when the isolated microorganism is inoculated into suitable laboratory animal.
- It should be possible to re-isolate the organism in pure culture from the lesions produced in the experimental animals.
- Antibody to the causative organism should be demonstrable in patient's serum.

Exceptions of Koch's postulates: Some bacteria that do not satisfy Koch's postulates are *Mycobacterium leprae* and *Treponema pallidum*.

Koch's Phenomenon

Robert Koch observed that guinea pigs already infected with tubercle bacillus developed a delayed hypersensitivity reaction when injected with tubercle bacilli or its protein.

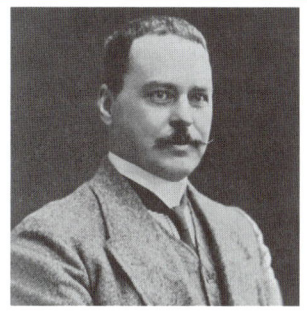

Sir Ronald Ross

Important Contributions
Awarded Noble Prize in the year 1902 for his contribution for development of life cycle of malarial parasite in mosquito.   • Ross developed mathematical models for the study of malaria epidemiology   • Established the developmental stages of malaria parasites in anopheline mosquitoes; and described the complete life cycles of *P. falciparum*, *P. vivax* and *P. malariae*

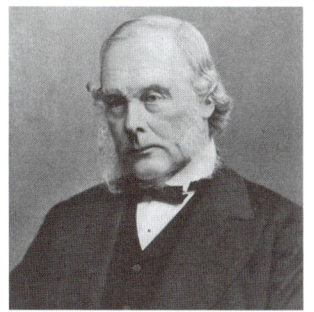

Joseph Lister
(Father of Antiseptic Surgery)

Important Contributions
Joseph Lister known as 'Father of Antiseptic Surgery'.   • Observed that postoperative infections were greatly reduced by using disinfectants, such as diluted carbolic acid during surgery to sterilize the instruments and to clean the wounds.   • He instructed surgeons under his responsibility to wear clean gloves and wash their hands before and after operations with 5% carbolic acid solutions.

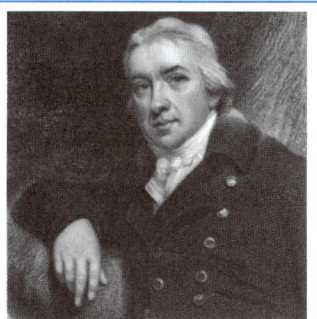

Edward Jenner
(Father of Immunology)

Important Contributions
Edward Jenner known as ' Father of Immunology'.   • Developed the first vaccine of world, the smallpox vaccine.   • Used cowpox virus (*Variola vaccinae*) to immunize children against smallpox from which the term 'vaccine' was derived

TERMINOLOGY IN MICROBIOLOGY

- **Microorganism:** These are extremely small organisms which we cannot see by our naked eyes (without microscope). The word **"microbe"** has been derived from French and was introduced in 1878 by a French Surgeon, **CE Sedillot**.
- **Microscope:** An instrument which is used to see microorganisms.
- **Health:** A state of complete physical, mental and social well-being and not merely the absence of disease or deformity.
- **Disease:** Any harmful deviation from the normal structural or functional state of an organism, generally associated with certain signs and symptoms and differing in nature from physical injury.
- **Plasmid:** This is an extrachromosomal double-stranded circular DNA having tendency to replicate independently.
- **Mutation:** It is defined as random, unidirectional heritable variation caused by change in the nucleotide sequence of the genome of cell.
- **Transformation:** It is defined as the random uptake of free or naked DNA fragment from surrounding medium/environment by bacterial cell and incorporation of this DNA fragment into its chromosome.
- **Transduction:** It is defined as the transmission of a portion of DNA from one bacterium to another by bacteriophage.
- **Bacteriophage:** It is a virus which infects and multiplies inside bacteria.
- **Conjugation:** It is defined as transfer of genetic material from one bacterium to another bacterium by mating/conjugation tube formation.
- **Decontamination:** It refers to the reduction of pathogenic microbial population to a level at which items are considered as safe to handle without protective attire.
- **Sterilization:** It is a process by which all living and dead microorganisms, including viable spores are either destroyed or removed from an article, body surface or medium.
- **Bactericidal:** It is an agent (e.g., antibiotics) capable of killing bacteria.
- **Bacteriostatic:** It is an agent that inhibits growth of bacteria.
- **Disinfectants:** It is the process that destroys or removes all the pathogenic organisms but not bacterial spores.
- **Antiseptics:** It is an agent that can be safely applied on the skin or mucous membrane to prevent infection by inhibiting the growth of bacteria.
- **Antibiotics:** These are the antimicrobial agents that destroy microorganisms within the body.
- **Viruses:** Smallest unicellular organisms that are obligate intracellular.
- **Virion:** The entire virus particle is called as virion.
- **Epidemiology:** It is defined as the study of distribution and determinants of infection related health state in specific population and also its application to control the disease.
- **Infection:** It is defined as a process in which pathogenic organism enters, establishes itself, multiplies and invades normal anatomical barriers of host resulting in disease.
- **Communicable disease:** Infectious disease that is capable of directly transmitting to humans from person to person, animal or environment is called communicable disease.
- **Outbreak:** It is defined as the sudden/acute rise in number of cases in disease in a particular geographical area.
- **Epidemic:** It is defined as the infection which occurs at much higher rate than normal in particular area. It affects large number of people or region.
- **Pandemic:** It is defined as the infection that spreads quickly to huge areas of the globe, e.g., COVID-19.
- **Endemic:** It is defined as a disease that occurs as persistent at low levels at certain areas, e.g., typhoid fever.
- **Sporadic:** It is defined as infection that occurs at irregular intervals or only in few places.
- **Incidence:** It is defined as the number of new cases of disease that occur in a defined population during particular time period. Incidence = No. of new cases in every year/population at risk during that period × 100
- **Prevalence:** It is defined as total cases of disease (new and old) that exist at particular time. Prevalence = No. of all current cases (old + new) existing at given time/estimated population at that point of time × 100
- **Case fertility rate:** It is defined as the number of deaths that occurred due to disease as compared to the total number of cases of disease.
- **Secondary attack rate:** It is defined as the number of exposed persons who developed disease within the range of incubation period after their exposure/contact with primary cases.
- **Eradication:** It means complete or permanant reduction of disease worldwide to zero new cases.
- **Elimination:** It means reduction to zero of new cases.
- **Control:** It means reduction of disease to locally acceptable level.
- **Infective dose:** It is defined as the minimum required amount/inoculum size of pathogenic organism to initiate an infection.
- **Source:** It means a person, environment, etc., from which organism is transmitted to host.
- **Reservoir:** It is the natural habitat where organism lives and multiplies.

- **Carrier:** It is the person with infectious agent but no clinical symptoms and shed organism from body through sneezing.
- **Convalescent carrier:** It refers to the person who had recovered from disease but continuously harbor disease and shed organism from his body.
- **Temporary carriers:** They shed pathogenic organism for <6 months.
- **Chronic carriers:** They shed pathogenic organism for long periods (usually indefinite periods).
- **Zoonoses:** The disease transmitted to man from animals is called zoonoses.
- **Droplets:** These are large particles having >5 μm in size
- **Aerosols:** These are small particles having less generated by infectious person during coughing, e.g., less than 5 μm in size.
- **Microbiota:** Community of microbes that live in and on an individual; can vary substantially between environmental sites and host niches in health and disease.
- **Prebiotic:** Food ingredient that supports the growth of one or more members of the microbiota.
- **Probiotic:** Live organism that, when ingested, is believed to provide benefit to the host.
- **Period of communicability:** It is also known as infectivity period. It is defined as a period during which a pathogenic organism may be transferred from infected person to other person directly or indirectly, e.g., influenza from -1 day to +1 week of onset of symptoms.
- **Immunity:** It is the resistance of body towards any foreign agent (microorganisms, etc.).
- *Lesions* are the characteristic changes in tissues and cells produced by disease in an individual or experimental animal.
- **Pathogenesis:** Mechanism by which the lesions are produced (i.e., 'how' of disease).
- **Symptoms:** Functional implications of the lesion felt by the patient.
- **Syndrome** is used for a combination of several clinical features caused by—altered physiologic processes.
- **Acute:** A disease with sudden onset of signs and a short course.
- **Chronic:** A condition with slow onset, mild but continuous manifestations and long-lasting, often progressive effects.
- **Abscess:** A localized collection of pus in a cavity formed by disintegration of tissues.
- **Agglutination:** Clumping together of cells or particles.
- **Anaphylaxis:** The immediate immunologic (allergic) reaction initiated by the combination of antigen (allergen) with mast cell cytophilic antibody. Anaphylactic shock—life-threatening respiratory distress, vascular collapse and shock; manifesting extremely great sensitivity to foreign protein or other material.
- **Hypersensitivity:** A state of altered reactivity in which the body reacts with an exaggerated immune response to a foreign agent.
- **Necrosis:** The morphological changes indicative of cell death caused by progressive enzymatic degradation.
- **Nosocomial:** Pertaining to or originating in a hospital.
- **Pyogenic:** Producing pus.
- **Pyrexia:** A fever or febrile condition.
- **Pyrogen:** A fever-producing substance.
- **Rhinitis:** Inflammation of the nasal mucous membrane.
- **Sepsis:** The presence and multiplication of bacteria (pathogenic organisms) or their toxins in the blood or tissues.

SCOPE OF MICROBIOLOGY

The scope and importance of microbiology is vast and is relevant to different fields which can be summarized as following:
- Production of antibiotics
- **Productions of acids and enzymes:** For example, *Penicillium glaucum* (Gallic acid) and *Aspergillus oryzae* (amylase)
- **Baking industry:** Yeast is used in the manufacture of bread
- **Used in the production of dairy products:** Dairy products, such as curd, butter, cheese and ghee are manufactured from bacterial activity, e.g., *Lactobacillus lactis* for cheese
- Production of enzymes, vaccines, biosurfactants, and other pharmaceutical products
- Treatment of industrial waste material.
- Microbiological assays of antibiotics.

CHAPTER 2

General Characteristics of Microbes

Chapter Outline

- Bacterial Taxonomy
- Structure and Classification of Microbes
- Morphological Types
- Size and Form of Bacteria
- Motility
- Colonization
- Growth and Nutrition of Microbes
- Temperature
- Moisture
- Blood and Body Fluids
- Laboratory Methods of Identification of Microorganisms
- Types of Staining—Gram's AFB, Special and Capsular Staining, Spore, LPCB, KOH
- Culture and Media Preparation—Solid, Liquid
- Types of Media—Semi-synthetic, Synthetic, Enriched, Enrichment and Differential Media
- Pure Culture Techniques—Tube Dilution, Pour Spread, Streak Plate, Anaerobic Cultivation of Bacteria

BACTERIAL TAXONOMY

Taxonomy is the classification of organisms into ordered groups. Bacterial taxonomy comprises of three separate but interrelated important areas. There is no universally accepted bacterial classification. There are mainly three approaches—Phylogenetic, Adansonian and Genetic.

Bacterial Classification

The most recent taxonomic classification of bacteria is based on Cavalier and Smith's six kingdom classifications (1998). It is the most accepted classification at present, surpassed the previous five kingdom classification (Whittaker, 1969) and three domain classification (Woese, 1990).

Phylogenetic Classification

Phylogenetic classification groups that are related on evolutionary basis where several ranks are used: *Divisions, Classes, Orders, Families, Tribes, Genera and Species.* The genera and species are distinguished by less important properties, such as fermentation, nutritional requirement, etc. The full taxonomical position of *Salmonella typhi* is as follows in **Table 2.1**.

TABLE 2.1: Taxonomy of *Salmonella typhi*.	
Division	*Protophyta*
Class	*Schizomycetes*
Order	*Eubacteriales*
Family	*Enterobacteriaceae*
Tribe	*Salmonellae*
Genus	*Salmonella*
Species	*Salmonella typhi*

A phylogenetic classification of bacteria is very useful in compilation of names and descriptions and also as an aid to identification of newly isolated bacterial types. For identification and classification of bacteria, a minimum number of important characters are selected so that various members can be distinguished. These important characters include:
- Morphology
- Staining
- Cultural characteristics
- Biochemical reactions
- Antigenic structure
- **Guanine:** Cytosine ratio of DNA

Other Classifications
- Adansonian classification
- Genetic classification
- Intraspecies classification

INTRODUCTION TO PROKARYOTES AND EUKARYOTES

Microorganisms and all other living organisms are divided into two categories—prokaryotes and eukaryotes—based primarily on their cellular characteristics and mode of reproduction.

Prokaryotes are composed of prokaryotic cells and eukaryotes are composed of eukaryotic cells.

Prokaryotes include several kinds of microorganisms, such as bacteria and cyanobacteria. Eukaryotes include all other cellular microorganism such microorganisms as fungi, protozoa, and simple algae.

Other major distinguishing features of the two groups are that eukaryotes are diploid (possess two copies of their genes) and normally reproduce sexually. In contrast prokaryotes are normally haploid (possess one copy of the set of genes in the cell).

Distinguishing features of the two types of cells are tabulated in **Table 2.2**.

TABLE 2.2: Difference between prokaryotes and eukaryotes.

Structure	Prokaryotes	Eukaryotes
Nucleus		
Nuclear membrane	Absent	Present
Nucleolus	Absent	Present
Chromosome	One	More than one
Deoxyribonucleoprotein	Absent	Present
Division	By binary fission	By mitosis
Cytoplasm		
Mitochondria, Golgi apparatus, lysosomes, endoplasmic reticulum	All are absent	All are present
Chemical composition		
Sterols	Absent	Present
Muramic acid	Present	Absent

INTRODUCTION TO MICROBES

Size of the Microorganisms

Microorganisms are extremely small. Size of the bacteria is expressed in micrometers (1 μm = 10^{-3} mm) whereas viruses are measured in nanometers (1 nm = 10^{-3} μm).

Most of the bacteria of medical importance generally measure 2–5 μm in diameter and about 3–5 μm in length, while the majority of the human pathogenic viruses range 20–300 nm in diameter.

Because of the small size, microorganisms cannot be seen distinctly with unaided eye but need a microscope for visualization.

Most bacteria can be observed by light microscope whereas viruses need an electron microscope.

Bacteria

Bacteria are simple in structure, microscopic, single-celled organisms which exist in their infinite numbers, everywhere in environment, both inside and outside. They are prokaryotic organisms, which are simple unicellular organisms with no nuclear membrane, mitochondria, Golgi bodies, or endoplasmic reticulum, that reproduce by asexual division.

They can be motile as well as non-motile. Most bacteria have either a gram-positive cell wall with a thick peptidoglycan layer, or a gram-negative cell wall with a thin peptidoglycan layer and an overlying outer membrane.

Morphology of Bacteria (Fig. 2.1)

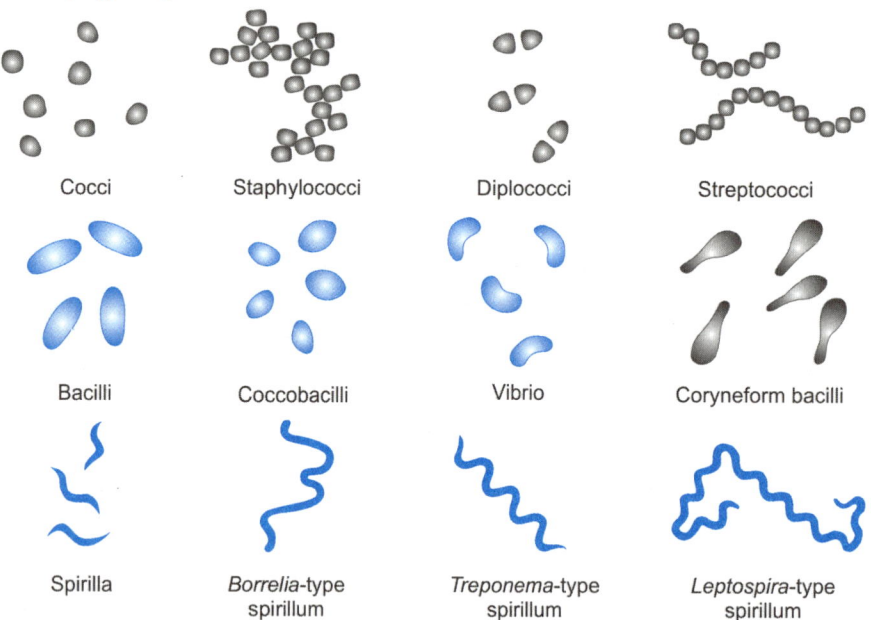

Fig. 2.1: Shapes and different arrangements of bacteria.

Various Shapes of Bacteria (Table 2.3)

Bacteria posses different shapes and accordingly they are so classified:
- **Cocci :** Singular is coccus . "Cocci" means oval or spherical cells
  These can exist in groups (clusters), chains or in pairs.
  On the basis of arrangement of individual organisms they may be:
  – *Micrococci:* Cocci that occurs singly.
  – *Diplococci:* Cocci that occurs in pairs (*diplo* meaning pair).
  – *Streptococcci:* Cocci that occurs in chains (*strepto* meaning chain).
  – *Staphylococci:* Cocci that occurs in bunches (*staphylo* meaning bunch).
  – *Tetrad:* Cocci that occurs in groups of four (*tetra* meaning four).
  – *Sarcinae (octad):* Cocci that occurs in group of eight (*octa* meaning eight).

TABLE 2.3: Morphological appearance of various bacteria.

Morphological form of bacteria	Example
Gram-positive	
Cluster	*Staphylococcus*
Chains	*Streptococcus*
Pairs, lanceolate shape	*Pneumococcus*
Pair or in short chains	*Enterococcus*
Gram-negative cocci	
Pairs, lens shaped	*Meningococcus*
Pairs, kidney shaped	*Gonococcus*
Gram-positive bacilli	
Chain (bamboo stick appearance)	*Bacillus anthrax*
Chinese letter or cuneiform pattern	*Corynebacterium diphtheriae*
Gram-negative bacilli	
Chains	*Streptobacillus*

- **Bacilli:** These are also called rods- or rod-shaped bacteria
  On the basis of arrangement of an individual organism they may be:
  - *Microbacilli:* Bacilli that occur singly.
  - *Diplobacilli:* Bacilli that occur in pairs.
  - *Streptobacilli:* Bacilli that occur in chains.
  - *Palisade arrangement:* Bacilli lined side-by-side like matchsticks and at angles to one another, e.g., *Corynebacterium diphtheriae* causing diphtheria.
  - *Comma-shaped:* Bacilli that are curved and looks like a comma, e.g., *Vibrio cholera* causing cholera
  - *Coccobacilli:* These are the bacteria which are intermediate to coccus and bacillus, e.g, *Brucella*
- **Spirochaetes:** These are spirally coiled bacteria, e.g., *Treponema*, is a causative agent of *Syphillis*
- **Actinomycetes:** These are branching filamentous bacteria resembling fungi. They have a rigid cell wall.
- **Mycoplasma:** These are the bacteria that lack cell wall and hence they possess no stable shape. They may occur as round or oval bodies and as interlacing filaments.
- **Rickettsiae and chlamydiae:** These are very small, obligate parasites. Due to their inability to grow outside living cells, they were previously considered as parasites.

Structure of Bacteria (Bacterial Anatomy)

Bacterial Cell Wall (Fig. 2.2)

It is the outer covering (if there is no envelope) of bacterial cell and is tough structure as well as rigid. Its usual thickness is about 10–25 nm. It cannot be seen by light microscope neither can be stained by simple stains **(Fig. 2.3)**. It has following functions:
- Gives protection to bacterial cell from external environment
- Maintains shape of bacteria
- It also takes part in bacterial cell division
- Protects bacteria from toxic substances, such as antibiotics, etc.
- Increases virulence of bacteria
- It is also used in vaccine preparation.

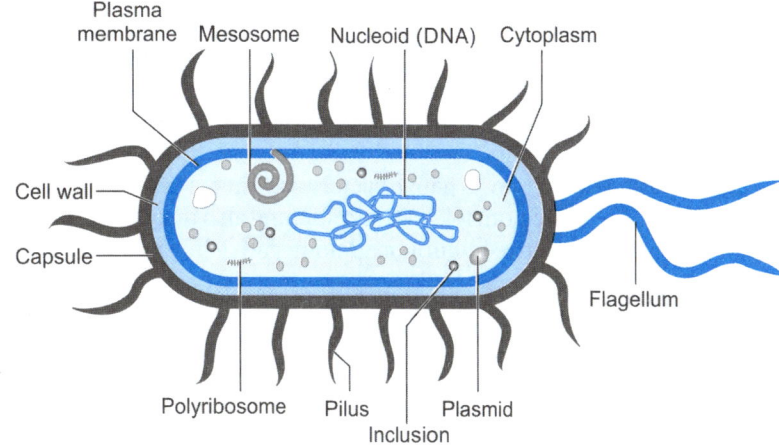

Fig. 2.2: Simple diagrammatic view of bacterial cell.

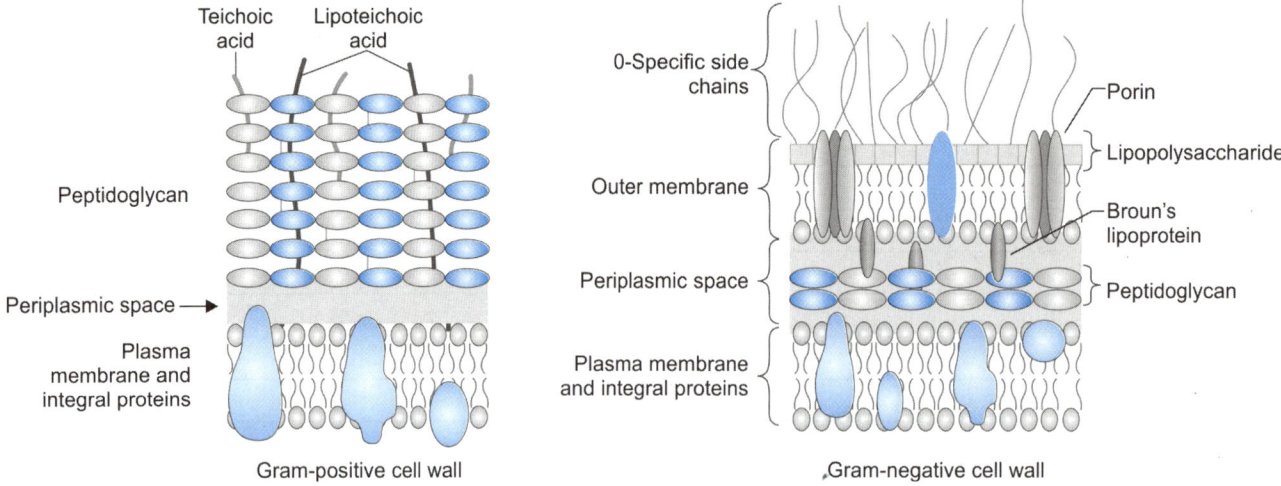

Fig. 2.3: Cell wall structure.

TABLE 2.4: Difference between cell wall of gram-positive and gram-negative bacteria.		
Composition/character	**Gram-positive cell wall**	**Gram-negative cell wall**
Complexity	Simple	More complex
Size	Thicker	Thinner
Layers	Single (homologous) usually	Multilayer
Composition	Peptidoglycan comprises up to 90% of cell wall Peptidoglycan is thicker 16–80 mm	Peptidoglycan comprises only 10% or less of cell wall Peptidoglycan is thinner 2 nm
Rigidity	Rigid	Less rigid
Teichoic acid	Present	Absent
Lipopolysaccharide	Absent	Present (endotoxin)
Amino acids	Present but few	Several
Response towards cell wall specific antibodies	More	Less
Toxic property of cell wall	No	Yes due to endotoxin
Content of lipid	Nil or scanty <5%	Present up to 20%
Aromatic amino acid	Absent	Present
Outer membrane	Absent	Present

Gram-positive and gram-negative bacteria vary in the cell wall. Both have different composition, thickness and complexity in their cell wall. The basic principle of Gram staining also relays on the composition of cell wall. There also certain antimicrobials which act on gram positive but not on gram negative due to this cell wall difference **(Table 2.4)**.

Cell wall demonstration can be done by:
- **Plasmolysis:** When bacteria is placed in a hypertonic saline, shrinkage of the cytoplasm occurs, while cell wall retains original shape and size
- Microdissection
- Differential staining
- Electron microscopy
- Specific antibody reaction

Cell Membrane

It is also known as **plasma membrane** or **cytoplasmic membrane and** lies beneath the cell wall.

Functions of cell wall:
- It is essential for survival of bacteria
- Being semi-permeable membrane, it acts as osmotic barrier.
- Being semi-permeable membrane, it allows only selective substances to pass through it.
- It also helps in nutrient uptake as proteins and other substances present in this membrane are involved in nutrient uptake and waste excretion.
- This is also the site of various metabolic process of bacteria, such as respiration, lipid synthesis, etc.
- It also helps bacteria to communicate with the external environment with the receptors present on it.

STRUCTURE OF CELL MEMBRANE

It is described by **Fluid Mosaic Model (Fig. 2.4).**

Size: Cell membrane is 5–10 mm in thickness.

Composition:
- It is composed of bilayered phospholipids having hydrophobic and hydrophilic ends.
- Bilayered phospholipids further contains various proteins in itself like integral and peripheral proteins.
- Sterol like cholesterol is absent (present in eukaryotic cell membrane) except mycoplasma membrane.
- There are carbohydrates attached to membrane proteins.

Cytoplasm

These are not membrane bound organelles as seen in eukaryotic cells. The plasma membrane within it is called **protoplast.**

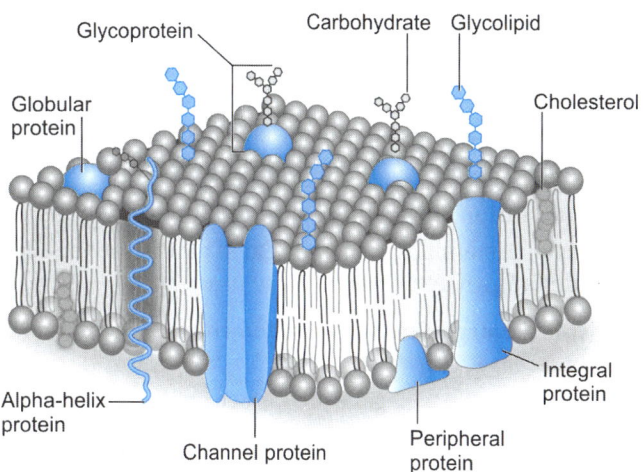

Fig. 2.4: Fluid mosaic model describing bacterial cell membrane.

Ribosome's:
• These are the site of protein synthesis
• They are composed of rRNA and proteins
Storage granules (inclusion bodies)
These are sources of stored energy and present in some species of bacteria. It is of two types:
1. Organic inclusion bodies, e.g., glycogen granules
2. Organic inclusion bodies, e.g., metachromatic granules found in *Corynebacterium diphtheriae*
Mesosomes
• These are actually the plasma membrane invaginations which are in the shape of vesicles, tubules or lamellae.
• They are common in gram-positive bacteria then gram-negative bacteria
Main functions
• This is the site of bacterial respiration
• Involved in cell wall formation
• Plays an important role in chromosome replication
Nucleoid:
• Genetic material is present irregularly shaped region which is called nucleoid
• Nuclear membrane is absent
• Nucleus absent
• In bacteria, there is a single haploid chromosome containing coiled circular double stranded DNA (ds-DNA) of 1 mm length
• **Plasmid** an extrachromosomal DNA is also present in bacteria

Cell Wall Appendages

Those parts of bacteria which are extending outwards from the cell wall of bacteria are termed as cell wall appendages. It includes the following parts of bacteria:
- Capsule and slime layer
- Flagella
- Fimbriae or pili

Capsule and Slime Layer

It is the amorphous viscid bacterial secretion which surrounds some bacteria as their outermost layer. When it diffuses into the surrounding medium and remains as a loose undemarcated secretion it is called as slime layer.

Composition: Usually, it is polysaccharide in nature (except *Bacillus anthracis* where it is polypeptide).

Function:
- Capsule enhances bacterial virulence by inhibiting phagocytosis
- Increases virulence of bacteria
- Prevents bacterial cell death due to various mechanisms
- Helps in biofilm formation to bacteria and also in adhesion.
- It also acts as a source of nutrients and energy.
- It can be also used in vaccine preparations in some cases.

Demonstration of capsule: Capsule can be seen/observed by
- Negative staining method (India Ink Preparation)—for *Cryptococcus*
- Quellung's reaction—for *Pneumococcus*

Capsulated organisms are: *Streptococcus pneumoniae, Klebsiella species. Bacillus anthracis, Haemophilus influenzae, Cryptococcus neoformans.*

Flagella (Fig. 2.5): Flagella are known as the organ of locomotion of bacteria as they make bacteria motile. These are thin thread like appendages which arise from the cell wall of bacteria. They arise from cytoplasmic membrane and pass out through cell wall. Length is 5–20 µm and thickness is 0.02 µm.

Structure:
- **Basal body:** It constitutes the extreme basal part of the flagellum attached with plasma membrane.
- **Hook:** It represents a broader and thicker basal region of flagellum and passes out through the cell wall.
- **Filament:** It is the thinner, elongated and terminal part of flagellum.

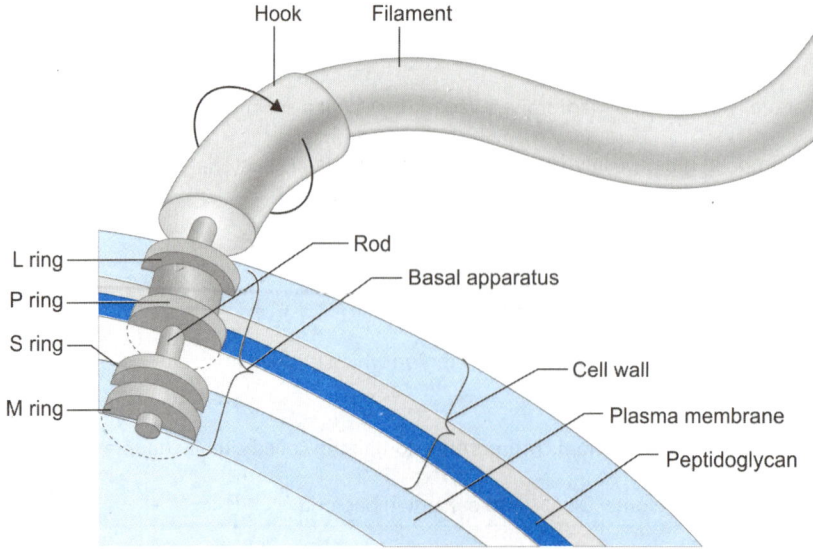

Fig. 2.5: Ultrastructure of flagella.

Motility of Bacteria

Not all bacteria exhibit self-propelled motion, i.e., motility, under appropriate circumstances. Motion can be achieved by one of three mechanisms:
1. Most motile bacteria move by the use of flagella (singular, flagellum), rigid structures 20 nm in diameter and 15–20 μm long which protrude from the cell surface (e.g., *Chromatium*).
2. Spirochetes are helical bacteria which have a specialized internal structure known as the axial filament which is responsible for rotation of the cell in a spiral fashion and consequent locomotion (e.g., *Rhodospirillum*).
3. Gliding bacteria all secrete copious slime, but the mechanism which propels the cells is not known.
4. Classification of bacteria on the basis of arrangement of flagella is shown in **Table 2.5**.

Note: *Proteus mirabilis* **swarming** behavior is characterized by the development of concentric rings of growth that are formed as cyclic events of swarm cells differentiation, swarming migration, and cellular differentiation are repeated during colony translocation across a surface.

TABLE 2.5: Classification of bacteria on the basis of arrangement of flagella.

Type	Arrangement of flagella	Image
Atrichous	Bacteria with no flagellum	
Monotrichous	Bacteria with single polar flagellum	
Lophotrichous	Bacteria with tuft of flagella at one pole	
Amphitrichous	Bacteria with single polar flagellum or tuft of flagella at both poles	
Peritrichous	Bacteria with flagella distributed all round the cell	
Amphilophotrichous	Bacteria with tuft of flagella at both poles	

Different types of motility with example	
Type of motility	**Bacteria**
Tumbling motility	*Listeria*
Gliding motility	*Mycoplasma*
Stately motility	*Clostridium*
Darting motility	*Vibrio cholerae*, *Campylobacter*
Cockscrew, flexion extension motility	*Spirochete*

Detection of Motility of Bacteria

Method

Hanging-Drop Method

Procedure
- Vaseline is applied to the four corners of a clean coverslip.
- Using a sterile loop, a loopful of the given suspension is placed on the center of the coverslip.
- A cavity slide is inverted over the cover slip so that the drop of suspension is in the center of the cavity.
- The slide is quickly and carefully turned over so that the coverslip is on the top with the drop hanging into the cavity.
- The microscope is adjusted for reduced light by lowering the condenser, and using the concave mirror.
- The edge of the drop is focussed under low power. The microscope is then turned to high power to observe the morphology and motility of the bacteria in the given suspension.

Result

| Motile organisms | Detected by presence of directional movement |
| Non-motile organisms | No movement |

Fimbriae or Pili

- Fimbriae (pili)—are hair-like structures on the outside of bacteria, and they are composed of protein subunits (pilin).
- Fimbriae can be morphologically distinguished from flagella because they are smaller in diameter (3–8 nm versus 15–20 nm) and usually are not coiled in structure.
- In general, several hundred fimbriae are arranged peritrichously (uniformly) over the entire surface of the bacterial cell. They may be as long as 15–20 μm or many times the length of the cell.
- Fimbriae represent the type of pill that help in adhesion.
- Fimbriae promote adherence to other bacteria or to the host. The tips of the fimbriae may contain proteins (lectins) that bind to specific sugars (e.g., mannose).
- Fimbriae are an important virulence factor for colonization and infection of the urinary tract by *E. coli, Neisseria gonorrhoeae*, and other bacteria.

Types of Pili

1. **F pili (sex pili):** They bind to other bacteria and form a tube for transfer of large segments of bacterial chromosomes between bacteria. These pili are encoded by a plasmid (F).
2. **Common pili or fimbriae:** They help in bacterial adhesion to host surfaces (epithelial surfaces, red blood cells, etc.) thus helping in colonization.

Functions of Fimbriae (Table 2.6)

- **Adhesion:** Fimbriae are organs of adhesion. This property enhances the virulence of bacteria.
- **Transfer of genetic material:** Sex pili are present in male bacteria. These pili are longer (18–20 μm) in size and 1–4 in number. They help male cells to attach with female cells in forming "conjugation tubes" through which genetic material is believed to be transferred from the donor to the recipient cell.

Detection/Demonstration Methods

- Electron microscopy
- Hemagglutination

TABLE 2.6: Difference between flagella and fimbriae.

Flagella	Fimbriae
They are thicker and larger in size	Thinner and smaller in size
They are helical and never straight	Non-helical and always straight
They arise from cytoplasmic membrane but not attached to cell wall	Attached to cell wall
They are present only in motile species	Present in both motile and non-motile species
They are organs of movement (motility)	Organs of adhesion and conjugation

Colonization

Colonization is defined as the entry and multiplication of the pathogen (bacteria) in host surface without invasion of the surface, which neither causes disease nor generates specific immune response.
- Different bacteria colonize different parts of the body. This may be closest to the point of entry or caused by the presence of optimal growth conditions at the site.
- Colonization requires special bacterial structures and functions to remain at the site, survive, and obtain food.
- Bacteria may use specific mechanisms to adhere to and colonize different body surfaces. For example, if the bacteria can adhere to epithelial or endothelial cell linings of the bladder, intestine, and blood vessels, then they cannot be washed away, and this adherence allows them to colonize the tissue.
- Many of these adhesin proteins are present at the tips of fimbriae (pili) and bind tightly to specific sugars on the target tissue.

Bacterial Spore
- The spore is a dehydrated multi-shelled structure that protects and allows the bacteria to exist in suspended animation.
- Spores are highly resistant resting stage formed in unfavorable conditions presumed to be related to the depletion of exogenous nutrients.
- The structure of the spore protects the genomic DNA from intense heat, radiation, and attack by most enzymes and chemical agents. In fact, bacterial spores are so resistant to environmental factors that they can exist for centuries as viable spores.
- Spores also are difficult to decontaminate with standard disinfectants or autoclaving conditions. The endospores are resistant to ordinary boiling, heating and disinfectants. They can withstand boiling up to 3 hours, dry heat at 150°C for 1 hour. However, they can be destroyed by autoclaving at 121°C for 15–20 minutes.
- Spore within the bacterial cell are called endospores.
- The location of the spore within a cell is a characteristic of the bacteria and can assist in identification of the bacterium.

Examples of spore forming bacteria
- *Bacillus anthracis*—obligate aerobes
- *Clostridium tetani, Clostridium botulinum*—obligate anaerobes

Uses of Spores and Various Shape and Position of Spores (Fig. 2.6)

Spores of various bacteria are used as an indicator/sterilization control in various sterilization processes (also as in bioterrorism, e.g., anthrax spores in 2001 in USA). For example, *Geobacillus stearothermophilus* in autoclave, *Bacillus atrophaeus* in hot air oven.

Demonstration/detection spore: This can be done by:
- Gram staining
- Modified Ziehl-Neelsen staining

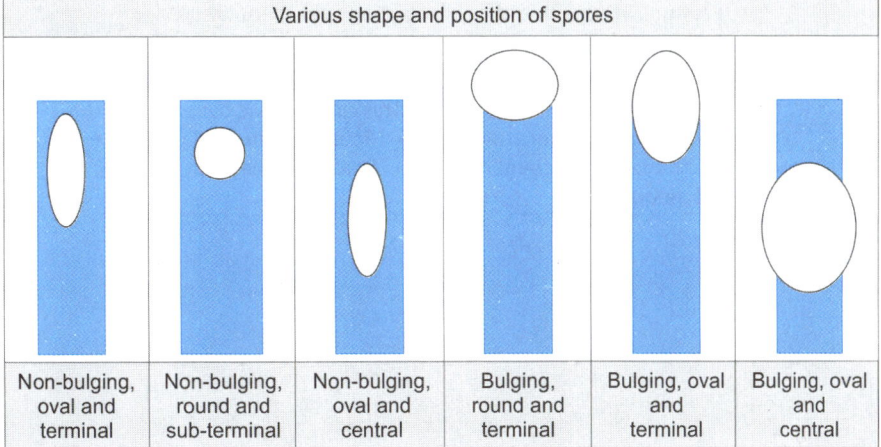

Fig. 2.6: Various shape and position of spores: Spores may be spherical or oval and may be central, sub-terminal or terminal in position.

GROWTH AND NUTRITION OF BACTERIA

Nutrition of Bacteria

The minimum nutritional requirement for growth and multiplication of bacteria includes sources as follows:
- **Water:** It constitutes about 80% of bacterial cell.
- Carbon, nitrogen, hydrogen, oxygen, inorganic salts (such as sulfur, phosphorus, sodium, potassium, magnesium, iron, manganese, etc., in small amounts).
- **Bacterial vitamins or growth factors:** Some fastidious bacteria require vitamins, such as thiamine, nicotinic acid, riboflavin, pyridoxine, folic acid and vitamin B12 for their growth also.

Bacterial Growth

Bacterial replication is a coordinated process in which two equivalent daughter cells are produced. For growth to occur, there must be sufficient metabolites to support synthesis of the bacterial components and especially the nucleotides for DNA synthesis.

Bacterial Cell Division

Bacteria divide by binary fission. Nuclear division occurs before cytoplasmic division. When a bacterial cell reaches a critical mass in its cellular constituents, the cell division starts. Bacteria nucleus or chromosome is a circular double stranded DNA molecule.

The nuclear division precedes bacterial cell division. During replication, the two strands of DNA are separated and new complementary strands are formed. Thus two identical double stranded DNA molecules are formed.

Generation Time

It is the time required by bacterium (singular) to give rise to two new cells (daughter cells) under optimal conditions. It varies in bacteria, for example:
- *Escherichia coli:* 20 minutes
- *Mycobacterium tuberculosis:* 20 hours
- *Mycobacterium leprae:* 20 days

Bacterial Count

It means to count the number of bacteria present in the given specimen. It can be total count or viable count.

Total count	Viable count
It represents total number of bacteria which will be present in the given specimen/culture, irrespective of whether they are dead or alive	It represents only viable (living) bacteria which will be present in the given specimen/culture
This is done by bacterial counting under microscope with the help of counting chamber	This can be done by: • Pour plate method • Spreading method

Bacterial Growth Curve (Fig. 2.7)

When bacteria is put in a suitable media (i.e., inoculated), its growth passes though several stages. When bacterial count of such culture is determined at different intervals and plotted in relation to time, a growth curve is obtained. This bacterial growth curve has the following characteristic four stages:

1. **Lag phase:**
   - After inoculation of the culture medium, multiplication usually does not begin immediately. The period between inoculation and beginning of multiplication is known as lag phase. During this period, the organisms adapt to the new environment, during which necessary enzymes and intermediate metabolites are built up in adequate quantities for multiplication to proceed.
   - There is increase in the size of the cells but there is no increase in numbers.
   - The duration of lag phase varies with the species, nature of culture medium and temperature, etc.
2. **Log phase:**
   - In this phase, the bacteria starts multiplying exponentially.
   - Bacteria are smaller in number (being immature).
   - It is the best stage to perform biochemical reactions.
   - It is the best stage to perform Gram staining as bacteria are uniformly stained.
3. **Stationary phase:**
   - In this phase, accumulation of toxic products, nutritional deficiency, etc., starts due to which the bacteria growth stops to some extent.
   - The number of new bacterial cells formed are equal to the number of cells dying, hence growth curve becomes plain.
   - The number of viable cells remain stationary as there is almost a balance between the dying cells and newly formed cells.
4. **Decline phase or death phase:**
   - In this phase, due to accumulation of the toxic products and exhaustion of nutrition, due to the death of cells.
   - Bacteria in this phase stops multiplying completely.
   - In this phase, the viable (living) cell count decreases but not total count.
   - In this phase, involution forms are also seen.

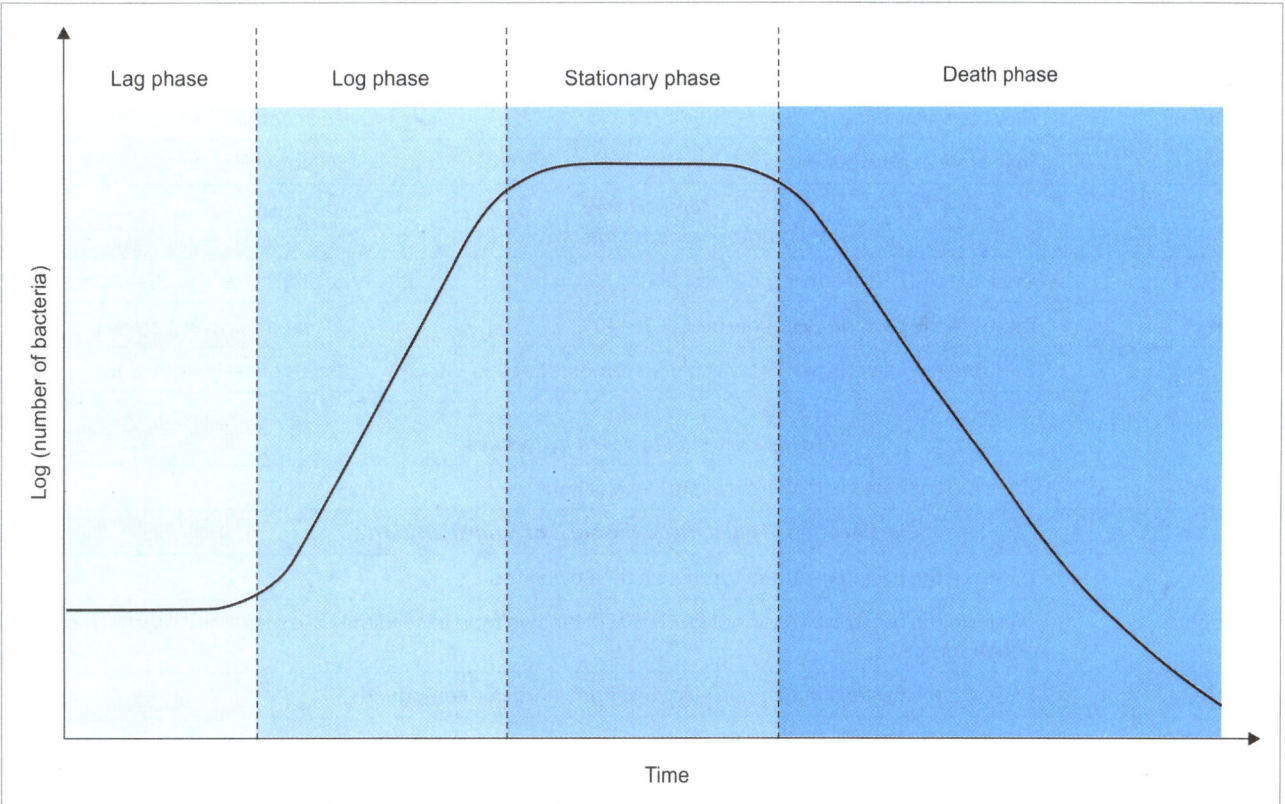

Fig. 2.7: Growth curve.

Factors that Affect Bacterial Growth (Table 2.7)

- Oxygen
- Carbon dioxide
- Temperature
- pH
- Light: Bacteria grow well in darkness except phototrophs.
- Osmotic conditions
- Moisture: It is one of the important factor require for bacterial growth.

TABLE 2.7: Factors that affect bacterial growth and classification of bacteria on those factors.

Classification	Definition	Example
Oxygen		
Obligate aerobes	These bacteria grow only in presence of oxygen	*Mycobacterium tuberculosis, Pseudomonas aeruginosa*
Facultative aerobes	These are aerobes but can also grow anaerobically	*Escherichia coli*, etc.
Facultative anaerobes	These are anaerobes but they can also grow aerobically	*Lactobacillus*, etc.
Microaerophilic bacteria	These are the bacteria which can grow in presence of low oxygen, i.e., 5–10% of oxygen	*Helicobacter*, etc.
Obligate anaerobes	These bacteria grow only in absence presence of oxygen	*Clostridium*, etc.
Aerotolerant anaerobes	These bacteria can tolerate oxygen for some time but they do not use the oxygen	*Clostridium histolyticum*, etc.
Carbon dioxide		
Capnophilic bacteria	These are the bacteria that require carbon dioxide in higher amounts (5–10%) for their growth	*Streptococcus pneumoniae*, etc.
pH **Most pathogenic bacteria grow at pH 7.2–7.6**		
Acidophiles	They grow at acidic pH	*Lactobacillus*, etc.
Alkaline pH	They grow at pH around 9	*Vibrio cholerae*, etc.
Temperature **Most pathogenic bacteria grow at 37°C**		
Psychrophiles	These are the bacteria that grow best below 20°C	Saprophytes, e.g., *Pseudomonas*, etc.
Mesophiles	These are the bacteria that grow best at 25–40°C	Most pathogenic bacteria
Thermophiles	These are the bacteria that grow at higher temperatures 55–80°C	*Geobacillus stearothermophilus*, etc.
Light **Mainly bacteria grow well in darkness**		
Phototrophs	These are the bacteria that grow in presence of light	
Classification of bacteria on the basis of mode nutrition		
Autotrophs	These are the bacteria that can synthesize their own food	
Heterotrophs	These are the bacteria that cannot synthesize their own food instead they use preformed organic molecule as carbon source	
Lithotrophs	These are the bacteria that obtain electrons from inorganic compounds	
Organotrophs	These are the bacteria that obtain electrons from organic compounds	
Chemotrophs	These are the bacteria that gain energy from external chemical compounds	
Phototrophs	These are the bacteria that obtain energy from light	

LABORATORY IDENTIFICATION OF MICRO-ORGANISMS

1. Catalase Test

Principle: The enzyme catalase decomposes hydrogen peroxide (H_2O_2) into water and nascent oxygen. The presence of enzyme in a bacterial isolates is evident when a small inoculum is introduced into H_2O_2 and the rapid elaboration of oxygen bubbles occurs. The lack of catalase enzyme is evident by a lack of or weak bubble.

Procedure: With an inoculating needle or a wooden applicator stick, transfer growth from the center of a colony to the surface of a glass slide. Add a drop of 3% hydrogen peroxide and observe the bubble formation. This test is used to differentiate *Staphylococcus* spp. and *Streptococcus* spp.

Interpretation: The rapid and sustained production of bubbles or effervescence constitutes a positive test because of the production of enzyme catalase.

Quality Control (Fig. 2.8)
- Positive control: *Staphylococcus aureus*
- Negative control: *Streptococcus pyogenes*.

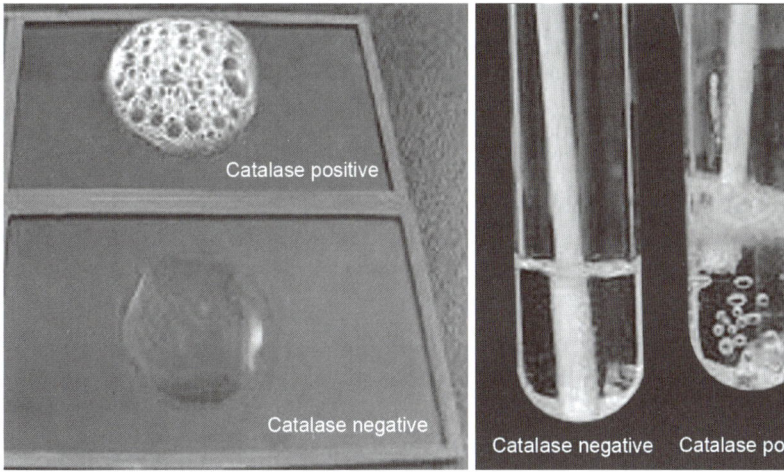

Fig. 2.8: Catalase test.

2. Oxidase Test

Principle: Cytochromes are iron-containing hemoproteins that act as the last link in the chain of aerobic respiration by transferring electrons (hydrogen) to oxygen, with formation of water. The cytochrome system is found in aerobic, microaerophilic and facultatively anaerobic organisms. The dye 1% solution of tetra methyl-para-phenylene-diamine dihydrochloride is oxidized to indophenol blue producing deep purple color.

Procedure: Wet filter paper method is used in this test. Strips of Whatman No.1 filter paper is soaked with a little freshly made 1% solution of tetra methyl-para-phenylene-diamine dihydrochloride and then with a help of sterile glass rod a single colony from the medium is rubbed over the strip.

Interpretation: A positive reaction is indicated by an intense deep purple blue color appearing within 5–10 seconds and a negative reaction by absence of coloration or by coloration later than 60 seconds.

Quality Control (Fig. 2.9)
- Positive control: *Pseudomonas aeruginosa* ATCC 27583
- Negative control: *Escherichia coli* ATCC 25922

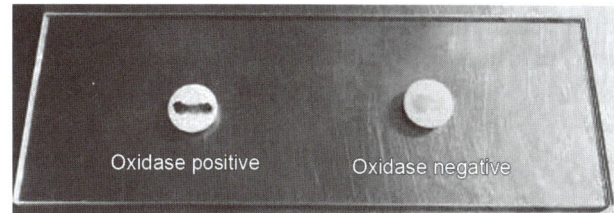

Fig. 2.9: Oxidase test.

3. Coagulase Test

This test is done to differentiate between *Staphylococcus* species. Both slide and tube coagulase test is done. Coagulase is present in two forms, bound and free, each having different properties that require the use of separate testing procedures.

Slide Coagulase Test

Principle: Slide coagulase test detects bound coagulase which is attached to the bacterial cell wall and is not present in culture filtrate. Fibrin strands are formed between the bacterial cells when suspended in plasma (fibrinogen), causing them to clump not visible aggregates.

Procedure: A smooth milky suspension of the growth is made in normal saline over a clean glass slide. Make similar suspension of control positive and negative strains to confirm the proper reactivity of the plasma. To the test suspension a loop full of undiluted human plasma is added and the suspension is observed for the appearance of coarse clumps.

Interpretation: It is read as positive when a coarse clumping of cocci is visible to the naked eye within 10 seconds. Negative is read when there is absence of clumping **(Fig. 2.10)**.

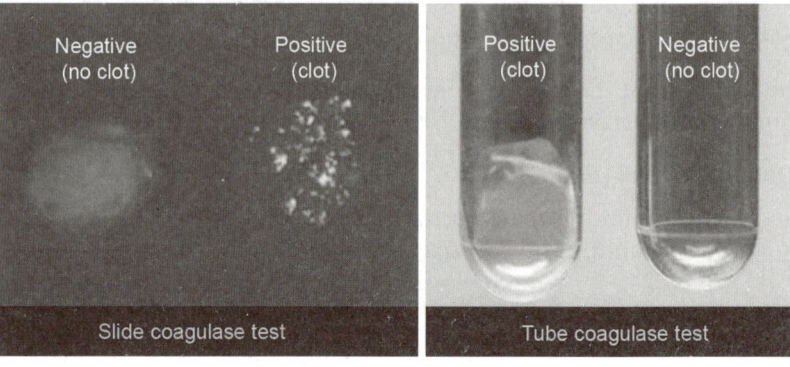

Fig. 2.10: Coagulase test.

Tube Coagulase Test

Principle: Coagulase is a protein that has prothrombin-like activity which can convert fibrinogen to fibrin. A visible clot is seen. Heat labile protein secreted free into the medium and clots the rabbit plasma in presence of factor known as coagulase reactive factor (CRF), which is similar to prothrombin present in plasma and converts fibrinogen into fibrin.

$$\text{Free coagulase + CRF} \longrightarrow \text{CRF coagulase}$$
$$\text{Fibrinogen} \longrightarrow \text{Fibrin}$$

4. Indole Test

Principle: This test is done to demonstrate the ability of certain bacteria that possess enzyme tryptophanase, which are capable of hydrolyzing and demeaning tryptophan with the production of indole, pyruvic acid and ammonia. Indole, a benzyl pyrrole, is one of the metabolic degradation products of amino acid tryptophan.

Procedure: Kovac's reagent method is employed. Kovac's reagent preparation.

Amyl or isoamyl alcohol: 150 mL
p-dimethylaminobenzaldehyde: 10 g
Concentrated HCl: 50 mL

Individual colonies are inoculated on to peptone water and incubated at 37°C for 18–24 hours. To this 0.5 mL of Kovac's reagent is added and gently shaken.

Interpretation: Appearance of bright fuschia pink colored ring at the interface of reagent and the broth within seconds after adding the reagent is indicative of the presence of indole and is a positive test.

Quality Control (Fig. 2.11)

- Positive control: *Escherichia coli* ATCC 25922
- Negative control: *Klebsiella pneumonia*.

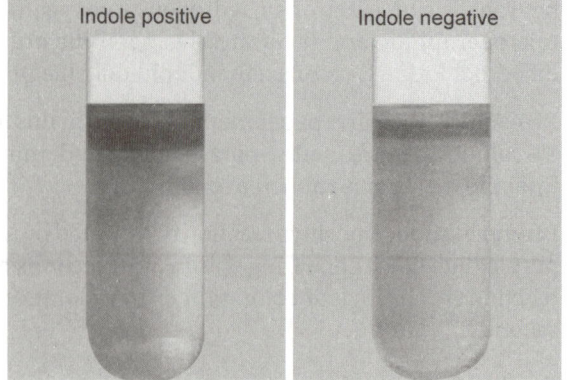

Fig. 2.11: Indole test. *(For color version, see Plate 1)*

5. Urease Test

Principle: Urease is an enzyme possessed by many species of microorganisms. This test is done to determine the ability of bacteria to decompose urea into ammonia. Christensen's urea agar medium is used. Indicator used is Phenol red.

Procedure: Inoculate heavily over the entire surface of Christensen's urea agar medium with the peptone water culture and incubate at 37°C. Examine after 4 hours and then overnight incubation.

Interpretation

- **Positive:** When the indicator turned to pink-purple.
- **Negative:** No change in color.

Quality Control (Fig. 2.12)

- **Positive control:** *Proteus* species
- **Negative control:** *Escherichia coli*.

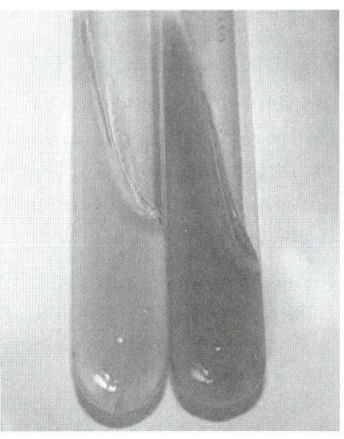

Fig. 2.12: Urease test. *(For color version, see Plate 1)*

6. Triple Sugar Iron Agar Test

Principle: This is done to determine ability of bacteria to ferment carbohydrates incorporated in a growth medium and production of hydrogen sulfide. Triple sugar iron (TSI) agar medium contains 10 parts lactose, 10 parts sucrose, 1 part glucose and peptone. Phenol red and ferrous sulphate serve as indicator of acidification and H_2S production respectively. With a sterile straight inoculating wire, touch the top of a well with isolated colony.

Procedure: Inoculate TSI slant by first stabbing through the center of the medium to the bottom of the tube and then streaking the surface of the agar slant. Incubate the tube at 37°C for 18–24 hours. The result is interpreted as follows:

Interpretation (Fig. 2.13):

Slant/butt	Color	Utilization
Alkaline slant/acid butt (K/A)	Red/yellow	Glucose only fermented; peptone is utilized
Acid slant/acid butt (A/A)	Yellow/yellow	Glucose, lactose and/or sucrose fermented
Alkaline butt/alkaline butt (K/K)	Red/red	No fermentation of glucose, lactose or sucrose

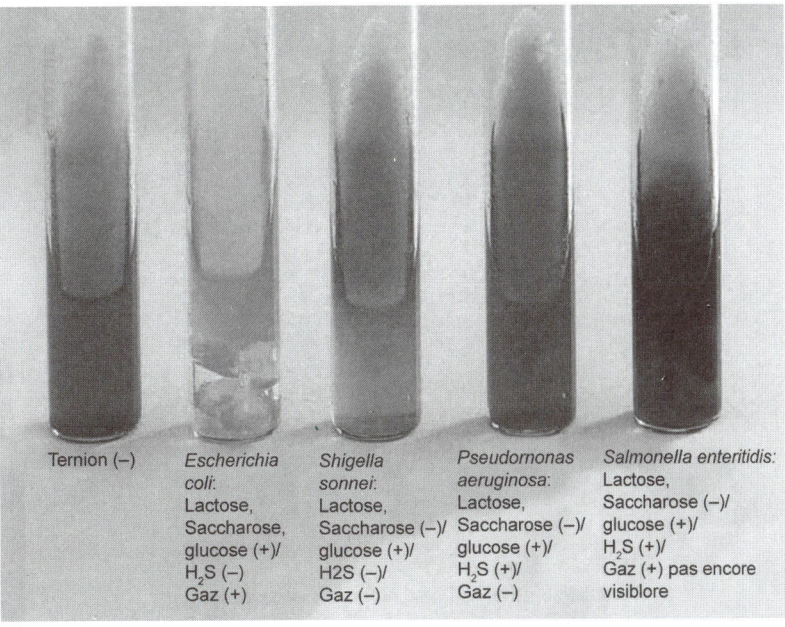

Fig. 2.13: Triple sugar iron agar test. *(For color version, see Plate 1)*

A black precipitate in the butt indicates production of ferrous sulfide and H_2S gas. Bubbles or cracks in the media indicate the production of CO_2 or H_2.

7. Citrate Utilization Test

Principle: The utilization of citrate by a test bacterium is detected in a citrate medium by the production of alkaline by products. To determine the ability of certain bacteria to obtain energy in a manner by utilizing citrate as a sole source of carbon for its growth. Simmon's citrate medium is used to know the utilization of citrate. Indicator is bromothymol blue.

Procedure: The citrate slant is inoculated with the suspected single colony and medium is incubated at 37°C for 24 to 48 hours. A positive reaction is indicated by the blue color and streak of growth. A negative reaction if original green color persists and no growth along the streak line.

Quality Control (Fig. 2.14)

- **Positive control:** *Enterobacter aerogenes*
- **Negative control:** *Escherichia coli.*

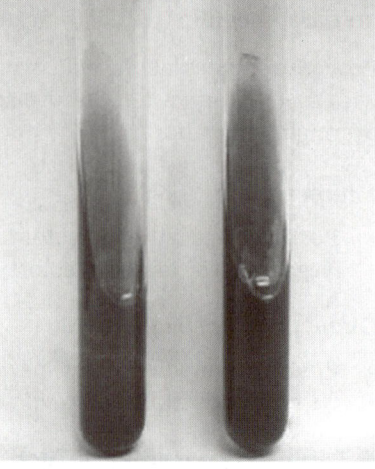

Fig. 2.14: Citrate utilization test. *(For color version, see Plate 1)*

8. Methyl Red Test

Principle: Methyl red is quantitative test for production of acid, requiring positive organism to produce string acids (lactic acid, acetic acid, formic acid) from glucose through the mixed acid fermentation pathway. This test is to determine the ability of bacteria which can maintain the low pH after prolonged incubation.

Procedure: Inoculate the glucose phosphate broth with a pure culture of test organism and incubate at 37°C for 48 hours (no fewer than 48 hours). To this, add about five drops of the methyl red reagent. Mix and read immediately.

Interpretation: Development of stable red color in the surface of the medium indicates sufficient acid production to lower the pH to 4.4 and constitutes a positive test.

Quality control (Fig. 2.15):

- **Positive control:** *Escherichia coli*
- **Negative control:** *Enterobacter aerogenes.*

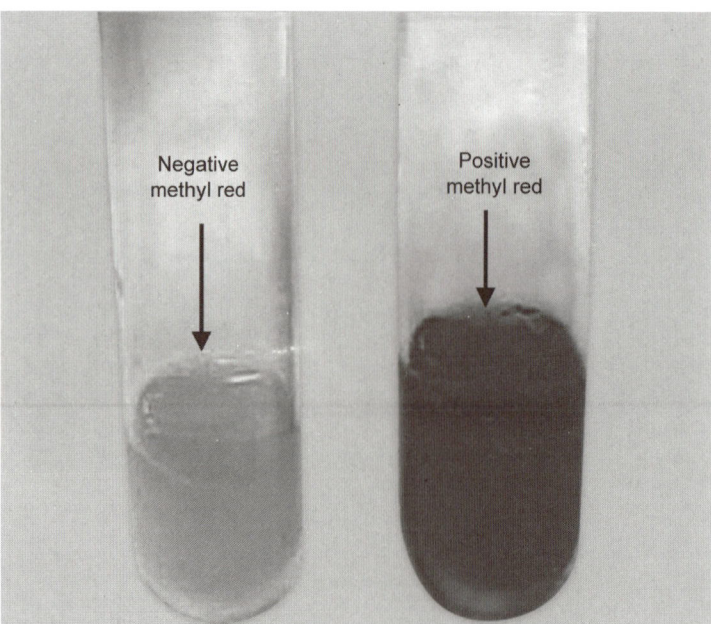

Fig. 2.15: Methyl red test. *(For color version, see Plate 1)*

9. Voges-Proskauer Test

Principle: Pyruvic acid is a pivotal compound formed in the fermentative degradation of glucose, further metabolized through various metabolic pathways, depending upon the enzyme systems possessed by different bacteria, where the end-product is acetoin (acetyl methyl carbinol). In the presence of atmospheric oxygen and 40% potassium hydroxide, acetoin is converted into diacetyl and alpha-naphthol serves as a catalyst to bring out a red complex.

Procedure: Inoculate the glucose phosphate peptone broth with a pure culture of test organism and incubate at 37°C for 48 hours. To this add 0.6 mL of 5% α-naphthol followed by 0.2 mL of 40% potassium hydroxide. Shake the tube gently to expose the medium to atmospheric oxygen and allow to remain it undisturbed for 10–15 minutes.

Interpretation: A positive reaction is indicated by the development of a red color in 15 minutes, indicating the presence of diacetyl, the oxidation product of acetoin. It turns crimson red in color in 30 minutes.

Quality control (Fig. 2.16):
- **Positive control:** *Enterbacter aerogenes*
- **Negative control:** *Escherichia coli*

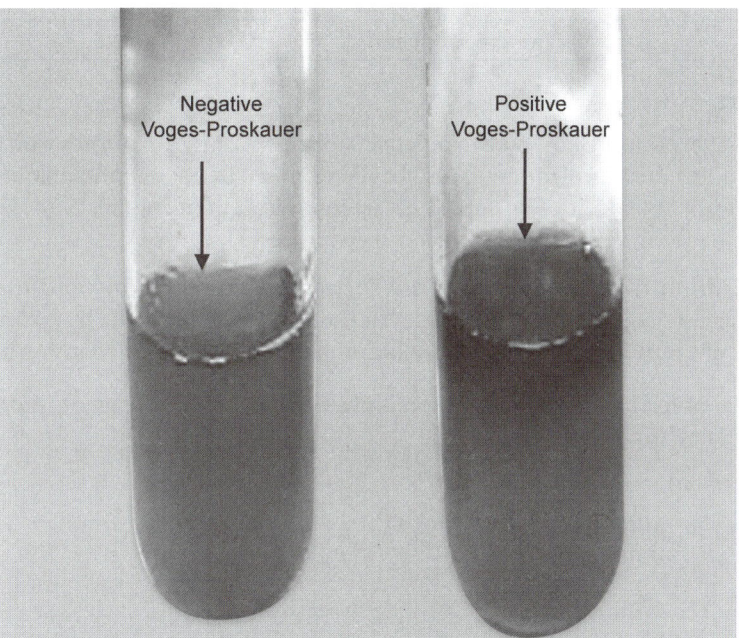

Fig. 2.16: Voges-Proskauer test. *(For color version, see Plate 2)*

10. Sugar Fermentation Test

Principle: This test is done to determine the ability of an organism to ferment a specific carbohydrate that is incorporated in a basal medium, thereby producing acid with or without visible gas.

Procedure: The test is performed on conventional culture media with test sugars. The common sugar fermentation media used are glucose, lactose, sucrose, maltose, mannose, arabinose and xylose. From the peptone water tube (which was incubated for 2 hours after inoculation) all the sugar fermentation media are inoculated with the help of a Pasteur pipette. After the different media are inoculated, these are incubated at 37°C for 18–24 hours. After 24 hours the sugar media are examined for the production of acid indicated by pink color and gas (presence of an air bubble inside the Durham's tube).

Interpretation: Positive test is indicated by change in color to pink with or without gas formation in Durham's tube. Negative test is indicated by growth, but no change in color.

11. Oxidation/Fermentation Test (Modified Hugh and Leifson)

Principle: This test is done to know the organism uses carbohydrate substrate to produce acid by products either oxidatively or fermentatively.

Procedure: Hugh-Leifson basal medium is prepared and carbohydrate to be added is sterilized separately and added to give final concentration of 1%. The medium is then tubed to a depth of about 4 cm.

Duplicate tubes of medium were inoculated by stabbing. One tube is promptly covered with liquid paraffin to a depth of 1 cm and is incubated at 37°C for 18–24 hours.

Interpretation: Acid production is detected in the medium by the appearance of a yellow color. In the case of oxidative organisms, color production may be first noted near the surface of medium. Following are reaction patterns:

Open tube	Covered tube	Metabolism
Acid (yellow)	Alkaline (green)	Oxidative
Acid (yellow)	Acid (yellow)	Fermentative
Alkaline (green or blue)	Alkaline (green or blue)	Non-saccharolytic

12. Nitrate Reduction Test

Principle: The test is used to determine the ability of an organism to reduce nitrate to nitrites which is used for the identification of family *Enterobacteriaceae*. The reduction of nitrate to nitrite is determined by adding sulfanilic acid and alpha-naphthylamine. The sulfanilic acid and nitrate forms a diazonium salt. The diazonium salt then couples with α-naphthylamine to produce a red, water soluble azo dye.

Procedure: This liquid medium is inoculated with the suspected single colony and the medium is incubated for 18–24 hours. Add 0.1 mL of the test reagent to the test culture. The test reagent is prepared by mixing equal volumes of solution A (8.0 g of sulfanilic acid in 1 L of acetic acid 5 mol/L) and solution B (5.0 g of α-naphthylamine in 1 L of acetic acid 5 mol/L).

Interpretation: Development of red color within 30 seconds after adding the test reagents indicates the presence of nitrites and represents a positive reaction for nitrate reduction.

Quality control (Fig. 2.17)
- **Positive control:** *Escherichia coli*
- **Negative control:** *Acinetobacter baumannii.*

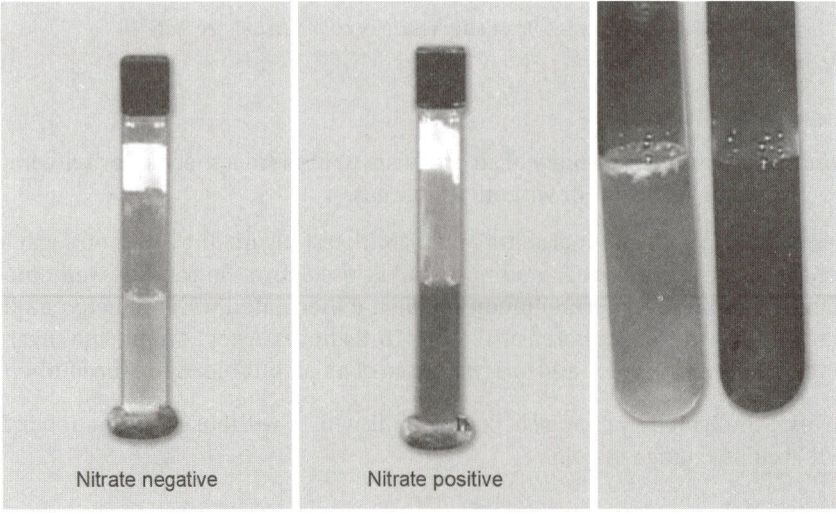

Fig. 2.17: Nitrate reduction test. *(For color version, see Plate 2)*

13. Phenylalanine Deaminase Test (PPA)

Principle: To determine the ability of bacteria to deaminate phenylalanine to phenyl pyruvic acid (PPA). Of the *Enterobacteriaceae*, only members of the *Proteus, Morganella and Providencia* genera possess the deaminase enzyme.

Procedure: This test was done to know the ability of the organism to deaminate phenylalanine with the production of phenyl pyruvic acid, which reacts with ferric salts to give green color. Inoculate it with pure growth and incubate 37°C for 18–24 hours. After incubation, allow a few drops of 10% solution of ferric chloride to run over the growth on the slope.

Interpretation: The immediate appearance of an intense green color indicates the presence of phenyl pyruvic acid and a positive test.

Quality control (Fig. 2.18)
- **Positive control:** *Proteus* species
- **Negative control:** *Escherichia coli.*

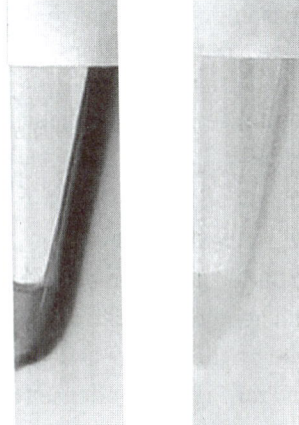

Fig. 2.18: Phenylalanine deaminase test. *(For color version, see Plate 2)*

14. Amino Acid Decarboxylases

Principle: Decarboxylases are group of substrate specific enzymes that are capable of reacting with the carboxyl portion of amino acids, forming alkalinel-reacting amines. The conversion of arginine to citrulline is a dehydrolase, in which an NH_2 group is removed from arginine. Citrulline is next converted to ornithine, which then undergoes decarboxylation to form putrescine.

Procedure: Two Moller decarboxylases broth base is used. The amino acid to be tested is added to the decarboxylase base before inoculation with the test organism. A control tube, consisting only the base without the amino acid, must also be set up in parallel. Both tubes are anerobically incubated by overlaying the mineral oil. Incubate at 37°C for 18–24 hours. At initial stages of incubation, both the tubes turn yellow, owing to the fermentation of small amount of glucose in the medium. If amino acid is decarboxylated alkaline amines are formed and the medium reverts to original purple color. Indicators are cresol red and bromocresol purple.

L-lysine ─────────── lysine decarboxylase ─────────→ cadaverine + carbon dioxide
Bromocresol purple ─────────── cadaverine ─────────→ bromocresol purple
(yellow)   (lavender purple)

Interpretation: Conversion of the control tube to a yellow color indicates that the organism is viable and that the pH of the medium has been lowered sufficiently to activate the decarboxylase enzymes. Reversion of the tube containing the amino acid to a blue-purple color indicates a positive test owing to the formation of amines from the decarboxylation reaction.

Quality control

Amino acid	Positive control	Negative control
Lysine	Enterobacter aerogenes	Enterobacter cloacae
Ornithine	Enterobacter cloacae	Klebsiella pneumoniae
Arginine	Enterobacter cloacae	Enterobacter aerogenes

STAINING METHODS

Simple Staining

Morphology of bacteria by using simple stains.

Requirements: Loeffler's methylene blue, dilute carbol fuchsin, normal saline, compound microscope and cedarwood oil.

Staining: Staining is an auxiliary technique used in microscopy to enhance contrast in the microscopic image. Different types of staining are simple staining, negative staining, differential staining.

Smear preparation: Place one single colony of solid bacterial growth and emulsify in one drop of normal saline in the center of a clean slide. Now, with your inoculating loop, mix the specimen with the saline completely and spread the mixture out to cover about half of the total slide area. Air dry it and fix it by passing over Bunsen burner. The smear is now ready for the staining procedure.

Principle: Simple staining is performed by a watery solution of a single basic dye, such as methylene blue, methyl violet and basic fuchsin. Positive charged cation of the basic dye combines firmly with the negatively charged radicals in the bacterial protoplasm.

The staining provides color contrast and impart the same color to all the bacteria. Hence, it is used to see the morphology of organisms.

Procedure:
- The slide is placed on the rack and is flooded with Loeffler's methylene blue/dilute carbol fuchsin.
- The stain is allowed to act for 3 minutes and for 30 seconds for methylene blue and for dilute carbol fuchsin respectively.
- The slide is then washed with distilled water and gently blotted to dry.
- A drop of cedarwood oil/liquid paraffin is placed on the smear.
- The microscope is adjusted for increased light by raising the condenser, and the slide is examined with the oil immersion objective using the plane mirror.

Gram's Staining (Fig. 2.19)

Principle: Certain bacteria are stained with aniline dyes, such as Gentian violet. When it is subsequently treated with a solution of iodine, mordanting action occurs. This prevents the subsequent decolorization of bacteria on treatment with acetone or alcohol. Other bacteria after similar treatment are readily decolorized. The theories behind it are:

- ***pH theory*:** Cytoplasm of gram-positive bacteria is more acidic (pH 2–3), hence can retain the basic dye (pH 4–5), (crystal violet) for longer time. Iodine serves as mordant as it combines with the primary stain to form a dye-iodine complex which gets retained inside the cell.
- ***Cell wall theory*:** Gram-positive cell has a thick peptidoglycan layer, which are tightly cross linked to each other. Peptidoglycan, acts as a permeability barrier preventing loss of crystal violet. Alcohol, thus shrinks the pores of thick peptidoglycan. Gram-negative cell wall is more permeable, hence allowing crystal violet to flow out easily. It is so because:
    - The thin peptidoglycan layer in the cell wall of gram-negative is not tightly cross linked.
    - Presence of lipopolysaccharide layer in the cell wall of gram-negative bacteria, which gets disrupted easily by the action of acetone or alcohol; thus allowing the primary stain to come out of the cytoplasm.
    - After mordanting with Gram's iodine, bigger die-iodine complex is formed. After decolorization, due to more lipid content in gram-negative bacterial cell wall gets dissolved leading to formation of larger pores through which the dye-iodine complexes escape.
- ***Magnesium ribonucleate theory*:** A compound of magnesium ribonucleate and basic protein concentrated at the cell membranes helps gram-positive bacteria to retain the primary dye. Gram-negative bacteria do not possess this substance.

Requirements: Gentian violet, Gram's iodine, alcohol/acetone, dilute carbol fuchsin/safranine, distilled water, fixed smears, compound microscope and cedarwood oil.

Procedure:
- **Primary staining:** Cover the smear with Gentian violet for one minute. Gentian violet is a basic dye which combines with the acidic cytoplasm of bacterial cells.
- **Mordanting:**
    - Gram's iodine is a mordant. The smear is covered with Gram's iodine for 1 minute. Gram's iodine forms a dye iodine complex.
    - The cell wall of gram-positive organism is impermeable to this dye iodine complex.
- **Decolorization:**
    - The slide is kept in slanting position.
    - Add acetone/absolute alcohol, drop by drop till the solution which comes out of the slide is almost colorless (30 seconds)
    - Gram-positive organism retains primary dye (Gentian violet) while the gram-negative organisms gets decolorized.
- **Counter staining:**
    - Smear is covered with diluted carbol fuchsin/Safranine for 30 seconds and wash with water.
    - Gram-positive organisms remains violet, gram-negative organisms take up the counter stain and turns pink.
    - Using filter paper the slide is gently blotted to dry.
    - A drop of cedarwood oil/liquid paraffin is placed on the smear.
    - The microscope is adjusted for increased light by raising the condenser, and the slide is examined under the oil immersion objective (100x) using the plane mirror.

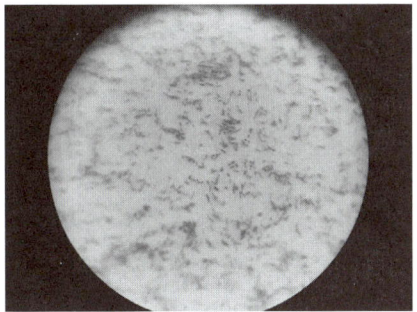 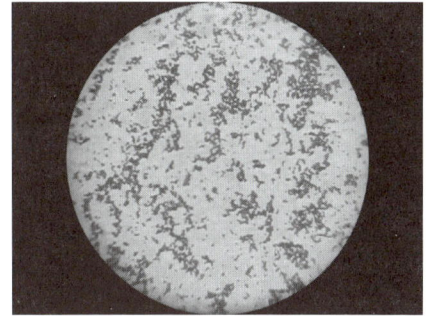

Gram-negative bacilli   **Gram-positive cocci**

Fig. 2.19: Gram staining (negative and positive). *(For color version, see Plate 2)*

ALBERT'S STAINING (FIG. 2.20)

Diagnosis of *Corynebacterium diphtheriae*, by Albert's technique.
Requirements: Albert's I solution, Albert's II solution, distilled water, fixed smears, compound microscope and cedarwood oil.
Composition of reagents:

Albert's I solution		Albert's II solution	
Toluidine blue	1.5 g	Iodine	6 g
Malachite green	2.0 g	Potassium Iodide	9 g
Glacial acetic acid	900 mL	Distilled water	10 mL
95% ethyl alcohol	20 mL		
Distilled water	1,000 mL		

Procedure: It consists of two steps.
1. **Staining:**
    - The slide is kept covered with Albert's I solution for 3–5 minutes.
    - Malachite Green in Albert's I solution stains the bacilli green, while toluidine blue stains the volutin granules metachromatically, a bluish black color.
2. **Mordanting:**

   The smear is covered with Albert's-II for 1 minute.

   Albert's iodine acts as a mordant.
    - The slide is then washed with water and blotted to dry.
    - A drop of cedarwood oil or liquid paraffin is placed on the smear.
    - The microscope is adjusted for increased light by raising the condenser, and the smear is examined under the oil immersion objective.

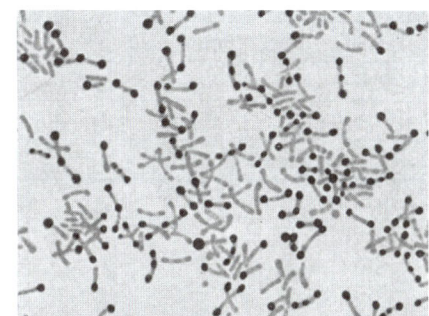

Fig. 2.20: Albert staining.

ZIEHL-NEELSEN'S STAINING (FIG. 2.21)

Aim: To stain the given fixed smear of sputum by Ziehl-Neelsen's technique for detection of *Mycobacterium*.

Principle: Aniline dye solutions do not readily penetrate the substance of the tubercle bacilli and therefore it is not suitable for staining. With strong staining solution that contains phenol and with the application of heat, which act as a mordant, it can be made to penetrate the bacillus. Once stained the tubercle bacillus will withstand the action of powerful decolorizing agents, thus retaining the stain.

Requirements: Strong carbol fuchsin, 20–25% H_2SO_4, 95% alcohol or acid alcohol, methylene blue solution, distilled water, spirit lamp, compound microscope and cedar wood oil/liquid paraffin.

Composition of strong carbol fuchsin:
- Basic fuchsin: 5 g
- Absolute alcohol: 50 mL
- Phenol (crystalline): 25 g
- Distilled water: 500 mL

Procedure:

- **Primary staining and mordanting:**
  - The fixed smear is flooded with strong carbol fuchsin for 5 minutes and heated intermittently. Until the steam rises, taking care to see that the stain does not boil and smear does not get charred. Smear is then washed well with distilled water.
  - The basic fuchsin in strong carbol fuchsin is a basic stain, while carbolic acid acts as a mordant. On heating, the mycolic acid in the cell wall of the acid fast organisms is liquefied and the basic stain imbibed by the organism is fixed by the mordant.

- **Decolorization:**
  - The slide is then covered with 20–25% H_2SO_4 for 2–3 minutes and washed with water. This step is repeated till the smear becomes colorless. With this, only acid fast organisms retain the basic stain, while the cells and other organisms are rendered colorless.
  - Decolorize it with 95% alcohol or acid alcohol. Decolorizing with alcohol; saprophytes can be differentiated from *Mycobacterium tuberculosis*, as saprophytes are only acid fast whereas *Mycobacterium tubercle* bacilli is acid as well as alcohol fast.

- **Counter staining:**
  - The slide is covered with methylene blue or 1–2 minutes, washed with water and blotted to dry.
  - Acid fast organisms remain red while the other organisms and cells, take up the counter stain and turn blue.
  - A drop of cedarwood oil or liquid paraffin is placed on the stained smear.
  - The microscope is adjusted for increased light by raising the condenser and smear is examined under the oil immersion objective.

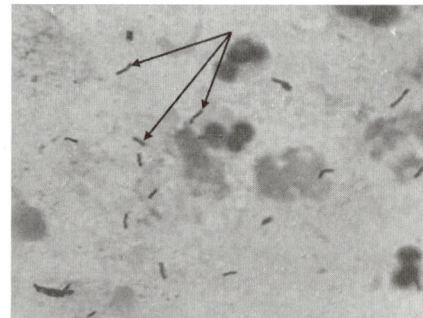

Fig. 2.21: Ziehl-Neelsen's staining.

National Tuberculosis Elimination Programme (NTEP)

Ziehl-Neelsen Staining Grading			
Finding	No. of fields	Grading	Result
No AFB in 100 oil immersion field	100	0	Negative
1–9 AFB per 100 oil immersion field	100	Scanty	Positive
10–99 AFB per 100 oil immersion fields	100	1+	Positive
1–10 AFB per oil immersion field	50	2+	Positive
>10 AFB per oil immersion field	20	3+	Positive

LACTOPHENOL COTTON BLUE STAINING (LPCB MOUNT)

Composition of Lactophenol Cotton Blue

- Phenol crystals   –   20 g
- Lactic acid   –   20 mL
- Glycerol   –   40 mL
- Distilled water   –   20 mL
- Cotton blue   –   0.075 g
  The phenol crystals are dissolved in the liquid by gently warming. Add dye to it.

Procedure (Fig. 2.22):

- A drop of lactophenol cotton blue is placed on the center of a clean slide.
- Using a sterile needle, a small portion of the pure fungal colony in the given culture is transferred to the drop of LCB slide.
- It is then teased apart with dissecting needles.
- A cover slip is carefully placed on the preparation avoiding air bubbles.
- After reducing the light, by lowering the condenser and using the concave mirror, the preparation is first screened under low power to visualize the hyphae and the conidia.
- It is then visualized under high power in order to identify the fungus.

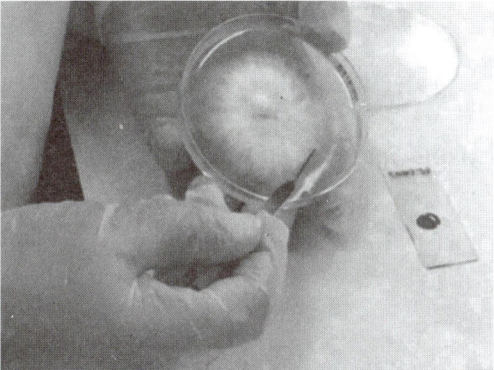

Fig. 2.22: LPCB mount preparation.

KOH MOUNT

KOH Mount

Potassium hydroxide (KOH) mount is a very useful test for the laboratory diagnosis of fungal infection of tissues especially skin, hair and nails. KOH separates the fungal elements from intact cells as it digests the protein debris and dissolves cement substances that holds the keratinized cells together and makes it easy to visualize under the microscope.

Requirements

- 10% KOH
- Coverslip
- Glass slide
- Needle
- Bunsen flame
- Specimen

KOH Procedure

- Place the specimens, such as epidermal scales, nail, hair, skin scrapping or tissue on a clean glass slide.
- Pour a drop of 10% KOH on the specimen and place a cover slip over it.
- Heat the slide gently over flame.
- Leave the slide for 5–10 minutes.

Examine the slide under microscope.

CULTURE AND MEDIA PREPARATION

Definition
Culture media are required to grow the organism from the infected material to identify the causative pathogen for their antibiotic susceptibility test. Basic constituents of solid culture media are:

- **Water:** Source of hydrogen and oxygen
- **Electrolyte:** Sodium chloride or other electrolytes
- **Peptone:** Complex mixture of partially digested proteins
- **Meat extract:** Contains protein degradation products, inorganic salts, carbohydrates and growth factors
- **Agar agar:** Prepared from sea weed (Algae-gelidium species). Used in conc. of 2–3%. It melts at 98°C and solidifies at 42°C. It is an inert substance, neither stimulate nor it inherit the growth.
- **Blood or serum:** Used for enriching culture media. 5–10% sheep blood is used for enriched media to provide extra nutrition to fastidious organisms.

Classification of Media

Based on Physical State
- Liquid media
- Semi-solid media
- Solid media

Based on Presence of Molecular Oxygen and Reducing Substances
- Aerobic media
- Anaerobic media

Based on Nutritional Factors
- Simple media
- Complex media
- Synthetic media
- *Special media:*
    - Enriched media
    - Enrichment media
    - Selective media
    - Differential media
    - Indicator media
    - Transport media

Chapter 2: General Characteristics of Microbes 33

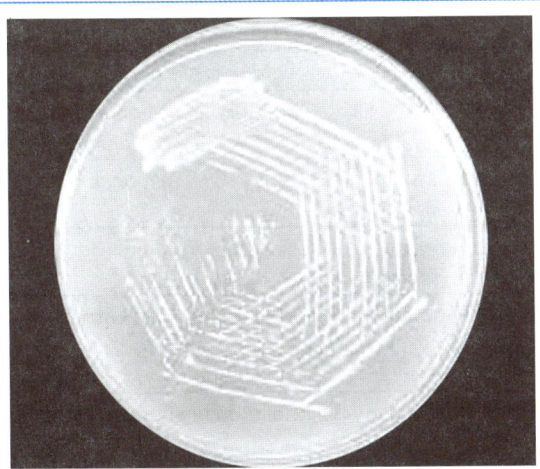

Nutrient agar. *(For color version, see Plate 3)*

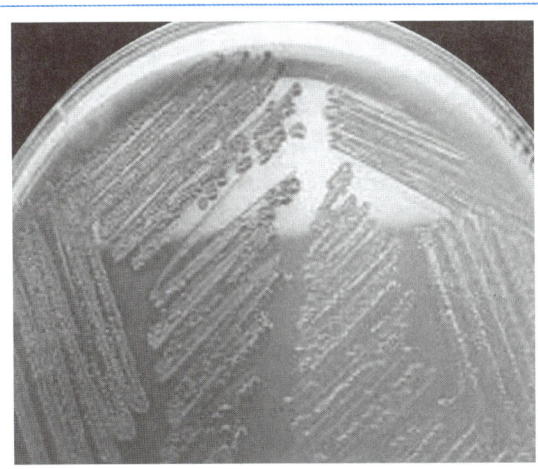

MacConkey's agar. *(For color version, see Plate 3)*

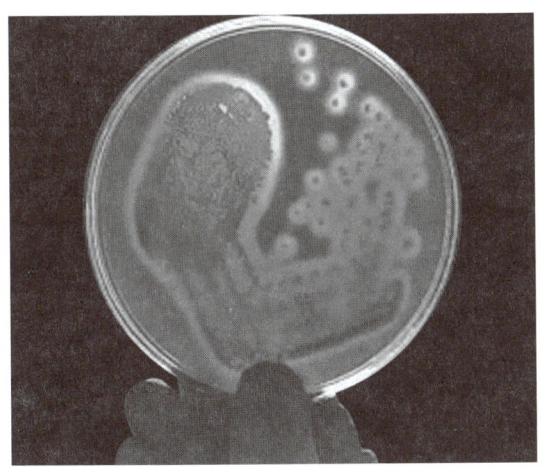

Blood agar. *(For color version, see Plate 3)*

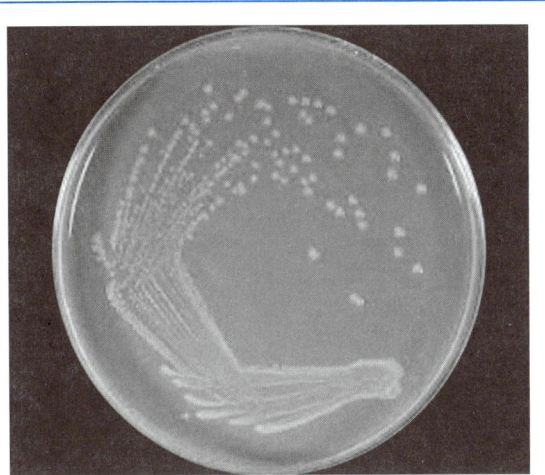

Chocolate agar. *(For color version, see Plate 3)*

CULTIVATION OF AEROBIC BACTERIA

Culture Media (Aerobic)

Solid media: Dispensed in petri dishes/McCartney bottles.

Type of medium	Name of medium	Composition	Laboratory use
A. Simple	Nutrient agar	Peptone + meat extract + agar + NaCl	Culture and demonstration of pigmentation of different bacteria
B. Complex/special			
i. Differential	MacConkey's agar	Lactose + peptone + NaCl + bile salts + neutral red + agar	Differentiate between lactose and non-lactose fermenters
ii. Enriched	a. Blood agar	Nutrient agar + 5% sheep blood	Differentiate between hemolytic and non-hemolytic bacteria
	b. Chocolate agar	Blood agar heated at 75°C for 10–15 minutes leads to release of X and V factors	*H. influenzae*, *Neisseria*
	c. Loeffler's serum slope	Nutrient broth + glucose + horse serum	*Corynebacterium diphtheriae*
C. Selective	1. Thayer-Martin medium	Agar base + Hb + growth factor + antibiotics, such as Vancomycin, Colistin + Nystatin	Isolation of *Neisseria gonorrhoeae*

Contd...

Contd...

Type of medium	Name of medium	Composition	Laboratory use
	2. Potassium tellurite agar	Blood agar + potassium tellurite	For *Corynebacterium diphtheriae*
	3. Wilson and Blair medium	Nutrient agar + glucose phosphate + brilliant green + bismuth sulfate	Isolation of *Salmonella* species
	4. Deoxycholate citrate agar (DCA)	Peptone + lactose + sodium deoxycholate + sodium citrate + neutral red	Isolation of *Salmonella* and *Shigella*
	5. TCBS medium (thiosulfate citrate bile salt sucrose agar)	Peptone + sodium thiosulfate + sodium citrate + NaCl + sucrose + ox bile + bromothymol blue	Isolation of *Vibrio cholerae*
	6. Lowenstein-Jensen medium	Egg + glycerol + NaCl + malachite green	Isolation of *Mycobacterium tuberculosis*
	7. Mueller-Hinton agar	Beef extract + casein hydrolysate + starch	For antibiotic susceptibility testing

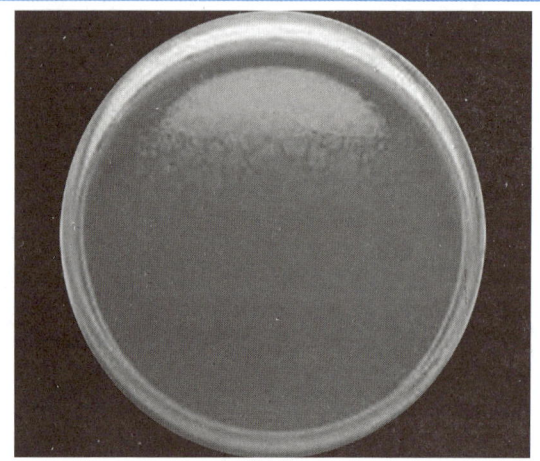

Wilson and Blair medium. *(For color version, see Plate 3)*

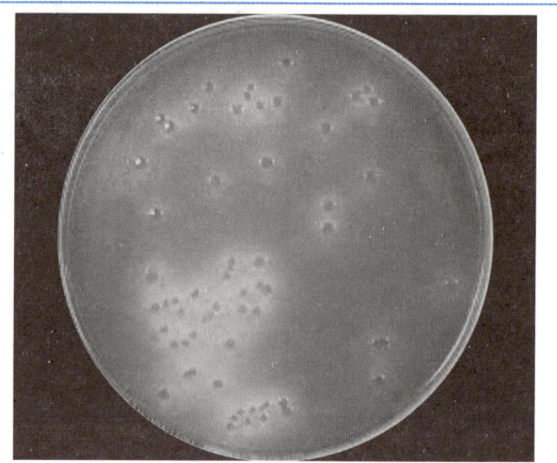

TCBS medium. *(For color version, see Plate 3)*

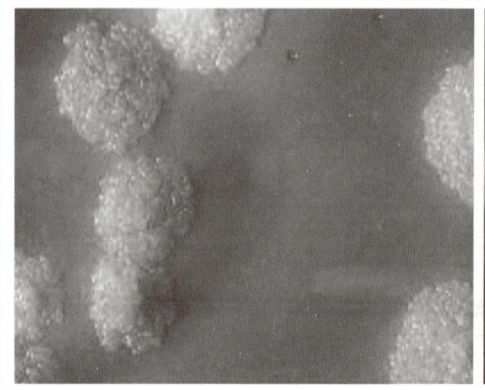 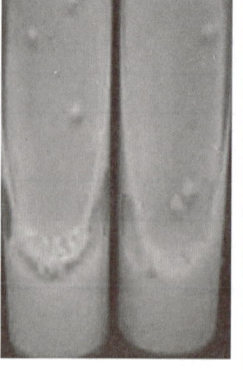

Lowenstein-Jensen medium. *(For color version, see Plate 3)*

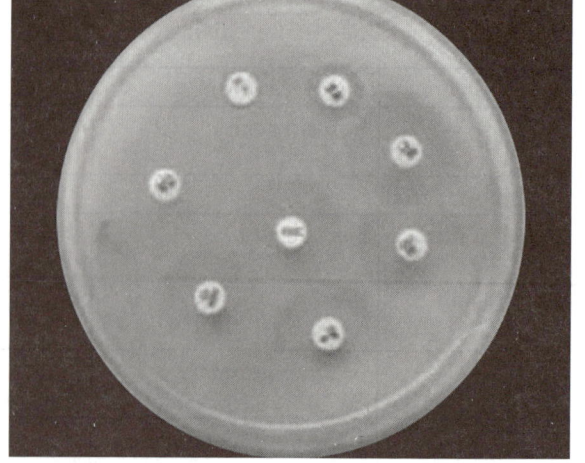

Mueller-Hinton agar.

Transport Media

It is devised to maintain the viability of a pathogen and to avoid overgrowth of other contaminants during transit of sample from patient to laboratory. It is available as sterile disposable swab kits **(Fig. 2.23)**.

Name of the medium	Composition	Laboratory use
Stuart transport medium	Sodium thioglycolate + sodium glycerophosphate + calcium chloride + agar + methylene blue + distilled water	For maintaining the viability of *Neisseria gonorrhoeae* on swab
Amie's transport medium	Sodium thioglycolate + NaCl + KCl + $CaCl_2$ + disodium hydrogen phosphate + potassium dihydrogen phosphate + charcoal + agar + distilled water	For maintaining the viability of *Neisseria gonorrhoeae* on swab
Pike's medium	Blood agar containing crystal violet + sodium azide	For *Strep. pyogenes*, *H. influenzae* swabs
Glycerol saline transport medium	Glycerol + NaCl + disodium hydrogen phosphate + phenol red 0.02% + water	For *Salmonella typhi* feces culture
Venkatraman Ramakrishnan medium	Crude sea salt + peptone + distilled water at pH 8.6–8.9	For *Vibrio cholerae*
Viral transport medium (VTM)	Modified Hank's Balanced Salt Solution supplemented with bovine serum albumin, sucrose, glutamic acid, and gelatin	For transporting H1N1, Novel Coronavirus (nCOVID) samples

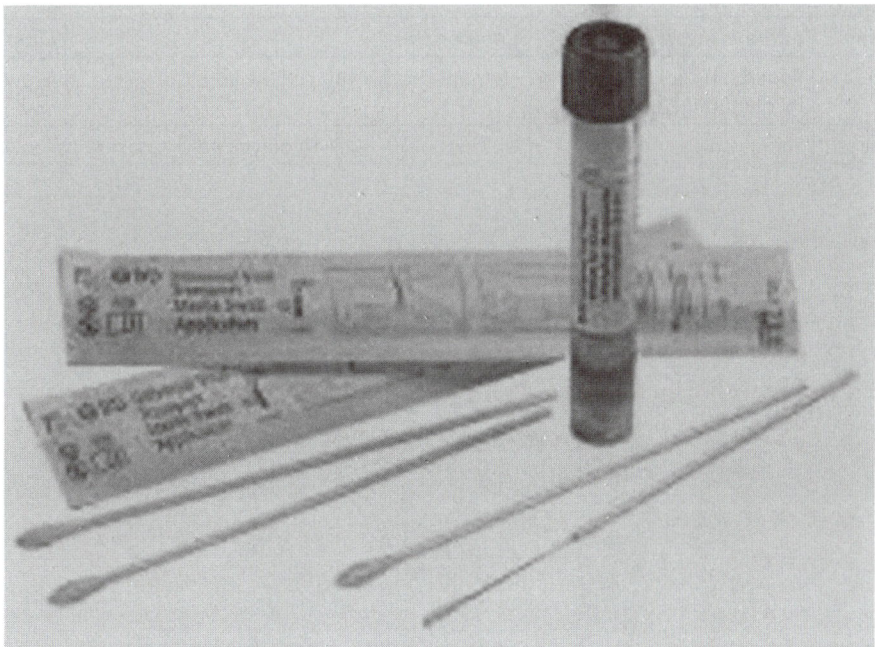

Fig. 2.23: Viral transport medium.

Liquid Media

Dispensed in tubes.

Type of medium	Name of medium	Composition	Laboratory use
A. Basal	Peptone medium	Peptone + NaCl + water	For sugar fermentation test
B. Special			
i. Enriched	1. Glucose broth	Nutrient broth + glucose	For Streptococcus
	2. Hiss serum	Serum + peptone water	For Corynebacterium
ii. Enrichment	1. Selenite-F broth	Peptone water + sodium selenite	Isolation of Salmonella and Shigella
For specimens other than blood	2. Tetrathionate broth	Nutrient broth + sodium thiosulfate + calcium carbonate + iodine solution	For Salmonella
	3. Alkaline peptone water	Peptone water pH = 8.6	For vibrio cholerae
Liquid media used for blood culture	1. Brain heart infusion broth	Nutrient broth + dehydrated heart meat	Blood culture
	2. Liver infusion broth	Nutrient broth + crushed lean liver of sheep	Blood culture of pyogenic bacteria and enteric bacilli
	3. Glucose broth	Nutrient broth + glucose	For pyogenic organism
	4. Bile broth	Nutrient broth + bile	For Salmonella

Biphasic Media

Dispensed in blood culture bottles.

Name of medium	Composition	Laboratory use
Casteneda medium	Brain heart infusion broth and agar	For blood culture for brucellosis

CULTIVATION OF ANAEROBIC BACTERIA

Culture Media (Anaerobic)

Sl. No.	Type of medium	Name of medium	Composition	Laboratory use
1.	Liquid medium	Robertson cooked meat medium (Fig. 2.24)	Nutrient broth + minced meat	Growth of anaerobic bacteria
2.	Thioglycolate broth	Thioglycolate medium	Nutrient broth + 1% thioglycolate + resazurin	Growth of anaerobic bacteria

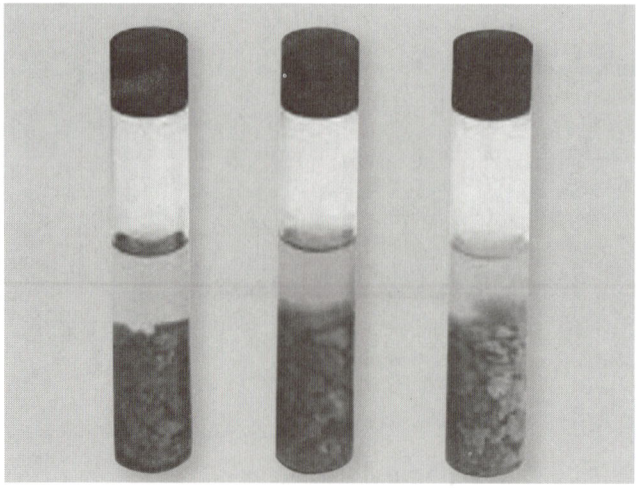

Fig. 2.24: Robertson cooked meat medium.

Inoculation Methods

Inoculation is done with a loop made of nichrome wire of 24 SWG size; loop 2–4 mm. In diameter with a wire 2 to 3" long and is sterilized in the Bunsen flame. Various methods of inoculation are employed:

Sl. No.	Name of method	Procedure	Indication
1.	Streak culture	Loop is sterilized on flame and inoculum is taken and smeared on a well	To get isolated colonies
		From there create a parallel streaks A, B, C and the tail	
2.	Lawn culture	Hooding the plate with liquid culture suspension	For antibiotic sensitivity pattern
3.	Stroke culture	Streaking on a nutrient agar slope	For pure culture of bacteria to perform slide agglutination test
4.	Pour plate method	Serial dilutions of bacteria into molten agar	Bacterial count and quantitative analysis of urine

Incubator

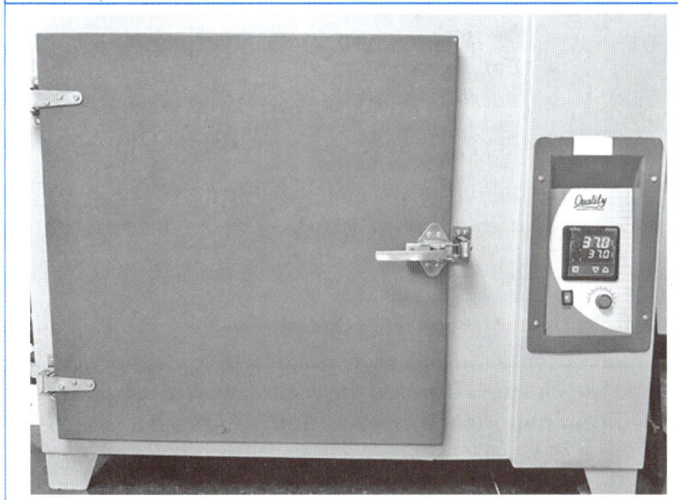

- In microbiology, an incubator is a device used to grow and maintain microbiological cultures or cell cultures.
- The incubator maintains optimal temperature, humidity and other conditions.
- For routine bacterial cultures, temperature is maintained at 37°C.

McIntosh and Filde's Anaerobic Jar

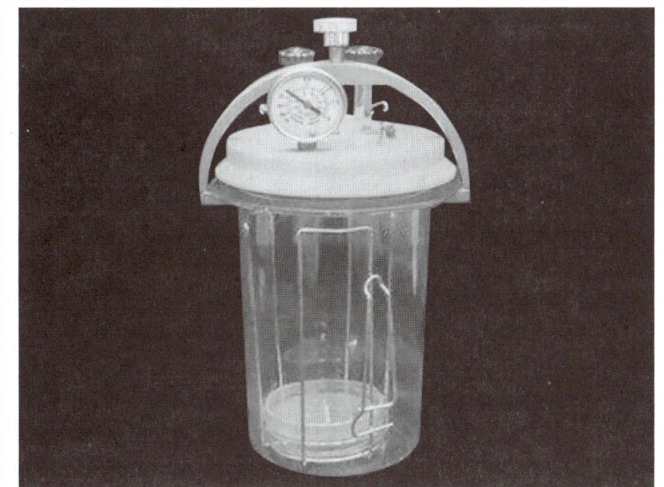

- **McIntosh and Filde's anaerobic jar** is an instrument used in the production of an anaerobic environment (anaerobiosis).
- Hydrogen gas is passed as the catalyst helps to combine hydrogen and oxygen.
- The presence of air is deleterious for many anaerobic bacteria and must be incubated in its absence. The inoculated culture plates are placed inside a metal jar and the lid clamped tight. The air inside is removed using a vacuum pump. The pressure inside the chamber is reduced to 100 mm below mercury.

CHAPTER 3

Pathogenic Organisms

Chapter Outline

- Bacteriology—Gram-Positive and Gram-Negative Bacteria
- Virology—DNA and RNA Virus
- Medical Mycology
- Medical Parasitology
- Medical Mycology
- Medical Parasitology
- *Neisseria*
- *Corynebacterium*
- *Bacillus*
- *Clostridium*
- *Enterobacteriaceae*
- *Vibrio*

STAPHYLOCOCCUS

Staphylococcus are gram-positive cocci arranged in grape like clusters. They are the commonest cause of suppuration. The genus *Staphylococcus* contains various species but the medically important species are *Staphylococcus aureus, Staphylococcus epidermidis, Staphylococcus sarprophyticus.*

I. Staphylococcus aureus

A. Morphology (Fig. 3.1)

They are gram-positive cocci arranged in grape-like clusters, non-motile, non-sporing approximately 1 μm in diameter. Cluster formation is due to sequential division of bacteria in three perpendicular planes with daughter cells remaining in close proximity.

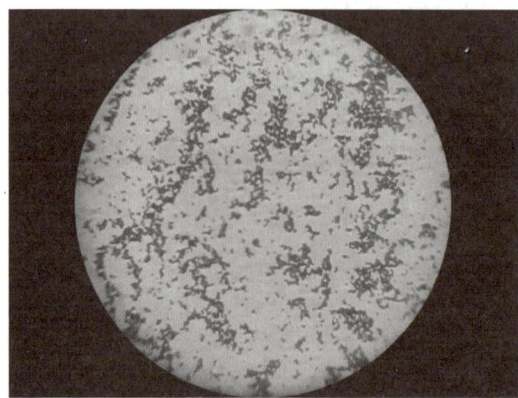

Fig. 3.1: *S. aureus*—gram-positive cocci in chains.

B. Culture

They grow readily on ordinary culture media within a temperature range of 10–42°, the optimal temperature being 37°C and pH 7.4–7.6. They are aerobes and facultative anaerobes.
- **Nutrient agar (Fig. 3.2A):** After overnight or 24 hours incubation, the colonies are 2–4 mm in diameter, circular, smooth, convex, opaque and easily emulsifiable. Most of the strains produce golden yellow pigment. The pigment is not diffusible into the medium.
- **Blood agar (Fig. 3.2B):** Colonies are similar to those on nutrient agar and in addition a beta type of hemolysis is seen.
- **Mannitol salt agar:** This is both a selective and an indicator medium. It contains nutrient agar with 1% mannitol, 7.5% sodium chloride and phenol red as indicator. Yellow colored colonies are seen on this medium due to fermentation of mannitol by most strains of *Staph. aureus*.
- **Liquid medium:** Uniform turbidity is produced in peptone water or nutrient broth.

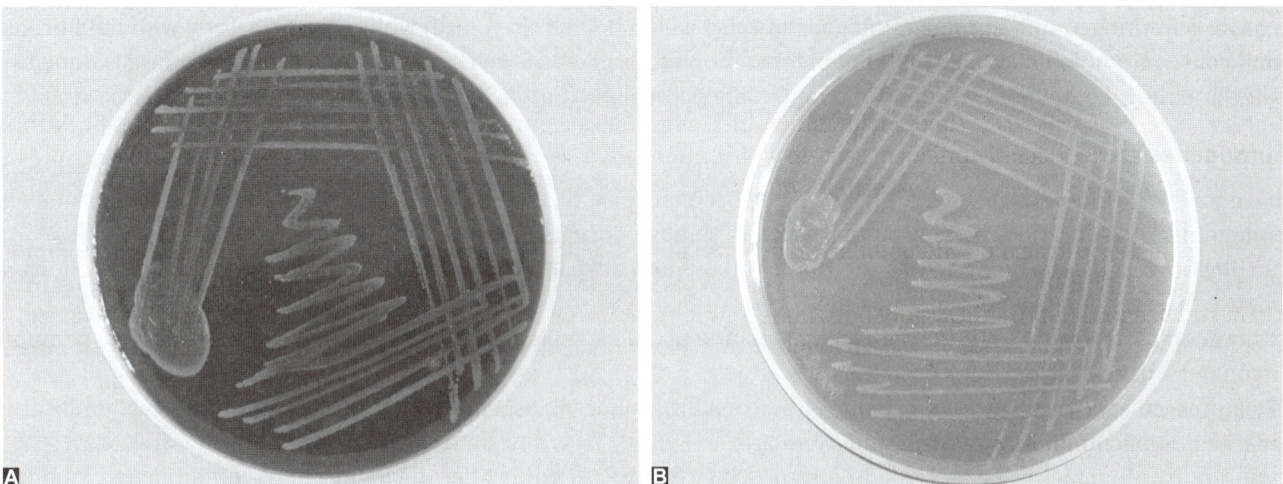

Figs. 3.2A and B: (A) *S. aureus*—golden yellow colonies on nutrient agar; (B) Blood agar.
(For color version, see Plate 4)

C. Biochemical Reactions

Staph. aureus is catalase positive (unlike streptococci) and oxidase negative. It ferments a number of sugars producing acid without gas.
- Coagulase production
- Mannitol fermentation
- Gelatin liquefaction
- Phosphatase production
- Production of enzyme deoxyribonuclease
- Tellurite reduction.

D. Resistance

Staphylococci are more resistant among the non-sporing bacteria. They survive in dried pus for 2–3 months. Most of the staphylococci are killed at 62°C for 30 minutes but some may require 80°C for one hour.

E. Antigenic Structure

- **Capsule:** Some strains of *Staph. aureus* possess capsule and inhibit phagocytosis. The capsule is composed of polysaccharide.
- **Peptidoglycan:** Peptidoglycan is a polysaccharide polymer that provides rigidity to the cell wall.
- **Teichoic acid:** It is a major antigenic determinant of all strains of *Staph. aureus*.
- **Protein A:** It is a cell wall component of most strains of *Staph. aureus* (especially Cowan I strain).

F. Toxins and Enzymes

Staph. aureus forms a number of toxins and enzymes. They are important virulence factors of the organism for producing a disease in the host.

- **Toxins:**
  - *Hemolysins:* Four antigenically distinct types called alpha, beta, gamma and delta haemolysins are produced by staphylococci. These are exotoxins.
  - Leucocidin
  - *Enterotoxin:* The toxin is responsible for staphylococcal food poisoning.
  - Toxic shock syndrome toxin (TSST)
  - Exfoliative (epidermolytic) toxin
- **Enzymes:** *Staph. aureus* produces a number of enzymes, coagulase, phosphatase and deoxyribonuclease which are related to virulence of the bacteria.

  Staph. aureus produces an enzyme coagulase. It has a property to clot human or rabbit plasma. Coagulase is secreted free into the culture medium. It requires a plasma factor (coagulase reacting factor, CRF) for its clotting action. Coagulase converts fibrinogen into fibrin clumping factor (also called bound coagulase) which reacts directly with the fibrinogen and causes clumping of cocci due to the precipitation of fibrin on the cell surface. The test for coagulase is done by the slide and the tube method. It is done to differentiate pathogenic (*Staph. aureus*) strain from non-pathogenic strains.

G. Pathogenesis

Staph. aureus is an important pyogenic organism and lesions are localized in nature in contrast to streptococcal lesions which are spreading in nature. Thick creamy pus is formed in staphylococcal infections.

Staphylococcal diseases may be classified as cutaneous and deep infections, food poisoning, nosocomial infections, skin exfoliative diseases and toxic shock syndrome.

- **Cutaneous infections:** Superficial infections include pustules, boils, carbuncles abscesses, styes, impetigo, pemphigus neonatorum, wound and burn infections.
- **Deep infections:** These include osteomyelitis, tonsillitis, pharyngitis. sinusitis, pneumonitis, empyema, endocarditis, meningitis, bacteremia, septicemia and pyemia.
- **Food poisoning:** Staphylococcal food poisoning may follow 2–6 hours after the ingestion of contaminated food which contains preformed enterotoxin of *Staph. aureus*
- **Nosocomial infections:** They are important cause of healthcare-associated infections.
- **Skin exfoliative diseases of hospital-acquired infections:** These diseases are produced by the strains of *Staph. aureus* that produce exfoliative toxin. Stripping of the superficial layers of the skin from the underlying tissue occurs in the various exfoliative syndromes caused by staphylococci (bullous impetigo, pemphigus neonatorum, Ritter's disease). Staphylococcal scalded skin syndrome (SSSS) is one example of exfoliative diseases in which toxin spreads systemically.

  Toxic shock syndrome (TSS): It is caused by toxin shock syndrome toxin (TSST-1). Although TSS became widely known in association with the use of tampons by menstruating women, it occurs in other situations also.

H. Antibiotic Sensitivity

Most of the strains of *Staph. aureus* are sensitive to Penicillin. Soon after penicillin came to be used clinically, resistant strains began to emerge Penicillin resistance in staphylococci is due to:

- Production of beta lactamase (penicillinase) which is plasmid coded and transmitted by transduction or the conjugation beta lactamase inactivates penicillin by splitting the beta lactam ring.
- **Methicillin resistant staphylococci:** There is reduction in affinity of penicillin binding proteins of the staphylococcal cell wall for β-lactam antibiotics. This change is normally chromosomal in nature. This type of resistance also occurs in beta lactamase resistant penicillins such as methicillin, nafcillin and oxacillin. They may cause outbreaks of hospital infection. These strains are called methicillin resistant *Staph. aureus* (MRSA). These are important of causes of postoperative wound infections and other hospital-acquired infections. Vancomycin or teicoplanin is used for treatment of infections with MRSA.

I. Laboratory Diagnosis

- **Specimens:** These are collected according to the nature of lesion as follows:
  - Pus—suppurative lesions
  - Sputum—respiratory infections
  - Blood—septicemia or PUO
  - Urine—urinary tract infection
  - CSF—meningitis
  - Feces—food poisoning
  - Food or vomit—food poisoning

- **Collection and transport:** Specimens should be collected in sterile containers under all aseptic conditions. In case of urine, midstream urine should be collected. Blood should be collected in blood culture bottles, comprising of glucose broth and taurocholate broth.
  Specimens should be transported immediately to the laboratory and processed.
- **Direct microscopy:** Direct microscopy with Gram-stained smears of pus or wound exudate is useful, where gram-positive cocci in clusters may be seen.
- **Culture:** The specimens are inoculated on following media:
  – Blood agar
  – Peptone water
  Specimens where staphylococci are expected to be scanty or outnumbered by other bacteria (e.g., feces), are inoculated on selective media
  The inoculated media are incubated at 37°C for 18–24 hours. Next day, culture plates are examined for morphology of bacterial colonies and other characters. Uniform turbidity is produced in liquid medium such as peptone water. Gram staining from colony on blood agar and hanging drop preparation from peptone water are done to further characterize the bacteria.
- **Colony morphology and Gram staining:** On blood agar, colonies are 2-4 mm in diameter, circular, raised, opaque and produce golden yellow pigment. Beta hemolysis is seen around these colonies.
  On Gram staining, they are gram-positive cocci (1 μm in diameter) arranged in grape like clusters. Non-motile cocci in clusters are seen in hanging drop preparation.
- **Biochemical reactions:**
  – *Catalase test:* All staphylococci (pathogenic and non-pathogenic) are catalase positive. This test distinguishes *Staphylococcus* from *Streptococcus* which is catalase negative.
  – *Coagulase test:* It is positive in *Staph. aureus* but negative in other staphylococci.
- **Antibiotic susceptibility antibiotic sensitivity can be determined by Kirby-Bauer method:** Benzyl penicillin is the most effective antibiotic in sensitive strains. Cloxacillins are used against for lactamase producing strains. Vancomycin is used in treatment of infections with MRSA strains. For mild superficial lesions, topical applications of bacitracin or chlorhexidine may be sufficient.

II. Coagulase Negative Staphylococci

Coagulase negative staphylococci (CONS) form the part of the normal flora of the skin. They are opportunistic pathogens which cause infection in debilitated or immunocompromised patients.

Staphylococcus epidermidis

It is a skin commensal and acts as opportunistic pathogen in prosthetic devices, e.g., prosthetic heart valves, intraperitoneal catheters, orthopedic prostheses and vascular grafts. It may cause septicemia and subacute bacterial endocarditis. It may produce stitch abscess. It mainly acts as pathogen in immunocompromised individual. Their etiological role may be proved by repeated isolation.

Staphylococcus saprophyticus

It acts as an opportunistic pathogen. It is an important cause of urinary tract infection in young, sexually active females. *Staph. saprophyticus* can also cause septicemia and endocarditis in patients with cardiac surgery. The etiological role is again by repeated isolation. Saprophyticus is Novobiocin resistant which distinguishes it from *Staph. epidermidis*.

III. Micrococci

Micrococci are free living in the environment. These are gram-positive cocci, catalase positive, coagulase negative, arranged in clusters which differ from staphylococci in attacking sugars oxidatively. They may appear in irregular clusters, groups of four or eight. They are often larger than staphylococci. Colonies are generally white in color. Their staining is often not uniform. They are saprophytes and commensals. They may rarely cause opportunistic infection.

STREPTOCOCCUS AND ENTEROCOCCUS

Streptococci are gram-positive cocci which are arranged in chains. They are part of the normal human flora. Some of them are important human pathogens causing pyogenic infections.

I. Classification

Streptococci are divided into aerobic streptococci, obligate anaerobes and facultative anaerobes. Aerobic and facultative anaerobic streptococci are classified on the basis of their hemolytic properties. Three types of hemolytic reactions (α, β and γ) are observed on blood agar medium.

A. Alpha (α) Hemolytic Streptococci

They produce a greenish discoloration around the colonies. This is due to partial hemolysis. The zone of lysis is small (1 or 2 mm wide) with presence of unlysed erythrocytes. Alpha hemolysis is seen with viridans group of streptococci and *Pneumococcus*.

B. Beta (β) Hemolytic Streptococci

These streptococci produce a clear, colorless zone of complete hemolysis (2–4 mm wide) around the colonies, within which erythrocytes are completely lysed. The lysis of erythrocytes is due to the production of two types of streptolysin by the organisms Streptolysin O and Streptolyson S. Most of the pathogenic streptococci fall into this group. *Streptococcus pyogenes* is the most important and is responsible for many important human infections.

C. Gamma (γ) or Non-hemolytic Streptococci

They produce no hemolysis and *Streptococcus faecalis* is a typical example.

The beta hemolytic streptococci were classified by Lancefield (1933) serologically into a number of broad groups based on the nature of a carbohydrate (C) antigen on the cell wall. These are known as Lancefield groups, 20 of which have been identified, named A-V (without I and J) by precipitation reaction performed with appropriate sera. Majority of streptococci that produce human infections belong to group A named as *Streptococcus pyogenes*. These are further subdivided by type specific antisera into approximately 80 Griffith serotypes (type 1, 2, etc.) based on their surface proteins (M, T and R).

II. Streptococcus pyogenes

A. Morphology (Fig. 3.3)

The individual cocci are spherical or oval, 0.5–1.0 μm in diameter and are arranged in chains. Chain formation is due to successive cell divisions occurring in one plane only and daughter cells failing to separate completely.

Streptococci are gram-positive, non-motile and non-sporing. Some strains of *Streptococcus pyogenes* have capsules composed of hyaluronic acid.

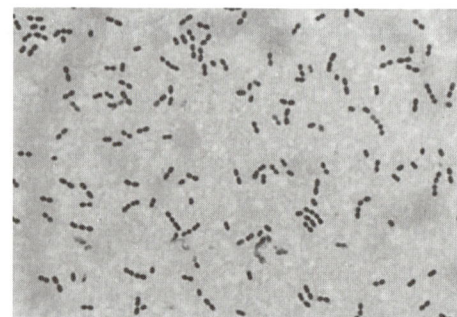

Fig. 3.3: *Streptococcus pyogenes* arranged in long chains. *(For color version, see Plate 4)*

B. Culture

They are aerobes and facultative anaerobes, growing best at a temperature of 37°C (range 22–42°C). These are most exacting in nutritive requirements, growth occurring only in media containing blood, serum or sugars. On blood agar, after overnight incubation, the colonies are small (0.5–1.0 mm, pin point), circular, semitransparent, low convex with a wide zone of beta hemolysis around them (Fig. 3.4). Growth and hemolysis are promoted by presence of 10% CO_2, in the environment. Selective media containing 1: 500,000 crystal violet (crystal violet blood agar) permit growth of streptococci but inhibit other bacteria especially staphylococci.

In liquid media, such as glucose broth, growth occurs as a granular turbidity with a powdery deposit. Bacterial chains being heavier settle down as deposit.

C. Biochemical Reactions

Streptococci are catalase negative, unlike staphylococci which are catalase positive.

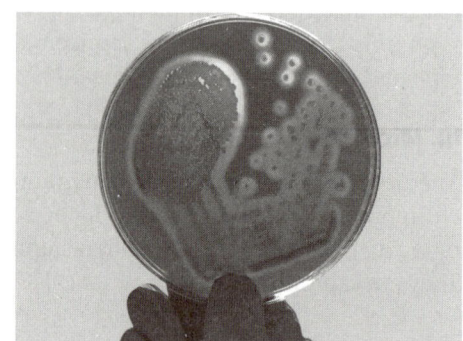

Fig. 3.4: *Streptococcus pyogenes* on blood agar. *(For color version, see Plate 4)*

D. Antigenic Structure

- **Capsular hyaluronic acid:** Capsule may be present on groups A and C streptococci. The capsule when present inhibits phagocytosis.
- **Group specific polysaccharide antigen:** The cell wall is composed of an outer layer of protein (fimbria containing protein) and lipoteichoic acid, a middle layer of group-specific C carbohydrate and inner layer of peptidoglycan (mucoprotein). The peptidoglycan is responsible for cell wall rigidity.
- **Type specific antigen:** The outer part of the cell wall contains protein antigens. *Streptococcus pyogenes* is further subdivided on the basis of their surface proteins M, T and R.

Toxins and Enzymes

Strep. pyogenes produces several exotoxins and enzymes which contributes to its virulence.

Toxins

Hemolysins: Streptococci produce two types of hemolysins, streptolysin "O" and "S". Streptolysin "O" is so named as it is oxygen labile. It is inactivated in the presence of oxygen. It lyses red cells and is also cytotoxic for neutrophils, platelets and cardiac tissue. It is antigenic antistreptolysin 'O' (ASO) regularly appears in sera with streptococcal infection. Streptolysin 'S' is an oxygen stable hemolysin and is responsible for the hemolysis seen around colonies of streptococci on the surface of blood agar plates.

Streptococcal pyrogenic exotoxin (SPE)
Toxin is responsible for streptococcal toxic shock syndrome and scarlet fever SPE is also called erythrogenic.

This toxin is responsible for Dick test and Schultz-Charlton reaction. When the toxin is injected intradermally into the skin of a susceptible child, erythematous reaction appears. This is called Dick test. In scarlet fever, when homologous antitoxin injected locally into the rash, blanching of the rash occurs, it is named as Schultz-Charlton reaction.

E. Enzymes

- **Streptokinase (fibrinolysin):** Streptokinase facilitates the spread of infection by asking down the fibrin barrier around the lesions.
- **Deoxyribonucleases (streptodornase):** Group A streptococci elaborate four antigenically distinct deoxyribonucleases (DNAases), A, B, C, and D of which, type B is the most antigenic in man.
- **Nicotinamide adenine dinucleotidase (NADase):** NADase acts on the coenzyme NAD and liberates nicotinamide from the molecule. It is believed to be leucotoxic.
- **Hyaluronidase:** It breaks down hyaluronic acid of the tissues and favors spread of streptococcal lesion along intercellular spaces (spreading factor).

F. Pathogenesis (Table 3.1)

Streptococcus pyogenes produces pyogenic infections with a tendency to spread locally. Non-suppurative sequelae of local infections include acute glomerulonephritis and rheumatic fever.

TABLE 3.1: Streptococcal diseases.

Streptococcus	Lesions
Streptococcus pyogenes Pyogenic infections	
Respiratory tract	Acute tonsillitis or pharyngitis (sore throat), scarlet fever
Skin infections	Infections of wounds, burns and skin lesions (eczema), erysipelas, impetigo
Genital infections	Puerperal sepsis
Streptococcal toxin shock syndrome	Bacteremia, necrotizing fasciitis
Deep infections	Bone and joint infections, lymphadenitis, septicemia, abscess in internal organs
Non-suppurative complications	Rheumatic fever, acute glomerulonephritis
Group B streptococci	Neonatal infections (septicemia and meningitis)
Streptococcus faecalis	Urinary tract infection, endocarditis
Viridans streptococci	Endocarditis, dental caries

1. Pyogenic Infections
- **Respiratory infections:** Sore throat (acute tonsillitis and/or pharyngitis) is the most common of streptococcal diseases. **Scarlet fever:** It consists of a combination of sore throat and a generalized erythematous rash. It is caused by a strain producing the erythrogenic toxin.
- **Skin infections:** Streptococcus pyogenes causes suppurative infections of the skin with a predilection to produce lymphangitis and cellulitis.
  The two typical streptococcal skin infections are—erysipelas and impetigo. These skin infections are the main cause leading to acute glomerulonephritis in children in the tropics.
- **Streptococcal toxic shock syndrome:** Streptococcal toxic shock syndrome (TSS) is a condition in which the entire organ system collapses, leading to death.
- **Other pyogenic infections:**
  – Puerperal sepsis *Streptococcus pyogenes* was an important cause of puerperal sepsis. It used to take a heavy toll of life before antibiotics became available
  – Sepsis, infections of skin lesions (eczema, psoriasis, scabies), wounds and burns
  – Pyemia, septicemia, abscess in internal organs (brain, lung, liver and kidney).

2. Non-suppurative Complications

Streptococcus pyogenes infections are sometimes followed by two important non-suppurative sequelae—acute rheumatic fever and acute glomerulonephritis. These complications occur 1-4 weeks after the acute infection. *Streptococcus pyogenes* is no longer detectable when these complications set in. The latent period suggests an immune response. Rheumatic fever is often preceded by sore throat while acute glomerulonephritis by the skin infection. These sequelae or complications are believed to be the result of hypersensitivity to some streptococcal components. Rheumatic fever may follow infection with any serotype of *Streptococcus pyogenes* while acute glomerulonephritis is caused by only a few nephritogenic types.

III. Laboratory Diagnosis

Diagnosis of acute suppurative infections is made by culture, while in the non-suppurative complications, diagnosis is mainly based on the demonstration of antibodies.

1. Acute Suppurative Infections
- **Specimens:** Specimen is collected according to the site of lesion, such as swab, pus/pus swab, or blood.
- **Collection and transport:** Specimens should be collected in sterile under all aseptic conditions. These should be immediately sent to the laboratory in Pike's medium (blood agar containing 1 in 1,000, violet and 1 in 16.000 sodium azide).
- **Gram staining of smears:** Gram-positive cocci (0.5–1.0 um in diameter is indicative of streptococcal infection. Smear examination is important such as pus.
- **Culture:** The specimen is inoculated on blood agar incubated at 37°C for 18–24 hours. Hemolysis is better under anaerobic conditions or in the 5–10% carbon dioxide. Crystal violet blood agar is a selective for *Streptococcus pyogenes*.
- **Colony morphology and staining:** The colonies of streptococci are small 0.5–1.0 μm pinpoint as compared to pinhead size of moist circular, low convex with a zone of β-hemolysis.
- **Biochemical reactions:** Streptococci are catalase negative which is a test to differentiate streptococci from staphylococci.
- **Identification of various groups of streptococci:** *Streptococcus pyogenes* (group A) is more sensitive (0.04 units/disc). Group 'B' streptococci can be identified by CAMP reaction (Christie-Atkins-Munch-Peterson).
- **Lancefield grouping:** Hemolytic streptococci are grouped by the Lancefield technique.
- **Antigen detection tests:** Agglutination tests are used to demonstrate Group A Streptococci antigen from throat swab.
- **Molecular methods:** Polymerase chain reaction (PCR), is more sensitive but it is expensive.

2. Non-suppurative Complications

Rheumatic fever and glomerulonephritis, serological tests provide retrospective evidence of streptococcal infection. The routine test done is antistreptolysin-O. A titer of 200 units or more is significant for rheumatic fever and is indicative of prior streptococcal infection.

ASO titer in glomerulonephritis, 300 or 350 which is significant. This test is useful for retrospective diagnosis of streptococcal infections.

Penicillin G is the drug of choice. In patients allergic to penicillin G, erythromycin or cephalexin is used.

Other Hemolytic Streptococci

Group B streptococci (GBS): *Streptococcus agalactiae* is an important pathogen of bovine in cattle. In recent years, it has been recognized as the most important pathogen in neonates causing septicemia and meningitis. It may also cause abortion and puerperal sepsis. *Streptococcus agalactiae* is present in female genital tract from where bacterial infection in neonates occur. Other group B infections includes osteomyelitis, arthritis, conjunctivitis, eye infections, endocarditis and peritonitis.

ENTEROCOCCUS

Enterococci are normal inhabitants of human intestinal tract and possess some distinctive properties as follows:
- They are relatively heat resistant and can withstand heat at 60°C for 30 minutes (heat test or heat resistance test)
- Their ability to grow in the presence of 6.5% sodium chloride
- Their ability to grow at 45°C and at pH 9.6.

On MacConkey's medium they grow as tiny deep pink colonies. On Gram's staining, enterococci appear as pairs of oval cocci and short chains. The identification of the species is based on biochemical reactions. *Enterococcus faecalis* is the most commonly isolated *Enterococcus* from human sources.

E. faecalis is frequently isolated from cases of urinary tract infection and wound infection. They may also cause other infections like subacute bacterial endocarditis, septicemia, peritonitis and infection of biliary tract. Strains resistant to penicillin and other antibiotics occur frequently. Vancomycin is the primary alternative drug to a penicillin for treating enterococcal infections. Vancomycin resistant enterococci (VRE) have also been isolated.

PNEUMOCOCCUS

Pneumococci are normal commensals of the upper respiratory tract. They are important pathogens of pneumonia and otitis media in children. They are reclassified as *Streptococcus pneumoniae*. They differ form streptococci in their morphology (diplococci), bile solubility, optochin sensitivity and by a specific polysaccharide capsule.

A. Morphology

Pneumococci are gram-positive, small (1 μm diameter), slightly elongated cocci arranged in pairs (diplococci) with the broad ends in apposition. Each coccus has one end broad or rounded and other pointed (flame shaped or lanceolate appearance). They are capsulated and the capsule encloses each pair. The capsule may be demonstrated as a clear halo in India ink preparation. They are nonmotile and nonsporing.

B. Culture

They are aerobes and facultative anaerobes and their growth is improved by 5–10% CO. The optimum temperature for growth is 37°C (range 25–42°C) and pH 7.8 (range 6.5–8.3).

On blood agar, after incubation for 18 hours, the colonies are usually small (0.5–1 mm), dome shaped, with an area of greenish discoloration (alpha hemolysis) around them. On prolonged incubation, the colonies become flat, with raised edges and central umbonation (due to autolysis occurring at center) which creates a draughtsman appearance (concentric ring when viewed from above). In liquid medium such as glucose broth, it produces uniform turbidity.

C. Biochemical Reactions

Pneumococci ferment several sugars which is tested in Hiss's fermentation of inulin.
Bile solubility test: Pneumococci are soluble in bile. Bile solubility test is important to differentiate *Pneumococcus* from other Streptococci.

Optochin Sensitivity Test

Pneumococci are sensitive to optochin (5 μg), a wide zone (14 mm or more) of inhibition occurs on incubation. This is very useful test to differentiate pneumococci from other streptococci which do not show zone of inhibition by optochin disc.

D. Antigenic Structure

The most important antigen of the *Pneumococcus* is capsular polysaccharide. Other antigens are somatic M protein and a group specific cell wall carbohydrate.
- **Capsular polysaccharide:** Capsular polysaccharide is type specific. Pneumococci are classified into types based on the nature of the capsular polysaccharide. More than 90 serotypes are recognized.

These are named 1, 2, 3, and so on. Serological typing of *Pneumococcus* is carried out by three methods:
1. Agglutination of organisms with type specific antiserum.
2. Precipitation of capsular polysaccharide with type specific antiserum.
3. Quellung reaction or capsule swelling reaction was described by Neufeld (1902). In this reaction, a suspension of pneumococci is mixed on a slide with a drop of specific antiserum. In presence of the homologous antiserum, the capsule around pneumococci reveals an apparent swelling, sharply delineated and refractile under the microscope.

- **M protein:** M protein is characteristic for each type of *Pneumococcus*.
- **Cell wall carbohydrate (C-substance):** Pneumococci contain a species specific carbohydrate antigen which is named as C-substance. It is present in all pneumococci. The C-substance is precipitated by an abnormal protein (μ-globulin), that appears in the acute phase sera of cases of pneumonia but disappears during convalescence. It is also detected in blood of patients with some other illnesses. This is known as the C-reactive protein (CRP). It is not an antibody of C substance. It is an 'acute phase' substance and its production is stimulated by bacterial infections, malignancies and tissue destruction.

E. Pathogenesis

Streptococcus pneumoniae is one of the most common bacteria causing pneumonia, both lobar and bronchopneumonia. *Streptococcus penumoniae* is the second most important cause of pyogenic meningitis after N. meningitidis. This disease is more common in children.

Pneumococcus may also produce empyema, pericarditis, otitis media, sinusitis, conjunctivitis, peritonitis and complications of pneumonia.

F. Laboratory Diagnosis

- **Specimens:** Clinical samples, such as sputum, cerebrospinal fluid (CSF), pleural exudate or blood are collected according to the site of lesion. Blood culture is useful in pneumococcal septicemia.
- **Collection and transport:** All the specimens should be collected in sterile containers under all aseptic conditions. They should be processed immediately. In case of delay, CSF specimen should never be refrigerated but kept at 37°C (*H. influenzae*, another causative agent of pyogenic meningitis, if present, may die at cold temperature).
- **Direct microscopy and antigen detection:** Gram staining of smear reveals a large number of polymorphs and typical organism. In case of meningitis, presumptive diagnosis may be made by finding gram-positive diplococci which may be intracellular as well as extracellular in CSF smear. Capsular polysaccharide antigen can be demonstrated by counterimmunoelectrophoresis. This has been employed in blood, urine and cerebrospinal fluid. Antigen may also be detected by immunochromatographic assay, latex agglutination or coagglutination.
- **Culture:** Specimen is inoculated on blood agar and incubated at 37°C for 24 hours in the presence of 5–10% CO_2. Typical colonies develop with α-hemolysis. Organisms from the isolated colony are identified by Gram staining and biochemical reactions.
- **Colony morphology and staining:** Colonies are usually small (0.5–1 mm), with alpha hemolysis around them. On prolonged incubation, colonies have draughtsman appearance.
- On Gram staining pneumococci are gram-positive, small (1 um diameter), diplococci **(Fig. 3.5)**. They are flame shaped or lanceolate in appearance. The capsule may be demonstrated as a clear halo in India ink preparation.
- **Biochemical reactions:** Important biochemical tests are inulin fermentation and bile solubility tests. Another test which has a great value is optochin sensitivity test.
- **Animal pathogenicity test:** From specimens where organisms are expected to be scanty, intraperitoneal inoculation in mice may be used. Inoculated mice die in 24–48 hours. Heart blood and peritoneal exudate of the animal show pneumococci.

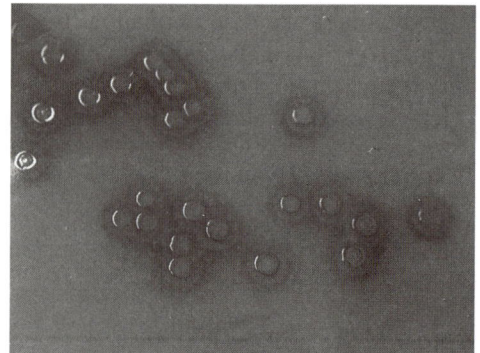

Fig. 3.5: *Pneumococcus* colonies on blood agar. (For color version, see Plate 4)

G. Treatment

The antibiotic of choice is parenteral penicil. Cephalosporin are indicated in case of Penicillin-resistant strains.

NEISSERIA

The genus *Neisseria* consists of gram-negative, aerobic, oxidase positive, nonmotile diplococci (arranged in pairs). They may be classified into pathogenic and non-pathogenic (commensals). The two pathogenic species are *N. meningitides* (causes pyogenic meningitis) and *N. gonorrhoeae* (causes gonorrhea). The non-pathogenic species include *N. flavescens*, *N. sicca*, *N. subflava* and other species.

I. *Neisseria meningitidis* (Meningococcus)

A. Morphology

They are gram negative, spherical or oval cocci, 0.6–0.8 µm in size arranged in pairs with the adjacent sides flattened **(Fig. 3.6)**. They are non-motile. The cocci are generally intracellular when isolated from lesions.

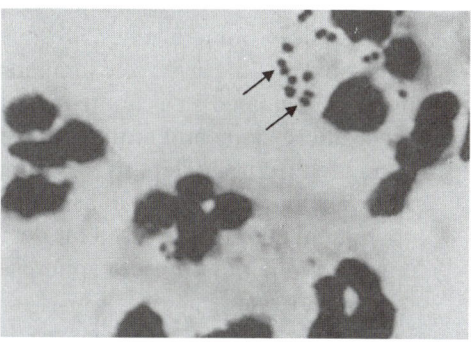

Fig. 3.6: *N. meningitidis*—gram-negative cocci in pairs.

B. Culture

They do not grow on ordinary media but have exacting growth requirements. Growth occurs on media enriched with blood or serum. Blood agar, chocolate agar and Mueller-Hinton agar are commonly used media. Thayer-Martin medium with antibiotics (vancomycin, colistin, nystatin and trimethoprim) is selective media used for its isolation.

They are strict aerobes and cannot grow anaerobically. The optimum temperature and pH for growth are 35–36°C and 7.4–7.6 respectively. A moist environment with 5–10% CO_2 is must for growth to occur.

On solid media, the colonies are small (1 mm in diameter), round, convex, gray, translucent and with entire edges. In liquid media, it produces a granular turbidity.

C. Biochemical Reaction

N. meningitidis is catalase and oxidase positive. The prompt oxidase reaction helps to identify *Neisseria* (both meningococci and gonococci) in mixed cultures. Glucose and maltose are fermented with acid production but no gas (gonococci ferment glucose but not maltose). They do not reduce nitrates to nitrites.

Oxidase Test

When freshly prepared oxidase reagent (1% tetramethyl-p-phenylenediamine dihydrochloride) is poured on the culture plate, *Neisseria* colonies can be picked up for subcultures immediately, as the organism dies on prolonged exposure to the reagent. The test may also be performed by rubbing bacterial growth with a loop on a filter paper strip moistened with the oxidase reagent (Kovac's method). A deep purple color is positive reaction.

D. Antigenic Structure

N. meningitidis has been divided into 12 serogroups on the basis of immunological specificity of the capsular polysaccharide. These serogroups are A, B, C, X, Y, Z, W-135, 29E, H, I, K, and L. Groups A, B and C are the most important.

E. Resistance

These are very delicate organisms, being highly susceptible to heat, desiccation and to disinfectants. They are susceptible to penicillin, ampicillin, chloramphenicol, macrolides and ciprofloxacin. Strains resistant to penicillin have now been reported from several countries.

F. Pathogenesis

N. meningitidis causes pyogenic meningitis in all ages, but is most common in children and young adults.

Meningococci are strict human pathogens. The infection is acquired by droplet spread via the reservoir of *N. meningitides*. The incubation period of the disease is about 3 days.

Meningococcemia presents as acute fever with petechial rash. A few develop fulminant meningococcemia (Waterhouse-Friderichsen syndrome) characterized by shock, disseminated intravascular coagulation and multisystem failure. It is usually a fatal condition.

G. Laboratory Diagnosis

- **Specimens:** The following specimens are collected depending on the clinical presentation:
  - CSF
  - Blood
  - Petechial lesions specimen
  - Nasopharyngeal swab—especially to detect carriers.
- **Collection and transport:** Collection of specimen is done under sterile conditions by lumbar puncture for CSF and by venipuncture for blood. Blood is injected into blood culture bottles (glucose broth and sodium taurocholate broth) through the hole in the bottle cap. Nasopharyngeal specimen is collected by using a sterile swab. All the specimens must be transported immediately. CSF should never be refrigerated as *H. influenzae* (another common causative agent of meningitis) may die at the cold temperature. The nasopharyngeal swab should be held in transport medium (e.g., Stuart's) until it is inoculated on a culture medium.
- **Direct microscopy and antigen detection:** CSF is divided into three portions. One portion is centrifuged and smear is prepared from the deposit for Gram staining. Meningococci are seen as gram-negative diplococci present mainly inside polymorphs (intracellular), but may also be present extracellularly. A large number of pus cells are also seen. The supernatant fluid may be used for detection of meningococcal antigen [capsular polysaccharide by rapid tests, such as countercurrent immunoelectrophoresis (CIEP)], coagulation or latex agglutination test. Antigen detection is useful when organism are scanty.

  The second portion of the CSF is used for direct culture. While the third portion of the CSF is incubated overnight after adding an equal volume of glucose broth and then subcultured on blood agar or chocolate agar. Culture of third portion of CSF may sometimes succeed when direct culture fails.
- **Culture:**
  - *CSF:* Centrifuged deposit is inoculated on blood agar or chocolate agar. The plate is incubated at 35–36°C under 5–10% CO_2. Colony morphology, Gram staining and biochemical reactions are performed.
  - *Blood:* Blood culture is often positive in meningococcemia and in early cases of meningitis. Blood culture bottles (glucose broth and sodium taurocholate broth) are incubated at 35–37°C for 24 hours. Subcultures are made from these broths on to blood agar and chocolate agar. These plates are again incubated at 35–37°C under 5–10% CO_2 for 18–24 hours. Identification of organisms is done by colony morphology, Gram staining and biochemical reactions are performed.
  - *Other specimens:* Other specimens (petechial lesions, nasopharyngeal swab, autopsy specimens) are inoculated on blood agar and chocolate agar and are processed in similar way as for CSF.
- **Colony morphology and Gram staining:** On solid media, colonies are small (1 mm in diameter), round, convex, gray, translucent and with entire edges. Smear is prepared from the suspected colony and Gram staining is done. On Gram staining, they are gram-negative, spherical or oval cocci, 0.6–0.8 µm in size, arranged in pairs (diplococcic) with the adjacent sided flattened.
- **Biochemical reactions:** *N. meningitidis* is catalase and oxidase positive. Glucose and maltose are catabolized with acid production but no gas. The breakdown of glucose and maltose occurs by oxidation and not by fermentation.
- **Slide agglutination:** Direct slides agglutination of the organism may be done with specific antisera.

H. Treatment

Meningococci are uniformly sensitive to penicillin. Chloramphenicol is used in persons allergic to penicillin. Cefotaxime or ceftriaxone are as effective as chloramphenicol and the possibility of blood dyscrasia may be avoided.

I. Prophylaxis

1. **Chemoprophylaxis:** It is indicated for close contacts of patients for elimination the bacteria from nasopharynx. Rifampicin or ciprofloxacin are recommended.
2. **Immunoprophylaxis:** Meningococcal vaccines prepared from polysaccharides of serogroups A, C, W-135 and Y are available. Single dose is given intramuscularly. The protection is group specific and lasts for at least 3 years.

II. Neisseria gonorrhoeae (Gonococcus)

N. gonorrhoeae causes the sexually transmitted disease, Gonorrhea.

A. Morphology

They are gram-negative oval cocci arranged in pairs (diplococci) with adjacent sides concave (paper or bean shaped). In smear from purulent material, they are intracellular with in polymorphs, some cells containing as many as a hundred cocci (**Fig. 3.7**).

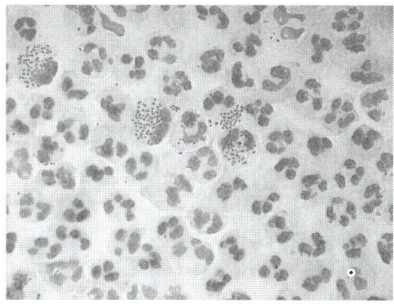

Fig. 3.7: *N. gonorrhoeae*—gram-negative cocci in pairs. *(For color version, see Plate 4)*

B. Culture

This organism is more difficult to grow than *N. meningitidis*. They are aerobic, but may grow anaerobically as well. They grow best at a temperature of 35–36°C in presence of 5–10% CO_2 and at pH 7.2–7.6. They require an enriched medium like chocolate agar for their growth. Selective medium is the Theyer-Martin medium that contains, nystatin and trimethoprim, which inhibits most contaminants including commensal *Neisseria*.

Colony Morphology

Colonies are small, round, gray translucent, convex with finely granular surface. They are easily emulsifiable.

C. Biochemical Reaction

N. gonorrhoeae is oxidase positive. Gonococci ferment glucose (with acid production only) and not maltose.

D. Antigenic Structure

The antigenic structure is complex. The surface structures of *N. gonorrhoeae* include the following:
1. **Capsule:** It is polyphosphate and not polysaccharide.
2. **Pili:** These are hair like structure extending from the surface. Pili enhance attachment of the organism to host cells and resist phagocytosis. They act as virulence factor. They are made up of pilin proteins.
3. **Lipopolysaccharide (LPS):** Toxicity in gonorrheae is largely due to the endotoxic effects of this component.
4. **Proteins:** The outer membrane antigens (proteins) are the porins.

E. Resistance

N. gonorrhoeae is a very delicate organism. Gonococci are readily killed by heat, drying and antiseptics. Formerly, they were highly susceptible to sulfonamides and penicillin but have steadily developed resistance to many antibiotics. PPNG (penicillinase producing *Neisseria gonorrhoeae*) strains are resistant to penicillin due to production of β lactamase (penicillinase) enzyme by these strains.

F. Pathogenesis

1. **Gonorrhea:** It is a sexually transmitted disease involving urethra in both sexes but in females, the endocervix is the primary site of infection. The incubation period is 2–8 days. The disease is an acute urethritis characterized by purulent urethral discharge. Asymptomatic infection is common in women. In males, the acute urethritis may extend to the prostate, testes, seminal vesicles and epididymis.
   The infection may spread to the periurethral tissues causing abscesses and multiple discharging sinuses (Watercan perineum). In females, the primary infection may spread from urethra and cervix to uterus, fallopian tubes, ovaries and may cause pelvic inflammatory disease resulting in sterility.
2. **Ophthalmia neonatorum:** It is a non-venereal gonococcal conjunctivitis in the newborn through infected birth canal.
3. **Gonococcal vulvovaginitis:** In women, the vagina usually is resistant to gonococcal infection because of the acidic pH of the vaginal secretions, but vulvovaginitis can occur in prepubertal girls.
4. **Other infections:** Sometimes, the disease may involve rectum or oropharynx following rectal intercourse or by orogenital contact respectively. Involvement of oropharynx may lead to gonococcal pharyngitis.

G. Laboratory Diagnosis

The diagnosis is readily made in acute stage, as urethral discharge contains large number of gonococci. It is difficult to detect gonococci from chronic cases.

1. **Specimens:** Urethral discharge and cervical discharge (in females) are collected in acute urethritis. In women, cervical swab is collected in addition to urethral discharge. High vaginal swabs are not satisfactory.
   In chronic urethritis, urethral discharge is observed only in few cases. In these cases, some exudates obtained after prostatic massage or morning drop of secretion may be examined. Centrifuged deposits of urine is examined in cases where no urethral discharge is available.
2. **Transport:** All the specimens should be transported and processed immediately. If this is not possible, specimens should be collected with charcoal coated swabs and transported to the laboratory in Stuart transport medium.
3. **Direct microscopy:** Gram staining of smear provides presumptive evidence of gonorrhea in men. Gram negative intracellular diplococci are found in smear of at least 95% cases of acute gonococcal urethritis in males. In females, diagnosis of gonorrhea by smear examination is unreliable as some of the normal genital flora have similar morphology. Fluorescent antibody tests are more sensitive and specific methods for diagnosis by microscopy especially in females.
4. **Detection of antigen or nucleic acid:** The gonococcal antigens can be detected by ELISA in clinical specimens. Nucleic acid can be directly detected in urethral discharge using DNA probe.
5. **Culture:** The specimens should be inoculated directly on preheated plates immediately on collection. Chocolate agar is used for culture of the specimens and incubated at 35–37°C under 5–10% CO_2 for 48 hours. In chronic cases, where mixed infection is usual, selective medium, such as Thayer-Martin medium is used.
6. **Colony morphology and Gran staining:** On solid medium, colonies are small, round, convex, gray, translucent with finely granular surface. They are easily emulsifiable. Smears are made from the colony and Gram staining is done. Gonococci are gram-negative cocci arranged in pairs (diplococci) with adjacent sides concave (pear or bean shaped).
7. **Biochemical reactions:** They are oxidase positive. They ferment glucose with acid only. They do not ferment maltose unlike meningococci.

H. Treatment

The organism is sensitive to large doses of penicillin (intramuscular) or doxycycline.
In penicillin-resistant gonorrheae, cefotaxime, ceftriaxone, ciprofloxacin, tetracycline or spectinomycin are used.

I. Prophylaxis

Control of gonorrheae consists of early detection of cases, tracing of contacts, health education and other general measures. Vaccination has no role in prophylaxis.

CORYNEBACTERIUM

Corynebacterium are gram-positive, non-acid–fast, non-sporing, non-motile bacilli. They frequently show club-shaped swellings (*coryne* means club shaped). The most important member of the genus is *C. diphtheriae* which causes diphtheria in humans.

I. *Corynebacterium diphtheriae*

A. Morphology

These are thin, slender, gram-positive bacilli and measure approximately 3–6 μm × 0.6–0.8 μm. They are pleomorphic. They are club-shaped due to the presence of metachromatic granules at one or both ends. With Loffler's methylene blue stain, granules take up a bluish purple color and hence they are named *metachromatic granules*. These granules are also called *volutin* or *Babes-Ernst granules*. The bacilli are usually seen in angular fashion resembling the letters V or L. This has been called *Chinese letter* or *cuneiform arrangement* (Fig. 3.8).

The bacilli look green and metachromatic granules appear bluish black when Albert stain is used. They are non-capsulated, non-acid-fast and non-motile.

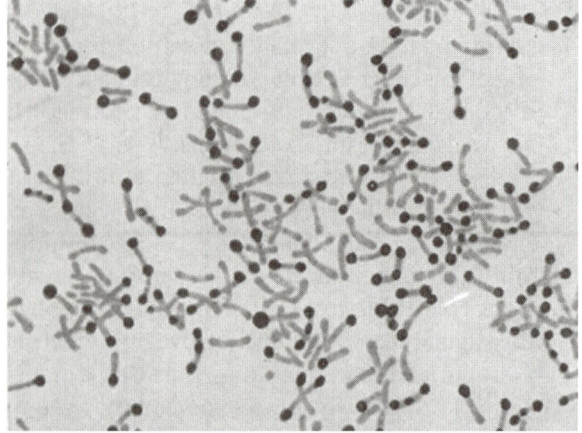

Fig. 3.8: *C. diphtheriae*—Chinese letter or cuneiform arrangement. *(For color version, see Plate 4)*

B. Culture Characteristics

C. diphtheria are grown best on media enriched with blood, serum or egg. Growth is scanty on ordinary media. They are aerobic and facultatively anaerobic. The optimum temperature for growth is 37°C (range 15–40°C) and optimum pH 7.2. The following are the usual media employed for cultivation of diphtheria bacillus.
1. **Hiss's serum water:** This is a liquid medium containing serum. Growth is seen as a turbidity and pellicle formation.
2. **Loeffler's serum slope:** Diphtheria bacilli grow on this medium very rapidly. Colonies appear after 6 to 8 hours of incubation, long before other bacteria grow. The colonies are small, circular, white or creamy and glistening.
3. **Tellurite blood agar medium:** It contains potassium tellurite (0.04%) which inhibits most other bacteria and thus acting as a selective agent. The organisms grow slowly on this medium and form gray or black colonies due to reduction of potassium tellurite to tellurium. The colonies may take two days to appear on this medium.

C. Biochemical Reactions

They ferment glucose and maltose with the production of acid but without gas. They do not ferment lactose, mannitol or sucrose.

D. Toxin

The pathogenicity is due to production of a very powerful exotoxin by virulent strains of diphtheria bacilli. Avirulent strains are frequent among convalescents, carriers and contacts.

Mode of Action

It acts by inhibiting protein synthesis. It inhibits polypeptide chain elongation in the presence of nicotinamide adenosine dinucleotide (NAD) by inactivating the elongation factor, EF-2.

E. Pathogenesis

Diphtheria is most commonly seen in children of 2–10 years. Infection is confined to humans only. The incubation period is 3–4 days, but may on occasion be as short as one day. Infection occurs by way of droplet spread. Diphtheria may be of following clinical types depending upon the site of infection:
1. Faucial
2. Laryngeal
3. Nasal
4. Conjunctival
5. Otitic
6. Vulvovaginal
7. Cutaneous mainly around mouth and nose.

The toxin has both local as well as systemic effects.

F. Laboratory Diagnosis

Laboratory confirmation of diphtheria is necessary for control measures and epidemiological studies, but not for the treatment of cases. Specific treatment should be started immediately after clinical diagnosis without waiting for laboratory reports. Laboratory diagnosis consists of isolation of organism and demonstration of its toxicity by virulence tests.

1. Isolation of Organism

- **Collection of specimen:** Two swabs from the lesions (throat nose, larynx, ear, conjunctiva, vagina, or skin) are collected. One swab is used for smear examination and other for culture. Local lesion is usually in the throat. Swabs are collected prior to start of antibiotics and application of antiseptics in form of gargles. The swabs are rubbed over the affected area and pseudomembrane, if formed, should be scraped with swab. If there is no definite localized lesion, the swabs should be rubbed over tonsils and the posterior pharyngeal wall without touching the mouth parts.
- **Direct microscopy:** Smears are staining with both Gram and Albert stain. Diphtheria bacilli show beaded slender green rods in typical Chinese letter pattern on Albert's staining. However, they cannot be confidently differentiated from some commensal corynebacteria "the organisms resembling *C. diphtheriae*" seen in direct smear examination. Gram staining is done to identify Vincent's spirochetes and fusiform bacilli (other causes of sore throat).

- **Culture:** The swabs are inoculated on the following culture media:
  - *Loeffler's serum slope* (**Fig. 3.9**)*:* Growth appears within 6–8 hours on this medium. Subculture from Loeffler's serum slope is made on tellurite blood agar and plate is incubated at 37°C for 48 hours.
  - *Tellurite blood agar:* These plates have to be incubated at 37°C for at least 48 hours before declaring these as negative, as growth may sometimes be delayed.
- **Colony morphology and staining:** On Loeffler's serum slope, the colonies are small, circular, white or creamy. *Diphtheria bacilli* grow as black or gray colored colonies on tellurite blood agar. Smears are prepared from suspected growth from various media. These smears are stained with Albert and Gram stain to confirm the morphology of *C. diphtheriae*. Albert staining shows green bacilli with bluish black metachromatic granules. Gram staining reveals gram-positive bacilli.
- **Biochemical reactions:** Hiss's serum water is used for testing fermentation of carbohydrates.

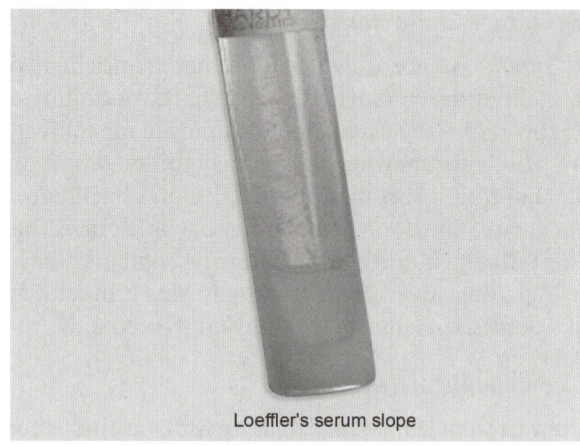

Fig. 3.9: *C. diphtheriae*—Loeffler's serum slope.

2. Virulence Tests

These tests demonstrate the production of exotoxin by bacteria isolated on culture. Virulence testing may be done by in vivo or in vitro methods.

In vivo tests: Two types of test are used viz., subcutaneous and intracutaneous.

a. **Subcutaneous test:** The growth from an overnight culture on Loeffler's serum slope is emulsified in 2–5 mL broth and 0.8 mL of the emulsion is injected subcutaneously into two guinea pigs, one of which has received an intramuscular injection of 500 units of diphtheria antitoxin 18–24 hours previously (this protected animal acts as control). If the stain is virulent, the unprotected animal will die within 2 to 3 days with evidence of hemorrhage in the adrenal glands which is the feature.

b. **Intracutaneous test:** Two guinea pigs (or rabbits) are injected intracutaneously with 0.1 mL emulsion from growth on Loeffler's serum slope, one of these animals is protected with 500 units of antitoxin the previous day (control) and the other is given 50 units of antitoxin intraperitoneally 4 hours after the skin test, in order or prevent death. If the strain is toxigenic (virulent), the inflammatory reaction at the site of injection progresses to necrosis in 48–72 hours in the test animal but there is no change in the control animal. An advantage in the intracutaneous test is that 8 to 10 strains can be tested at a time in a pair of animals and the animals do not die.

In vitro test

Elek's get precipitation test: This is an immunodiffusion test. A rectangular strip of filter paper soaked in diphtheria antitoxin (1000 units per mL) is placed on the surface of a 20% horse serum agar plate while the medium is still fluid. When the agar solidifies, the test strain is streaked at right angle to the filter paper strip. The positive and negative controls are also put up. The plate is incubated at 37°C for 24–48 hours.

G. Prophylaxis

1. **Active immunization:** Active immunization is started at 6 weeks of age by toxoid in combination with tetanus toxoid and pertussis vaccine (DPT, triple vaccine). Three doses of 0.5 mL each are given by intramuscular route at an interval of 4–6 weeks. Booster doses of DPT are given at months and at 5 years.
2. **Passive immunization:** This is an emergency measure when susceptible persons are exposed to infection, as when a case of diphtheria is admitted to pediatric wards. In such case 500–1000 units of antitoxin (anti-diphtheritic serum, ADS) is administered subcutaneously.

H. Schick Test

This test demonstrates immunity or susceptibility of a person's against diphtheria and is one example of neutralization test (toxin-antitoxin)

I. Treatment

C. diphtheriae is sensitive to penicillin, erythromycin and other antibiotics.

BACILLUS

Member of the genus *Bacillus* are ubiquitous, present in soil, dust, air and water and are frequently isolated as contaminants. *B. anthracis*, the causative agent of anthrax, is the most important pathogen of the group. *B. cereus* can cause food poisoning. They are generally motile with peritrichous flagella except the anthrax bacillus which is non-motile.

I. Bacillus Anthracis

It is the causative agents of anthrax, a disease primarily of animal, and man gets infected secondarily.

A. Morphology

Bacillus anthracis is a gram-positive, non-acid-fast, non-motile large (3–10 μm × 1–1.6 μm), rectangular, spore forming bacillus. The spore are refractile, oval and central in position and are of the same width as the bacillary body so that they do not cause bulging of vegetative cell. The ends of the bacilli are truncated or often concave and somewhat swollen so that a chain of bacilli presents a bamboo stick appearance.

B. Culture

B. anthracis is an aerobe and facultative anaerobic with a temperature range for growth being 12–45°C (optimum 34–37°C)
- **Nutrient agar media:** Colonies are round 2–3 mm in diameter raised opaque and grayish white. Under low power of the microscope the edges of the colony is found to be composed of long interlacing chains of bacilli resembling locks of matted hair called the 'Medusa head appearance'.
- **Blood agar media:** The colonies are non-hemolytic, though occasional strains produce a narrow zone of hemolysis.
- **Selective medium:** A selective medium (PLET medium) consisting of heart infusion agar with polymyxin lysozyme ethylene diamine tetraacetic acid (EDTA) and thallous acetate has been devised for isolation of *B. anthracis* from mixture containing other spore bearing bacilli.

C. Pathogenesis

Anthrax is primarily a disease of animals, such as cattle and sheep, and less often of horse and swine. Infected animals discharge large number of bacilli from the mouth nose and rectum. These bacilli sporulate in soil and remains as the source of infection.

Human Anthrax

Humans are secondarily infected from diseased animals. There are three clinical type of disease based on route of infection—cutaneous, pulmonary and intestinal anthrax. All types lead to septicemia, cutaneous anthrax follows entry of the spores through the skin. This is commonly found in farmers and persons handling carcasses. The cutaneous anthrax may resolve spontaneously, but may sometimes lead to fatal septicemia.

Pulmonary anthrax occurs due to inhalation of the dust or filaments of wool from infected animals, particularly in wool factories. This is also called wool sorter's disease.

D. Laboratory Diagnosis

- **Specimens:** Swabs, fluid or pus from pustules; sputum and blood from pulmonary and septicemic anthrax are generally collected.
- **Microscopy:** Gram staining smear from the specimen shows often chains of large gram-positive bacilli. Capsule appears as a clear halo around the bacterium by India-ink staining.
- **Culture:** Specimen is inoculated on nutrient agar medium, and incubated at 37°C for overnight. Medusa head colonies appear on the medium. Smears made from these colonies show typical gram-positive spore bearing bacilli.
- **Animal inoculation:** While mouse or guinea pigs are injected with exudates or culture. Animal dies in 36–48 hours. Smears made from heart blood and sputum show bacilli.

II. Anthracoid Bacilli

Aerobic spore bearing bacilli resembling *B. anthracis* are called anthracoid or pseudoanthrax bacilli. Some of them are frequent laboratory contaminants and have to be differentiated from *B. anthracis*.

III. Bacillus cereus

B. cereus has assumed importance as a cause of food poisoning. It is widely distributed in nature, such as soil, vegetables, milk, cereals, spices, meat and poultry. Some spore survive cooking and germinate into vegetative bacilli which produce enterotoxin that cause food poisoning.

Type of Food Poisoning

1. **Short incubation period type (1–5 hours):** It is characterized by acute nausea and vomiting 1–5 hours after the meal. Diarrhea is not common. It is usually associated with consumption of cooked rice, usually fried rice from Chinese restaurants.
2. **Long incubation period type (8–16 hours):** It is characterized by acute abdominal pain and diarrhea, 8–16 hours after ingestion of contaminated food. Vomiting is rare.

CLOSTRIDIUM

I. Classification

Clostridia of medical importance can be classified on the basis of diseases they produce:
A. Tetanus   *C. tetani*
B. Gas gangrene   *C. perfringens*
C. Food poising
   1. Gastroenteritis   *C. perfringens*
   2. Necrotizing enteritis   *C. perfringens*
   3. Botulism   *C. botulinum*
D. Acute colitis   *C. difficile*

II. Clostridium perfringens (Clostridium welchii)

C. perfringens is the most important and common etiological agent of gas gangrene. It also produce food poising and necrotizing enteritis in man.

C. perfringens is a commensal in the large intestines of man and animals. The spores are commonly found in soil and dust.

A. Morphology

It is a large, stout, gram-positive bacillus measuring 4–6 µm × 1 µm with subterminal spore **(Fig. 3.10)**. It is capsulated and non-motile.

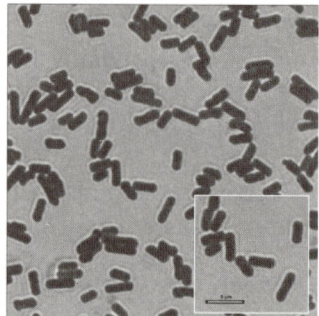

Fig. 3.10: *C. perfringens*—on Gram staining.

B. Culture

It grows on blood agar, Robertson cooked meat broth (RCMB) and thioglycollate broth within 24–48 hours. It is anaerobic and grows over a pH range of 5.5–8.0 and wide temperature range of 20–50°C. The optimum temperature for growth is 37°C.

On blood agar, colonies of most strains show a target hemolysis, resulting from a narrow zone of complete hemolysis caused by theta-toxin and a much wider zone of incomplete hemolysis due to alpha toxin. In Robertson cooked meat medium, the meat pieces turn pink but are not digested.

C. Biochemical Reaction

C. perfringens is predominantly saccharolytic but also have mild proteolytic action (gelatin liquefaction). It ferments glucose, lactose, sucrose and maltose with the production of acid and gas.

In litmus milk, lactose fermentation leads to formation of acid, which changes the color of litmus from blue to red. The acid coagulates the casein (acid clot) and the clotted milk is disrupted due to vigorous gas production and this is known as stormy fermentation.

D. Resistance

Spores are usually destroyed within five minutes by boiling but those of the 'food poisoning' strains resist boiling for 1–3 hours. Autoclaving at 121°C for 15 minutes is lethal. Spores are resistant to commonly used antiseptics and disinfectants.

E. Toxins

C. perfringens produce at least 12 distinct toxins but four major toxins include alpha, beta, epsilon and iota.

Alpha (α) Toxin

It is produced by all types of *C. perfringens*. Chemically, it is a phospholipidase (lecithinase C) and is responsible for profound toxemia in gas gangrene.

Nagler's Reaction

C. perfringens is grown on a medium containing 6% agar, 5% fluids, peptic digest of sheep blood and 20% human serum or 5% egg yolk in a plate. To one half of the plate, antitoxin is spread on the surface. The inoculated culture plate without the antitoxin will be surrounded by opacity while colonies on the other half with antitoxin shows no opacity, due to specific neutralization of the alpha toxin. Alpha toxin (lecithinase) splits lecithin into phosphorylcholine and a diglyceride (lipid). The lipid deposits around the colonies resulting on opacity.

Other Major Toxins

Beta (β), epsilon (ε) and iota (ι) toxins have lethal and necrotizing properties.

Enterotoxin

Some strains produce enterotoxin which causes diarrhea and other symptoms of food poisoning.

F. Pathogenesis

C. perfringens produces the following human infections:
1. Gas gangrene
2. Food poisoning
3. Necrotizing enteritis

G. Laboratory Diagnosis

The diagnosis of gas gangrene must be made primarily on clinical grounds and the laboratory only confirms the clinical diagnosis. The specimens to be collected are exudates from wound, necrotic tissue and muscle fragments.
1. **Direct microscopy:** Gram stained smears give presumptive diagnosis. Large number of gram-positive bacilli without spores is strongly suggestive of *C. perfringens*.
2. **Culture:** The specimens are inoculated on fresh and heated blood agar and cooked meat (CMB) broth. Growth in CMB is subcultured on blood agar plates after 24–48 hours. The blood agar is incubated anaerobically for 48–72 hours. Most strains produce beta hemolysis on blood agar and few are non-hemolytic. A plate of serum or egg yolk agar is used for Nagler's reaction. The bacterial isolates are identified by morphology, cultural characteristics and biochemical reaction. Toxigenicity of the strain can be done by animal pathogenicity.

III. *Clostridium tetani*

C. tetani is the causative agent of tetanus. It is widely distributed in soil and intestine of man and animals.

A. Morphology

It is a gram-positive, slender bacillus (measuring 4–8 μm × 0.5 μm) with spherical, terminal spore giving the bacillus the characteristic drumstick appearance **(Fig. 3.11)**. It is non-capsulated and motile (except *C. tetani* type VI) with peritrichous flagella.

B. Culture

It is an obligate anaerobe which grows on ordinary media. Growth is improved by the addition of blood or serum. The optimum temperature for growth is 37°C and pH 7.4. It can grow well in Robertson cooked meat broth (RCMB), thioglycollate broth, nutrient agar and blood agar. In RCMB, growth occurs as turbidity and there is also some gas formation. The meat is not digested but becomes black on prolonged incubation. The bacilli produce a swarming (thin spreading film) growth on blood agar.

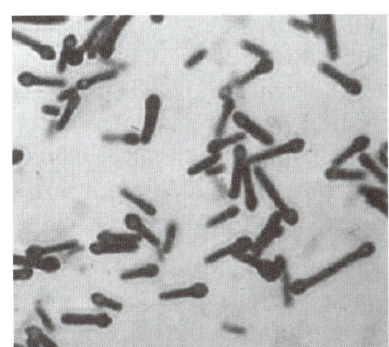

Fig. 3.11: *C. tetani*—on Gram staining.

C. Biochemical Reactions

C. tetani has slight proteolytic, but no saccharolytic property. Gelatin liquefaction occur very slowly. It does not ferment and sugar.

D. Resistance

Most of the strains are killed by boiling for 10–15 minutes but some boiling for three hours. However, autoclaving (at 121°C for 20 minutes) kills the spores of most strains. The spore may survive in soil for years.

E. Toxins

C. tetani produce two distinct toxin-tetanolysin (hemolysin) and tetanospasmin (neurotoxin).

F. Pathogenesis

Tetanus develops following the contaminants of wound with *C. tetani* spores. The cause of infection may be soil, dust, feces, etc. Infection strictly remains localized in the wound. Pathogenic effects are mainly due to tetanospasmin (neurotoxin) of *C. tetani*.

G. Laboratory Diagnosis

The diagnosis of tetanus should always be made clinically and laboratory tests are done only to confirm it. Laboratory diagnosis can be made by demonstration of bacilli by microscopy, culture or by animal inoculation. Specimens generally collected are wound swab, exudates or tissue from the wound.

1. **Microscopy:** Gram staining may show gram-positive bacilli with drumstick appearance.
2. **Culture:** Specimen is inoculated on freshly prepared blood agar and incubated at 37°C for 24–48 hours under anaerobic condition. *C. tetani* produces a swarming growth. Gram stained smear from culture shows typical gram-positive bacilli with drumstick appearance.
3. **Toxigenicity test:** Pathogenicity of the isolated organisms is established with demonstration of toxin production. It is best tested in animals.

H. Prophylaxis

The available methods are:

Surgical

It aims at removal of foreign body, blood clots, etc., in order to prevent anaerobic conduction favorable for the bacillus.

Antibiotics

Antibiotics destroy or inhibit tetanus bacilli and other pyogenic bacteria in wounds and thus the production of toxin is prevented. Long-acting penicillin injection or erythromycin may be given.

Immunization

Tetanus is preventable disease.

Active immunization

It is the most effective method of prophylaxis. Tetanus toxoid (formal toxoid) is commonly used for active immunization. Three doses of 0.5 mL tetanus toxoid each are given intramuscularly, with an interval of 4–6 weeks between first two doses and 6–12 months between the second and third dose. A full course of three doses confers immunity for a period of at least 10 years. A 'booster dose' of toxoid is recommended after 10 years.

Tetanus toxoid is given along with Diphtheria toxoid and Pertussis vaccine (DPT) in children. Pertussis vaccine acts as adjuvant. Three doses are given intramuscularly at interval of 4–6 weeks, starting at age as early as a weeks. Booster doses are given at age of 18 months and then at five years.

Passive immunization

Antitetanus serum (ATS), prepared by immunizing horse with toxoid, has been used for preventing tetanus. Being a horse serum, it carries the risk of hypersensitivity reaction.

Homologous serum prepared from humans, human antitetanus immune-globulins (HTIG), is now being used without the risk of hypersensitivity.

IV. Clostridium botulinum

Clostridium botulinum causes a severe form of food poisoning named botulism. It is a widely distributed saprophyte and is found in soil, animal manure, vegetables and sea mud.

A. Morphology

It is a gram-positive, non-capsulated bacillus about 5 μm × 1 μm, motile by peritrichous flagella and produces subterminal, oval, bulging spore.

B. Culture

It is a strict anaerobe and can grow on ordinary media. Optimum temperature is 35°C. Commonly used media is Robertson cooked meat broth (RCMB). Colonies are large, irregular, semitransparent, with fimbriate border. On blood agar, hemolysis around the colonies is observed **(Fig. 3.12)**.

C. Resistant

The spores are highly resistant, and can withstand heat for several hours at 100°C and for up to 10 minutes at 120°C.

D. Toxin

C. botulinum forms a power exotoxin. The toxin differs from other exotoxins in that it is not released during the life of the bacterium. It is produced intracellular and appears in the medium on autolysis of the cell. It is a neurotoxin and acts slowly, therefore, takes several hours to kill.

E. Pathogenesis

C. botulinum is non-invasive and its pathogenicity is due to the action of preformed toxin, the manifestations of which are collectively is called as botulism. Botulism is of three types—foodborne, infant and wound botulism.

Foodborne Botulism

It is due to preformed toxin contaminated with *C. botulism*. The source of botulism is usually various preserved foods—meat, fish, vegetables, etc.

The symptoms appear 12–36 hours after ingestion of contaminated food. Vomiting, thirst, constipation, ocular paresis, difficulty in symptoms. Diarrhea is not a symptom.

Infant Botulism

It affects infants, usually below 6 months. It is a disease due to ingestion of food contaminated by spores of *C. botulism*.

Wound Botulism

It is a very rare condition which results from wound infection with *C. botulism*.

F. Laboratory Diagnosis

Diagnosis may be confirmed by demonstration of the bacillus or the toxin in suspected residual food or on feces.

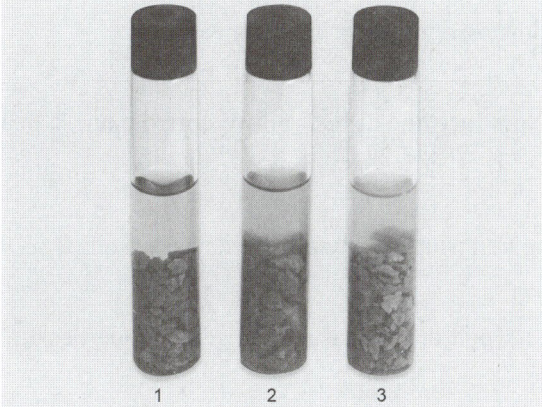

Fig. 3.12: Robertson cooked meat medium. (1) *Cl. tetanus*, (2) *Cl. perfringens*, (3) Control.

ENTEROBACTERIACEAE

Members of the family *Enterobacteriaceae* are aerobic and facultative anaerobic gram-negative enteric bacilli. They are motile by peritrichous flagella or are non-motile. They grow readily on ordinary media, ferment glucose with production of acid or acid and gas, reduce nitrates to nitrites, oxidase negative and catalase positive except *Shigella dysenteriae* type 1 which is catalase negative and *Plesiomonas* species, which is oxidase positive. They are non-capsulated and non-sporing.

I. *Escherchia coli*

A. Morphology (Fig. 3.13)

E. coli is a gram-negative bacillus measuring 1–3 µm × 0.4–0.7 µm. Most strains are motile. It is non-sporing and non-capsulated.

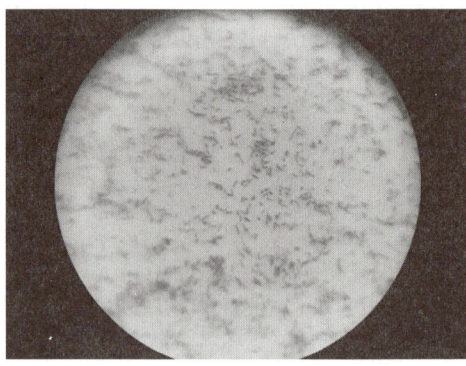

Fig. 3.13: Gram staining—gram-negative bacilli. *(For color version, see Plate 5)*

B. Culture (Fig. 3.14)

It is aerobe and facultative anaerobic and grows on ordinary culture medium at optimum temperature of 37°C (temperature range 10–40°C) in 18–24 hours. On MacConkey's medium, colonies are pink due to lactose fermentation (LF of lactose fermenter colonies). In general, colonies are circular. Moist smooth with entre margin and non-mucoid unlike colonies of *Klebsiella* which are mucoid. In liquid medium, growth occurs as uniform turbidity.

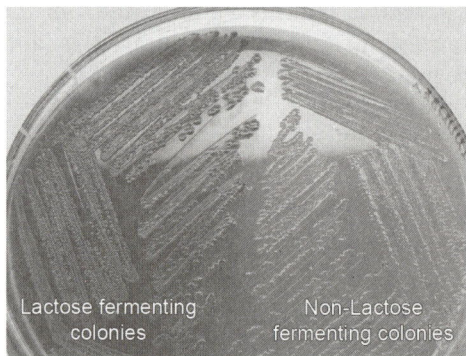

Fig. 3.14: MacConkey's agar—pink colored lactose fermenting colonies. *(For color version, see Plate 5)*

C. Biochemical Reactions

They ferment most of the sugars (glucose, lactose, mannitol, maltose) with production of acid and gas. Typical strains do not ferment sucrose. Indole and methyl red (MR) reaction are positive but Voges-Proskauer (VP) and citrate utilization tests ate negative (IMViC++--).

D. Antigenic Structure

Serotyping of *E. coli* is based on the presence of O (somatic antigen), K (capsular antigen) and H (flagellar antigen) antigens detected by agglutination reactions. Another antigen present is F (fimbrial) antigen.

E. Toxins

Some strains of *E. coli* produce enterotoxins, hemolysin and verocytotoxin.

Enterotoxins

Enterotoxins strains of *E. coli* (ETEC) produce one or both of two enterotoxins, a heat—labile toxin (LT) and a heat stable toxin (ST).

Hemolysin

Some strains of *E. coli* produce a hemolysin which can lyse erythrocytes of some species.

Verocytotoxin (VT)

It is also called *Shiga* like toxin (SLT). Biological, physical and antigenic properties of VT are similar to *Shiga* toxin produced by *S. dysenteriae* type 1.

F. Pathogenesis

E. coli forms a part of normal intestinal flora of man and animal. These are four major types of clinical syndromes which are caused by *E. coli:* (1) Urinary tract infection, (2) Diarrhea, (3) Pyogenic infections, and (4) Septicemia.

Urinary Tract Infection

E. coli is the most common organism responsible for urinary tract infections (UTI). *E. coli* that causes UTI often originates in the intestine of the patient.

Diarrhea

E. coli causing diarrheal diseases are of four groups. They produce diarrhea with different pathogenic mechanisms.

Enteropathogenic E. coli (EPEC)

EPEC adhere tightly to enterocytes, leading to inflammatory reaction and epithelial degenerative changes. EPEC are non-invasive and do not produce enterotoxins.

Enterotoxigenic E. coli (ETEC)

These are the strains that form a heat-labile enterotoxin (LT) or a heat-stable enterotoxin (ST) or both. They are now known to be a major cause of diarrhea in children in developing countries and are the most important cause of travelers diarrhea.

Enteroinvasive E. coli (EIEC)

Some strains of *E. coli* invade the intestinal epithelial cells as dysentery. These have been named enteroinvasive *E. coli* (EIEC). On instillation into the eyes, of guinea pigs, EIEC cause keratoconjunctivitis, this diagnostic test for EIEC is called Sereny test.

Enterohemorrhagic E. coli (EHEC) or Verocytotoxin producing E. coli (VTEC)

These strains cause hemorrhagic colitis (HC) and hemolytic uremic syndrome (HUS). Toxin responsible is called 'Verotoxin' because of its effect on vero cells in culture.

Pyogenic Infections

E. coli may cause wound infection, peritonitis, cholecystitis and neonatal meningitis. It is an important cause of neonatal meningitis.

Septicemia

E. coli is a very common cause of septicemia in many hospitals. This condition usually occurs in debilitated patients and mortality is very high.

G. Laboratory Diagnosis

Urinary Tract Infection

Normal urine is sterile, but during voiding may become contaminated with commensals of genital tract.

Specimen Collection

Midstream urine specimen (MSU): It is collected preferably prior to administration of antibiotics. Specimen is collected in a sterile container. Before collecting a sample, genitalia should be cleaned with soap and water and men are instructed to retract the foreskin of glans penis whereas women should keep the labia apart. The first portion of urine is allowed to pass, then without interrupting the urine flow, mid-portion of the stream is collected. The first portion of urine adequately flushes out the normal urethral flora.

Catheter urine specimen: Urine should be collected directly from the catheter and not from the collection bag. The catheter should not touch the container. Although a catheter specimen yields excellent results but catheterization to abstain urine is not justified because of risk of introducing infection.

Urine specimens from infants: A clean catch specimen after cleaning of genitalia is preferred.

Transport

As urine is a good culture medium, specimens after collection should reach the laboratory with minimum delay, if it is not possible, the specimen is to be refrigerated at 4°C.

Laboratory Methods

Part of the specimen is used for bacteriological culture and the rest is examined immediately under the microscope.

Microscopy: Urine is centrifuged and deposit is examined under the microscope for detection of pus cells, erythrocytes, epithelial cells and bacteria.

Culture: Most laboratories use a semiquantitative method (standard loop technique) for culture of urine specimens.

Standard loop technique

A standard calibrated loop is used to culture a fixed volume of uncentrifuged urine. Blood agar and MacConkey's agar are used and incubated at 37°C for 24 hours. Next day, the number of colonies grown is counted and total count per mL is calculated. The blood agar gives a quantitative measurement of bacterium, while MacConkey's medium enables the presumptive diagnosis of the bacterium.

Interpretation of results

Kass (1956) gave a criterion for active bacterial infection of urinary tract as follows:
- **Significant:** When bacterial count is more than 10^5/mL of a single species.
- **Doubtful significance:** Between 10^4 to 10^5 bacterial per mL. Specimen should be repeated for culture.
- **No significant growth:** $<10^3$ bacteria per mL and are regarded as contaminants.

II. Klebsiella

The genus *Klebsiella* consists of gram-negative, capsulated, non-sporing, non-motile bacilli that grows well on ordinary media, produce pink mucoid colonies on MacConkey's agar.

III. Proteus (Fig. 3.15)

The tribe Protease, in the family *Enterobacteriaceae*, contains three genera: *Proteus, Morganella, Providencia*. Proteus exhibits the phenomenon-'Swarming'. The single biochemical character, phenylpyruvic acid test (PPA test), distinguishes this tribe from all other member of *Enterobacteriaceae*. These bacteria are PPA test positive, i.e., they contain an enzyme phenylalanine deaminase which converts phenyl to phenylpyruvic acid (PPA) members of *Enterobacteriaceae*. These bacteria are PPA test positive, i.e., they contain an enzyme phenylalanine deaminase which convert phenylalanine to phenylalanine acid (PPA).

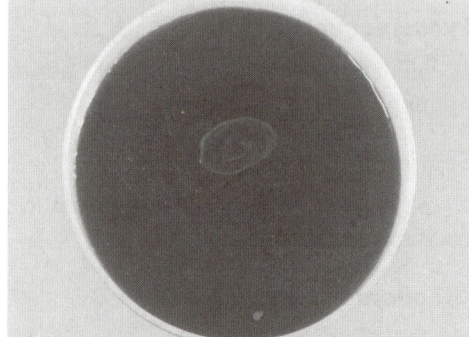

Fig. 3.15: On blood agar—Proteus swarming.

IV. Shigella

The organisms of genus *Shigella* are exclusively parasites of human intestine and other primates and cause bacillary dysentery in man.

Microscopy

Shigellae are short, gram-negative bacilli measuring about 1–3 μm × 0.5 μm. They are non-motile, non-capsulated and non-sporing.

V. Salmonella

The *Salmonella* are primarily intestinal parasites of vertebrates and which infect man, leading to enteric fever, gastroenteritis and septicemia. The most important member is *Salmonella typhi*, the causative agent of typhoid fever.

A. Morphology

Salmonellae are gram-negative bacilli measuring 1–3 μm × 0.5 μm. They are motile, non-sporing and non-capsulated. Motility is due to the presence of peritrichous flagella except *S. gallinarum* and *S. pullorum* which are non-motile.

B. Culture

Salmonellae grow on ordinary culture media at optimum temperature of 37°C (range 15–41°C), pH 6–8 and are aerobic and facultatively anaerobic. They produce colonies of 2–3 mm in diameter, circular, translucent, low convex and smooth. On MacConkey's agar and deoxycholate citrate agar (DCA), colonies with metallic sheen are formed due to non-lactose fermentation (NLF). On Wilson and Blair bismuth sulfite medium **(Figs. 3.16 and 3.17)** (selective medium for Salmonellae), jet black colonies with metallic sheen are formed due to formation of hydrogen sulfide. *S. paratyphi* A and other species which do not from H_2S produce green colonies. Xylose lysine deoxycholate (XLD) agar is another medium used for isolation of this organism. Most strains of *Salmonella* produce red colonies with centers, when grown on this medium. H_2S negative serotypes of *Salmonella* produce red colonies without black centers.

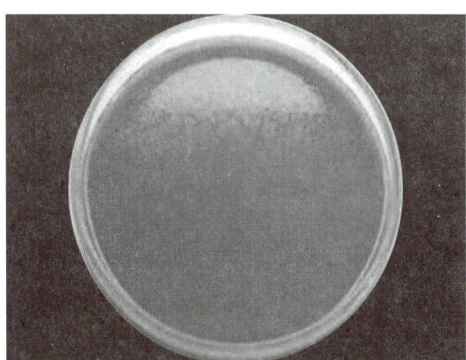

Fig. 3.16: Wilson and Blair medium.
(For color version, see Plate 5)

C. Biochemical Reactions

Salmonella ferments glucose, mannitol and maltose forming acid and gas except *S. typhi* which produce only acid and no gas. They do not ferment lactose or sucrose. Indole is not produced. Most salmonellae produce H_2S in triple sugar iron (TSI) agar except *S. paratyphi* A and *S. cholera* suis. They utilize citrate (except *S. typhi* and *S. paratyphi* A) and are MR positive and VP negative. Urea is not hydrolyzed.

D. Resistance

Salmonella are killed at 60°C in 15 minutes boiling, chlorination of water and pasteurization of milk destroy the bacilli. They survive in water, ice and snow for weeks and months.

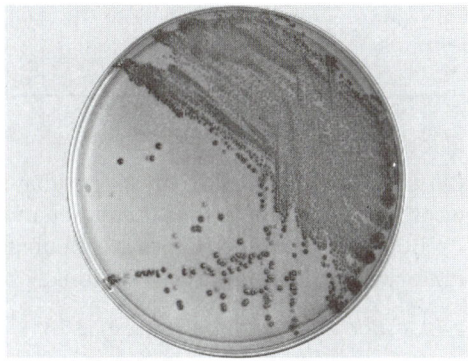

Fig. 3.17: Wilson and Blair medium—Jet black colonies of *Salmonella typhi*.
(For color version, see Plate 5)

E. Antigen Structure

Salmonellae posses three types of antigens based on which they are classified. These are (1) flagellar antigen 'H', (2) somatic antigen 'O', and (3) a surface antigen 'Vi', found in some species.

F. Pathogenesis

S. typhi, *S. paratyphi* A and usually *S. paratyphi* B are confined to human beings. The majority of other salmonellae are primarily infective for animals and human beings are secondarily infected.
Salmonellae cause three types of clinical syndrome in human beings, enteric fever, septicemia and gastroenteritis.

Enteric Fever
The term enteric fever includes typhoid fever (*S. typhi*) and paratyphoid fever (*S. paratyphi* A, B, C,). Infections due to *S. typhi* and *S. paratyphi* A are prevalent in India.
- Typhoid fever
- Paratyphoid fever

Septicemia
Salmonellae septicemia is commonly caused by *S. cholera suis* or *S. paratyphi* C and occasionally by other salmonellae. There is early invasion of blood stream and it produce local suppuration in different organs.

Gastroenteritis
Salmonellae gastroenteritis or food poisoning is caused by ingestion of food, such as meat, milk, egg contaminated by certain salmonellae which are primarily animal pathogens. Eggs and egg products are of great concern. *S. typhimurium* is the most frequently isolated in food poisoning. The incubation period is 12–24 hours.

G. Laboratory Diagnosis

Bacteriological diagnosis is enteric fever consists of:
- Isolation of bacilli.
- Demonstration of antibodies.

Isolation of Bacilli

This may be done by culture of specimens, such as blood, feces, urine, aspirated duodenal fluid, etc. Selection of relevant specimen depends upon duration of illness which is very important for the laboratory diagnosis of enteric fever **(Table 3.2)**.

TABLE 3.2: Relevance of examination of different specimens at different phases of enteric fever.		
Duration of disease	**Specimen examination**	**% Positivity**
1st week	Blood culture	90
2nd week	Blood culture Feces culture Widal test	75 50 Low titer
3rd week	Widal test Blood culture Feces culture	8–100 60 80

Blood Culture

Blood cultures are positive in approximately 90% of cases in first week of fever, 75% in the second week and 60% in the third week. Positivity rate decline thereafter and blood cultures remain positive in 25% of cases till fever subsides.

Both blood culture bottles are incubated at 37°C for overnight. The glucose broth is subcultured on blood agar and the taurocholate (bile) broth on MacConkey's agar.

Widal Tube Agglutination Test (Fig. 3.18)

- Timing of test is important, as antibodies begin to arise during end of first week. The titers increase during second, third and fourth week after which it gradually declines. The test may be negative in early part of first week.
- **Principle:** Patients' suffering from enteric fever would possess antibodies in their sera which can react and agglutinate killed, colored *Salmonella* antigens in a tube agglutination test.
- **Reading the results:** The control tubes must be examined first, where they should give no agglutination.
- Agglutination of O antigen appears as a "matt" or "carpet" at the bottom. Agglutination of H antigens appears loose, wooly or cottony. The highest dilution of serum that produces a positive agglutination is taken as titer. The titers for all the antigens are noted.
- Baseline titer of the population must be known before attaching significance to the titers. The antibody levels of individuals in a population of a given area give the baseline titer.
- A titer of 100 or more for O antigen is considered significant and a titer in excess of 200 or more for H antigens is considered significant.
- **Anamnestic response:** Those individuals, who had suffered from enteric fever in the past, sometimes develop anti-*Salmonella* antibodies during an unrelated or closely related infection. It can be differentiated from true infection by lack of any rise in titer on repetition after a week.

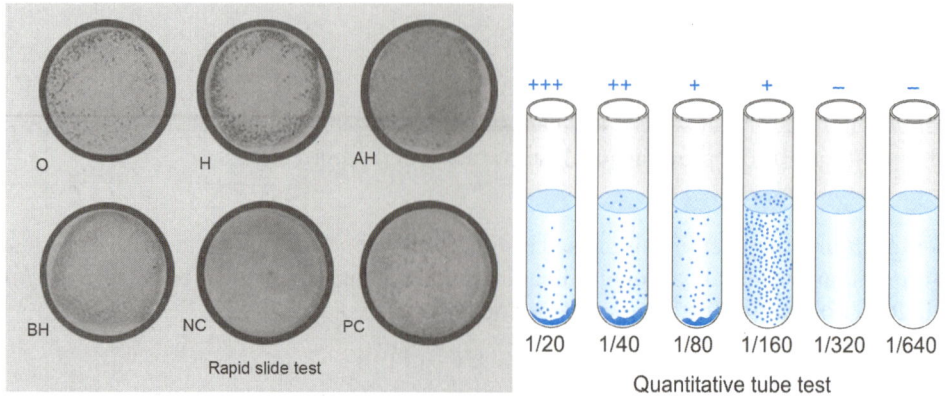

Fig. 3.18: Widal test.

VIBRIO

Vibrio are gram-negative oxidase positive, short, rigid, curved rods that are activity motile by a polar flagellum. The most important member of the genus is *Vibrio cholerae*. It is the causative agent of cholera.

I. *Vibrio cholerae*

A. Morphology

V. cholera is gram-negative, curved or comma-shaped rod, non sporing, non-capsulated, about 1.5 µm × 0.2 µm motile with a single polar flagellum and movement is named as darting motility.
 In stained mucus flakes of cholera cases, the vibrios are arranged in parallel rows, described by such as the 'fish in stream' appearance.

B. Culture

V. cholera is strongly aerobic. It grows within a temperature angle of 16–40°C but optimum pH being 8.2 (pH range 7.4–9.6).

Ordinary Media

Nutrient agar
After overnight incubation the colonies are moist, translucent, round disks, 1–2 mm in diameter, with a bluish tinge in transmitted light.

MacConkey's agar
The colonies are colorless or plate at first, but becomes reddish or pink on prolonged incubation due to late fermentation of lactose.

Blood agar
V. cholerae, classical biotype, does not produce hemolysis although some stains produce greenish discoloration around colonies which later becomes clear due to hemodigestion.

Peptone water
It grows as a surface pellicle because of its aerobic nature.

Special Media

The special media are classified as follows:
- Transport or holding media
- Enrichment media
- Plating media

Transport or holding media
Venkatraman-Ramakrishnan (VR) medium: It is a transport media for *Vibrio cholera* and its pH is 8.6–8.8. Vibrio do not multiply, but remain viable for several weeks.

Enrichment media
Alkaline peptone water (APW): It is a peptone water at pH 8.6. Besides enrichment medium, it is also as excellent transport medium.
Monsur's taurocholate tellurite peptone water: It contains peptone, sodium chlorite, sodium taurocholate in one liter of distilled water and pH is adjusted to 9.2. To this medium, sterile potassium tellurite solution is added. Like APW, it is not only a good enrichment medium but is transport medium as well.

Plating media
On TCBS agar: Yellow color colonies can be seen.
Alkaline bile salt agar (BSA) pH 8.2: It is modified nutrient agar medium containing 0.5% sodium taurocholate (bile salt). The colonies are similar to those on nutrient agar.
Monsur's gelatin taurocholate trypticase tellurite agar (GTTA) medium: pH 8.5: It is the most widely used selective medium for isolation of vibrios. It contains sodium thiosulfate, sodium citrate, bile salts, sucrose, bromothymol blue (indicator), yeast extract, peptone, sodium chloride, ferric citrate and water. *Vibrio cholerae* form yellow colonies due to sucrose fermentation, while non-sucrose fermenters, such as *V. parahaemolyticus* produce green colonies.

C. Biochemical Reactions

Carbohydrate breakdown is fermentative, producing acid, but no gas. It is catalase and oxidase positive. It ferments glucose, mannitol, sucrose, maltose and mannose, but not lactose, though lactose may be spilt very slowly. It is indole positive and reduces nitrates to nitrites. It is methyl red (MR) and urease negative. Gelatin is liquefied. It decarboxylates lysine and ornithine but do not utilize arginine. Voges-Proskauer (VP) reaction and hemolysis of sheep erythrocytes are positive in EL Tor biotype and both these tests are negative in classical biotype.

D. Antigen Structure

V. cholerae contain somatic 'O' and flagellar 'H' antigens. The 'H' antigen is shared by all the strains. On the basis of O antigen, it is divided into subgroups (now named O serogroups or serovars). Both classical and El Tor biotypes belong to serogroups O1 and are antigenically indistinguishable. These are referred as *V. cholerae* O1. On the basis of minor O antigens (A, B, C), *V. cholerae* O1 are subdivided into three serotypes—Ogawa (AB), Inaba (AC), and Hikojima (ABC).

At least 139 (O1 to O139) O serogroups are recognized. Serogroups O2 to O138 are called non-O1 *V. cholerae*. Since these organisms were not agglutinated by O-1 antiserum, they were called non-agglutinating.

Table 3.3 is depicts the serotype of cholera vibrios.

TABLE 3.3: Serotype of cholera vibrios.

Serotype	O antigen
Ogawa	AB
Inaba	AC
Hikojima	ABC

Direct Microscopy

For rapid diagnosis, the characteristic darting motility of the *Vibrio* and is inhibition by adding antiserum can be demonstrated under the dark field or phase contract microscope, using cholera stool.

Culture

Stool sample is directly cultured on following media:
- Selective media (BSA, TCBS or Monsur's GTTA) and non-selective media (blood agar and MacConkey's agar) are inoculated. These plates are incubated at 37°C for overnight.
- On TCBS agar: Yellow color colonies can be seen **(Fig. 3.19)**.
- Enrichment media, such as alkaline peptone water or Monsur's liquid media are inoculated. These media are incubated at 37°C for 6–8 hours before subculturing on to selective media.

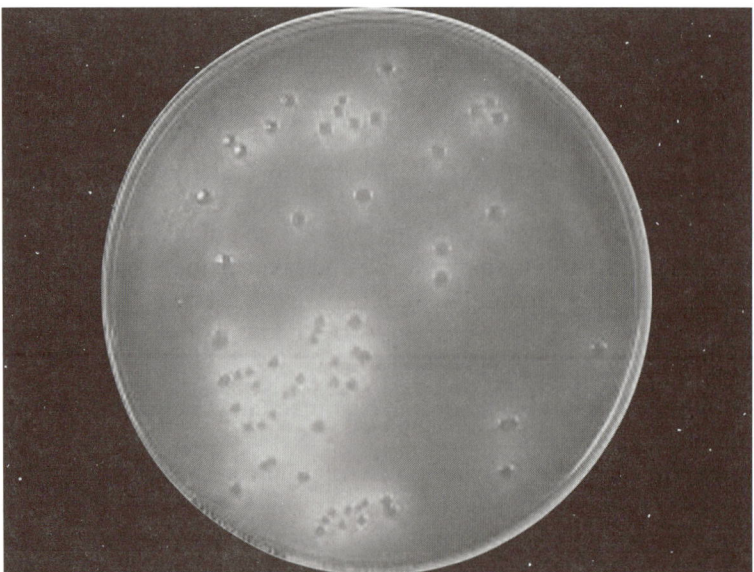

Fig. 3.19: On TCBS agar—yellow color colonies of *V. cholerae*.
(For color version, see Plate 5)

PSEUDOMONAS

The genus *Pseudomonas* belongs to the family *Pseudomonadaceae* which contains over 200 species. The most important among these is *Ps. aeruginosa*.

Pseudomonas aeruginosa

A. Morphology

It is slender, gram-negative bacillus, 1.5–3 um × 0.5 μm, non-capsulated, non-sporing and is actively motile by a polar flagellum.

B. Culture

It is a strict aerobe and grows well on ordinary media like nutrient broth and nutrient agar. The optimum temperature for growth is 37°C. But growth occurs at a wide range of temperature 5–42°C.
1. **Nutrient agar:** Colonies are smooth, large, translucent, low convex, 2–4 mm in diameter. The organism produces a sweetish aromatic odor. There is greenish blue pigment which diffuses into the medium.
2. **Blood agar:** Colony characters are similar to those on nutrient agar. Many strains are hemolytic on blood agar.
3. **MacConkey agar:** Colonies are pale or colorless (non-lactose fermenters, NLF).
4. **Cetrimide agar:** It is a selective medium for *Ps. aeruginosa*.
5. **Peptone water:** It forms a turbidity with a surface pellicle. *Pseudomonas* being a strict aerobe tends to collect at the surface for more oxygen hence forming surface pellicle.

C. Pigment Production

Ps. aeruginosa produces a number of pigments which diffuse into surrounding medium. These pigments are:
1. **Pyocyanin:** It is a bluish-green pigment. It is not produced by other species of the genus, hence, it is diagnostic of *P. aeruginosa*.
2. **Fluorescin (pyoverdin):** It is a greenish yellow pigment. It may be produced by many other *Pseudomonas* species also.
3. **Pyorubin:** It is a reddish brown pigment.
4. **Pyomelanin:** It is a brown colored pigment.

D. Biochemical Reactions

Ps. aeruginosa derives energy from carbohydrates by oxidative breakdown rather than a fermentative metabolism. It utilizes only glucose oxidatively with acid production. All strains of *Ps. aeruginosa* are oxidase positive and utilize citrate as the sole source of carbon.

E. Resistance

It is killed by heating at 55°C for one hour. It is resistant to the chemical disinfectants and can even grow in certain antiseptics like quaternary ammonium chloroxylenol and hexachlorophene. It is sensitive to 2 aqueous alkaline solution of glutaraldehyde compounds.

F. Pathogenesis

It causes infections more common in patients with neutropenia, cystic fibrosis, burns and those on ventilators. It is the most important agent causing nosocomial infections. It is due to its resistance to common antibiotics and antiseptics that it establishes itself widely in hospitals. Equipments such as respirators and endoscopes, articles such as bed pans, and antiseptic or disinfectant solutions may be frequently contaminated. The other common infections caused by it are:
1. Urinary tract infections.
2. Acute purulent meningitis.
3. Post-tracheostomy pulmonary infection.
4. Septicemia in debilitated patients.
5. Wound and burn infections.
6. Chronic otitis media and otitis externa.
7. Eye infections.
8. Infantile diarrhea.

G. Laboratory Diagnosis

1. **Specimens:** Pus, wound swab, urine, sputum, blood or CSF.
2. **Culture:** Specimens may be inoculated on nutrient agar, blood agar or MacConkey's agar and incubated at 37°C for 18–24 hours. On nutrient agar, there is bluish green pigment diffused in the medium. On MacConkey's agar they grow as pale colonies (NLF). In peptone water, surface pellicle and green pigment can be observed. Selective media such as cetrimide agar may be necessary to isolate *Ps aeruginosa* from faeces or other samples with mixed flora.
3. **Gram staining and motility:** They are gram-negative bacilli and are actively motile.
4. **Biochemical reactions:** The oxidase test is positive within 30 seconds. They are non-fermenter. They break down glucose oxidatively with acid production only.
5. **Antibiotic sensitivity test:** It is useful to select out proper antibiotic as multiple resistance to antibiotics is quite common in *Ps. aeruginosa*.

H. Treatment

It is intrinsically resistant to most of the commonly used antimicrobial agents. Ciprofloxacin, piperacillin, ticarcillin, azlocillin, cefotaxime, ceftazidime, gentamicin and tobramycin are used in treatment of *Ps. aeruginosa* infections.

MYCOBACTERIUM

Mycobacteria are slender bacilli that are difficult to stain, but once stained it resists decolourization with dilute mineral acids and are therefore called acid-fast bacilli or AFB. These organisms are aerobic, non-motile, non-capsulated and non-sporing. Growth is generally slow.

I. *Mycobacterium tuberculosis*

A. Morphology

M. tuberculosis is a slender, straight or slightly curved bacillus with rounded ends, occurring singly, in pairs or in small clumps. It measures 1.4 μm × 0.2 μm (average 3 μm × 0.3 μm) in size. These bacilli are acid-fast, non-sporing, non-capsulated and non-motile. Ziehl-Neelsen staining is useful to study the morphology of these organisms. With this stain, tubercle bacilli are seen bright red (acid-fast), while the tissue cells and other organisms are stained blue. Tubercle bacilli may also be stained with the fluorescent dyes (Auramine O, Rhodamine) and appear yellow luminous bacilli under the fluorescent microscope. They are gram-positive but are difficult to stain with the Gram stain.

B. Culture

M. tuberculosis is an obligate aerobe. The bacilli grow slowly (generation time is 20 hours) and colonies appear only in about 2 weeks and sometimes it may take up to 6–8 weeks. Optimum temperature for growth is 37°C (range 30–40°C). Optimum pH is 6.4–7.0. Tubercle bacilli can grow on a wide range of enriched culture media but Lowenstein-Jensen (LJ) medium is the most commonly used. This medium consists of beaten eggs, asparagine, mineral salts, malachite green and glycerol or sodium pyruvate.). Malachite green inhibits the growth of organisms other than mycobacteria and provides a color to the medium. *Mycobacterium tuberculosis* colonies are dry, rough, buff colored, raised, with a wrinkled surface. M. tuberculosis has a luxuriant growth (eugonic growth).

In liquid media, the bacilli grow as surface pellicle. Virulent strains tend to grow as serpentine cords in the liquid media, while avirulent strains grow in a more dispersed manner.

C. Biochemical Reactions

Mycobacterium species can be identified by several biochemical tests. Niacin test and nitrate reduction test are two important biochemical tests, which are positive in *M. tuberculosis*.

D. Pathogenesis

Tuberculosis may involve lungs (pulmonary) or site-other than lungs (extrapulmonary). The infection is commonly acquired by inhalation of infected droplets coughed or sneezed into the air by a patient with pulmonary tuberculosis).

Tubercle bacilli are engulfed by macrophages but they survive and multiply in macrophages. The cell-mediated immunity (CMI) plays a major role to interact with these macrophages whereas humoral immunity appears to be irrelevant.

E. Koch's Phenomenon

The response of a tuberculous animal to reinfection was best explained by Robert Koch. When a healthy guinea pig is inoculated subcutaneously with virulent tubercle bacilli, the puncture site heals quickly and there is no immediate visible reaction. After 10–14 days, a nodule appears at the site of injection which ulcerates and the ulcer persists, till the animal dies of progressive tuberculosis. The regional lymph nodes are enlarged and caseous. If on the other hand, virulent tubercle bacilli are injected in a guinea pig, which had received a prior injection of tubercle bacilli 4–6 weeks earlier, an indurated lesion appears at the site of injection in a day or two which undergoes necrosis in another day or so to form a shallow ulcer. This ulcer heals rapidly without involvement of the regional lymph nodes or tissues. This is called Koch's phenomenon. This phenomenon is a combination of hypersensitivity and immunity.

F. Laboratory Diagnosis

Bacteriological diagnosis can be established by microscopy, culture examination or by animal inoculation test.

1. **Specimen:** Specimen collection depends on the site of involvement. Tuberculosis may involve lungs (pulmonary) or sites other than lungs (extrapulmonary).
    i. *Pulmonary tuberculosis:* Sputum is the most common specimen. It is collected in a clean wide-mouthed container. A morning specimen may be collected on three consecutive days. If sputum is scanty, a 24-hour specimen may be collected. When sputum is not available, laryngeal swab or bronchial washings are collected. In children, gastric washings may be examined as they tend to swallow sputum.
    ii. *Meningitis:* Cerebrospinal fluid (CSF) from tuberculous meningitis (TBM) often forms a spider web clot on standing. Examination of which may be more useful than of fluid.
    iii. *Renal tuberculosis:* Three consecutive days of urine are examined.
    iv. *Bone and joints tuberculosis:* Aspirated fluid.
    v. *Tissue:* Biopsy of tissue.

2. **Direct microscopy:** Smear is made from the specimen and stained by the Ziehl-Neelsen technique. It is examined under oil immersion lens. The acid-fast bacilli (AFB) appear as bright red bacilli against a blue background. A negative report should not be given till at least 300 fields have been examined.

    However, grading of smears is done differently under Revised National Tuberculosis Control Programme (RNTCP) or National Tuberculosis Elimination Programme (NTEP).

3. **Concentration of specimens:** Concentration of a specimen is done to achieve:
    a. Homogenization of the specimen.
    b. Decontamination, i.e., to kill other bacteria present in the specimen.
    c. Concentration, i.e., to concentrate the bacilli in a small volume without inactivation.

    Such concentrate is used for culture and animal inoculation tests besides smear preparation. Several concentration methods are in use:
    a. **Petroff's method:** It is a simple and widely used technique. Sputum is mixed with equal volume of 4% sodium hydroxide and is incubated at 37°C with frequent shaking for about 30 minutes. It is then centrifuged at 3,000 rpm for 30 minutes. The supernatant fluid is poured off and the deposit is neutralized by adding 8% hydrochloric acid in presence of a drop of phenol red indicator the deposit is used for smear, culture and animal inoculation.
    b. **Other methods:** Mucolytic agents such as N-acetyl-L-cysteine with sodium hydroxide and pancreatin are used for concentration of specimens. In urine and CSF specimens centrifugation is done to concentrate the specimen. Centrifuged deposit is used for smear and culture examination.

4. **Culture:** Culture is a very sensitive method for detection of tubercle bacilli. It may detect as few as 10 to 100 bacilli per mL. The concentrated material is inoculated on two bottles of Lowenstein-Jensen medium The tubercle bacilli usually grow in 2–8 weeks. In a positive culture, characteristic colonies appear on culture medium. Smear is prepared from isolated colony and stained with Ziehl-Neelsen technique. When acid-fast bacillus (AFB) is slow growing, non-pigmented and niacin positive, it is regarded as *M. tuberculosis*, further confirmation is done by biochemical reactions.

    In radiometric method such as BACTEC, the growth may be detected in about a week by using ^{14}C labelled substrates. Culture media contains ^{14}C-labelled palmitic acid. Mycobacteria metabolize the ^{14}C-labelled substrates and release radioactively labelled $^{14}CO_2$.

5. **Serology:** Serology includes detection of anti mycobacterial antibodies in patient serum. Various methods such as enzyme-linked immunosorbent assay (ELISA), radioimmunoassay (RIA), latex agglutination assay have been employed. Diagnostic utility of these antibodies is equivocal.
6. **Molecular methods:** Polymerase chain reaction (PCR) is a rapid method in diagnosis of tuberculosis. It is based on DNA amplification and has been used to detect *M. tuberculosis* directly in clinical specimens.

   Gene Xert MTB/RIF: Gene Xpert MTB/RIF is an automated diagnostic test. It detects *M. tuberculosis* and rifampicin resistance by PCR. Results can be obtained from sputum specimen with 2 hours WHO has endorsed this test for use in tuberculosis endemic countries.

   Line probe assay (LPA) is used for identification of *M. tuberculosis* complex as well as detection of mutation in drug resistant genes.

G. Treatment

The antitubercular drugs include bactericidal agents such as Rifampicin (R), Isoniazid (H), Pyrazinamide (Z), Streptomycin and bacteriostatic agents include Ethambutol (E), Thiacetazone, ethionamide, paraamino-salicylic acid (PAS) and Cycloserine. Short course regimens of 6–7 months are used as resistant strains emerge readily by mutation and selection, combinations of two or more drugs are used.

A serious consequence of unchecked drug resistance has been the emergence of ***multidrug resistance tuberculosis*** **(MDR-TB)**. The term multidrug resistance refers to resistance to rifampicin and isoniazid, with or without resistance to one or more other drugs. MDR-TB is a global problem especially in HIV infected persons. The directly observed therapy under supervision (DOTS) is being used to prevent deterioration of resistance problem by ensuring the patient's compliance.

Another serious condition ***extensively drug resistant tuberculosis*** **(XDR-TB)** has emerged recently. XDR-TB is due to *M. tuberculosis* strains which are resistant to any fluoroquinolone and at least one of three injectable second line drugs (capreomycin, kanamycin and amikacin), in addition to isoniazid and rifampicin.

H. Prophylaxis

Protection from tuberculosis may be done by public health measures and BCG vaccination. General measures such as nutrition and health education are also important.

BCG Vaccine

Calmette and Guerin (1921) prepared an attenuated strain of *M. bovis*. The strain was attenuated by repeated subcultures. When the strain became incapable of producing tuberculosis in the susceptible guinea pig, it was named bacillus Calmette–Guérin (BCG).

Dose and Administration

Vaccine is given intradermally in a dose of 0.1 mL. BCG vaccine should be given soon after birth failing which it may be administered at any time during the first year of life.

National Tuberculosis Elimination Programme (NTEP)

Under NTEP any patient with cough for 2 weeks more is included for diagnosis of pulmonary tuberculosis. Diagnosis is mainly based on good quality microscopy include two sputum samples are collected from the patient. One early morning specimen and other is collected on spot when patient visits the chest clinic.

Both the sputum specimens are stained with Ziehl-Neelsen staining and observed for acid-fast bacilli (AFB). If one or both smears are positive then patient is diagnosed as sputum positive pulmonary tuberculosis and antitubercular treatment is started. If both smears are negative, diagnosis is done on resistant X-ray chest findings. In case of X-ray chest suggestive DR-TB of tuberculosis, patient is diagnosed as sputum negative pulmonary tuberculosis. Antitubercular treatment is started. Patient is declared not suffering from tuberculosis and when there is no finding suggestive of tuberculosis on X-ray chest.

II. Non-tuberculous Mycobacteria

Mycobacteria other than tubercle bacilli, that may occasionally cause human disease resembling tuberculosis is called as atypical mycobacteria. They normally exist as saprophytes of soil and water. They occasionally cause opportunistic disease in man and hence are also named opportunistic mycobacteria or non-tuberculous mycobacteria (NTM) or MOTT (mycobacteria other than tubercle bacilli).

A. Classification

On the basis of pigment production and rate of growth. Runyon (1959) classified non-tuberculous mycobacteria into four groups—Photochromogens, Non-photochromogens, Scotochromogens and Rapid growers.

B. Culture

Non-tuberculous mycobacteria grow in Lowenstein-Jensen (LJ) medium. Colonies appear within two to three weeks except in case of rapid growers which produce colonies in 4–5 days. Photochromogens form colonies that produce no pigment in the dark, but when colonies are exposed to light, a yellow orange pigment appears. The scotochromogens produce pigment in the dark non-photochromogens do not form pigment even on exposure to light. Rapid growers may be photo, scoto or non-photochromogens.

III. *Mycobacterium leprae*

Leprosy is a chronic mycobacterial disease of ancient world and is still afflicting patients in many parts of world—mainly Asia and Africa. It is caused by *Mycobacterium leprae*.

A. Morphology

M. leprae is a slender, slightly curved or straight bacillus, 1–8 um × 0.2–0.5 um. It is acid-fast, but less so than the tubercle bacillus and for which 5% sulphuric acid is used for decolorization after staining with carbol fuchsin. It is gram-positive and stains more readily.

The bacilli are seen singly and in groups, intracellularly or lying free outside the cells. Inside the cells they are present as bundles of organisms bound together by a lipid-like substance, the glia. These masses are known as globi. The parallel rows of bacilli in the globi give appearance of a cigar bundle. In tissue sections, the bacilli are arranged in clumps resembling cigarette ends. The globi are present in Virchow's lepra cells or foamy cells which are large undifferentiated histiocytes.

B. Cultivation

Lepra bacilli have not yet been grown on artificial culture media or tissue culture.

There have been many attempts to transmit leprosy to different experimental animals. The first breakthrough was achieved by Shepard (1960) when he showed that lepra bacilli could multiply in the foot pads of mice. The nine-banded armadillo (Dasypus novemcinctus) is highly susceptible to infection with *M. leprae*.

C. Pathogenesis

Leprosy is a chronic granulomatous disease of humans and the only source of infection is patient. The bacilli localize primarily in the skin, peripheral nerves and nasal mucosa but any tissue or organ may be involved. Due to preference of bacilli for lower temperatures, the superficial and cooler tissues are affected.

Incubation period is very long and variable. Sources of infection are nasal discharge and skin lesions of patients. Prolonged close contact with patients is necessary for transmission of the disease.

D. Ridley and Jopling's Classification

On the basis of clinical, histopathological and immunological findings. Ridley and Jopling have introduced a scale for classifying the spectrum of leprosy into five groups. These are tuberculoid (TT), borderline tuberculoid (BT), borderline (BB), borderline lepromatous (BL) and lepromatous (LL).

According to WHO, leprosy is divided into two groups, paucibacillary and multibacillary leprosy. This classification depends upon number of skin lesion and involvement of nerves. When there are ≤5 skin lesions and no/one nerve trunk involvement, it is called paucibacillary leprosy. In case of multibacillary leprosy, the patient have 6 or more skin lesions and more than one nerve trunk involvement. Paucibacillary includes all cases of tuberculoid types and some cases of borderline types and multibacillary includes all cases of lepromatous types and some cases of borderline type.

E. Lepromin Test

This reaction was first described by Mitsuda in 1919. The original antigen (lepromin) was a boiled, emulsified. lepromatous tissue rich in lepra bacilli. Nowadays, the lepromins used as antigens may be of human origin (lepromin-H) or armadillo derived (lepromin-A).

1. **Procedure:** The lepromin test is carried out by the intradermal injection of 0.1 mL of lepromin. The response to lepromin is typically biphasic consisting of early reaction of Fernandez and late reaction of Mitsuda.
    i. *Early reaction of Fernandez:* It consists of erythema and induration developing in 24–48 hours and usually remains for 3–5 days.
    ii. *Late reaction of Mitsuda:* It appears 1–2 weeks after the injection, reaching a peak in four weeks. The reaction appears in the form of a nodule that may ulcerate.
2. **Uses:**
    i. *Classification of leprosy:* The test is positive in tuberculoid leprosy and negative in lepromatous leprosy.
    ii. *Assessment of prognosis:* A positive lepromin test indicates a good prognosis and a negative one a bad prognosis.
    iii. *Assessment of resistance:* It is done to assess the resistance of an individual to leprosy. Resistance is indicated by positive lepromin test.

F. Laboratory Diagnosis

In lepromatous cases, bacilli are always found in large numbers but in tuberculoid cases, the bacilli are very few and found with great difficulty, or not at all.

1. **Specimens:** Specimens are collected from the nasal mucosa, skin lesions and ear lobules. The specimens from skin are obtained by slit and scrape method. About six different areas should be sampled, including the skin over the buttocks, chin, cheek, forehead and ears. Smears from the nose are made by scraping a little material from the nasal septum.
2. **Acid-fast staining:** Slit-skin smears from skin patches and ear lobes and nasal mucosal scrapings are stained by Ziehl-Neelsen method using 5% sulphuric acid as decolorizing agent. Acid-fast bacilli (AFB) arranged in parallel bundles within macrophages (Lepra-cell) confirm the diagnosis of lepromatous leprosy. The viable bacilli stain uniformly and the dead bacilli are fragmented, irregular or granular.

    The smears are graded, based on the number of bacilli as follows:

1-10 bacilli in 100 fields	= 1+
1-10 bacilli in 10 fields	= 2+
1-10 bacilli per field	= 3+
10-100 bacilli per field	= 4+
10-1000 bacilli per field	= 5+
More than 1,000 bacilli, clumps and globi in every field	= 6+

    i. *Bacteriological index (BI):* It is defined as number of total bacilli in a tissue.
    ii. *Morphological index (MI):* It is defined as the percentage of uniformly stained (viable) bacilli out of the total number of bacilli counted. It provides a method for assessing the progress of patients on chemotherapy.
3. **Skin and nerve biopsy:** These are useful in the diagnosis and accurate classification of leprosy lesion.

G. Treatment

Patients with paucibacillary (TT, BT) leprosy are given Rifampicin 600 mg once a month (supervised) and Dapsone 100 mg daily (unsupervised) for 6 months. For multibacillary (BB, BL, LL) leprosy, rifampicin 600 mg once a month (supervised), dapsone 100 mg daily (unsupervised), clofazimine 300 mg once a month (supervised), and 50 mg, clofazimine daily (unsupervised) are given for one year.

ZOONOSES

Introduction
Zoonoses are diseases and infections of animals; their causative agents are transmitted between animals and humans.

Etiology
Zoonotic diseases commonly occur in individuals which handle animals/animal products. The most common zoonotic diseases are listed in **Tables 3.4 and 3.5**.

TABLE 3.4: Common zoonotic diseases.

Bacteria	Rickettsia	Virus	Parasite	Fungus
Anthrax	Scrub typhus	Rabies	Taeniasis	
Plague				
Brucellosis	Murine typhus	Yellow fever	Echinococcosis	Zoophilic dermatophytes
Leptospirosis	Tick typhus	Japanese encephalitis	Leishmaniasis	
Salmonellosis	Q fever	KFD	Toxoplasmosis	
		Chikungunya		

TABLE 3.5: Laboratory procedures for bacterial zoonoses.

Disease	Sample	Microbiology	Culture	Serology	Other
Cutaneous anthrax	Fluid from eschar	Gram-positive bacilli (bamboo stick appearance)	Nutrient agar (Medusa head)	• Ascoli's thermoprecipitin test • CFT	Lysis by gammaphage
Pulmonary anthrax	Sputum Stool		Blood agar (string pearls)	ELISA	Direct fluorescent antibody test
Intestinal anthrax		McFadyean's reaction	Gelatin stab (inverted fir tree)		
Acute brucellosis (undulant fever)	Blood	Gram-negative coccobacilli	Casteneda method	• Standard agglutination test • ELISA • CFT	Skin test
Bubonic plague	Fluid from buboes	Gram-negative bacilli	Nutrient agar	Passive hemagglutination	PCR
Pneumonic plague	Sputum	Bipolar staining	Blood agar		
Septicemic plague	Blood	Safety pin appearance	Ghee broth ('stalactite' growth)		
Salmonellosis	• Stool • Food	Gram-negative bacilli	• MacConkey agar • Wilson and Blair medium	Widal test	
Leptospirosis	• Blood • Urine	Dark ground microscope; spirochete	Korthof's medium	Microscopic agglutination test	
Tuberculosis (*M. bovis*)	Sputum	Acid-fast bacilli	LJ medium		PCR

Laboratory Diagnosis
For the diagnosis of zoonoses. In humans and animals this based on:
- Isolation of causative agent
- Serology
- Autopsy

Collection of Specimens
Specimens are collected according to the site of lesion. **Tables 3.6 to 3.9** list the types of specimens to be collected and laboratory diagnosis tests for bacterial, rickettsial, viral, parasitic and fungal zoonoses, respectively.

TABLE 3.6: Laboratory procedure for ricketsial zoonoses.

Disease	Sample	Culture	Serology
Scrub typhus	Blood	Yolk sac of chick embryo	Weil-Felix test
Murine typhus	Blood	Yolk sac of chick embryo	Weil-Felix test
Tick	Blood	Yolk sac of chick embryo	CFT

TABLE 3.7: Laboratory procedures for viral zoonoses.

Disease	Sample	Microscopy	Culture	Serology
Rabies	• Antemortem—corneal impression smear skin biopsy; saliva • Postmortem-brain	• Immunofluorescence • Negri bodies	Tissue culture (WI 38, BHK 21)	
Yellow fever	Blood	Yolk sac of chick embryo		Hemagglutination inhibition
Japanese encephalitis	CSF	Intracerebral inoculation into suckling mice		• CFT • Neutralization
KFD				Immunofluorescence
Chikungunya		Tissue culture		ELISA

TABLE 3.8: Laboratory procedures for parasitic zoonses.

Disease	Sample	Microscopy	Serology
Taenia	Stool	Egg	ELISA
Echinococcus	Stool		• ELISA • Hemagglutination • Indirect fluorescent antibody
Leishmania	Blood	Peripheral blood, amastigote (LD bodies)	• Aldehyde test • Antimony test • CFT

TABLE 3.9: Laboratory procedures for fungal zoonoses.

Disease	Sample	Microbiology	Culture
Geophilic dermatophytes			
Microsporum canis	Skin scrapping	KOH preparation	SDA
Trichophyton verrucosum	Hair clipping		
T. equinum	Nail clipping		

MEDICAL VIROLOGY

Viruses are the smallest obligate intracellular infective agents containing one type of nucleic acid (DNA or RNA). Various DNA viruses are tabulated in **Table 3.10** and various RNA viruses are tabulated in **Table 3.11**.

TABLE 3.10: DNA viruses.

Sl. No.	Group	Morphology	Viruses	Disease	Route of infection	Diagnosis
1.	Poxviruses	• Brick shaped • Can be seen by light microscopy • DNA genome	• Variola • Molluscum contagiosum	• Smallpox • Benign wart	• Respiratory tract • Sexually transmitted	• Grows in chorioallantois membrane (CAM) of chick embryo and tissue culture
2.	Herpesviruses	• Enveloped • Double stranded DNA • DNA genome • 100–200 nm in diameter	• Herpes simplex virus (HSV)	• Acute gingivostomatitis • Herpes labialis • Keratoconjunctivitis • Eczema herpeticum • Genital herpes • Neonatal herpes • Aseptic meningitis	• Respiratory tract • Skin lesions • Sexually transmitted • Birth canal	• Direct examination to observe inclusion bodies • Tissue culture • Polymerase chain reaction (PCR)
			• Varicella zoster	• Chickenpox	• Respiratory tract	• Direct examination to observe inclusion bodies • Tissue culture • Polymerase chain reaction (PCR)
			• Cytomegalovirus	• Congenital infection	• Sexually transmitted • Blood transplantation • Organ transplantation	• Cytomegalic cells demonstration • Tissue culture • Antigen detection • PCR • Serology
			• Epstein-Barr virus (EBV)	• Infection mononucleosis • Burkitt's lymphoma • Nasopharyngeal carcinoma	• Oral contact (kissing)	• Atypical lymphocytes demonstration in blood • Paul-Bunnell test • Antigen detection • PCR
3.	Adenoviruses	• Non-enveloped • Double stranded DNA genome • 70–75 nm in diameter	• Adenovirus	• Respiratory infections • Eye infection • Urinary tract infection	• Through conjunctiva • Through nasal mucosa • Feco-oral route	• Virus particles seen by electron microscope • Viral antigens demonstration by immunofluorescence • Tissue culture

Section I: Applied Microbiology

TABLE 3.11: RNA viruses.

Sl. No.	Group	Morphology	Viruses	Disease	Route of infection	Diagnosis
1.	Picornaviruses	• Non-enveloped • Single stranded • 27–30 nm in diameter	• Poliomyelitis	Poliomyelitis	• By ingestion • By respiratory secretions	• Direct demonstration of virus in feces by electron microscopy • Tissue culture
2.	Orthomyxoviruses	• Enveloped • Single stranded RANA genome • 80–120 nm in diameter	Influenza virus	Influenza	Through respiratory tract	• Demonstration of viral antigens in nasopharyngeal secretions by immunofluorescence • Isolation of virus in chick embryo • Serology and PCR
3.	Rhabdoviruses	• Bullet shaped • Single stranded RNA genome • 75 x 180 nm	Rabies virus	Rabies	By bite of rabid dog or other animals	• Demonstration of viral antigen in corneal smear by immunofluorescence • Demonstration of Negri bodies in brain. • Isolation of virus by intracerebral inoculation in mice.
4.	Arboviruses	• Enveloped • Single stranded RNA genome • 40–50 nm in diameter • Enveloped • Singles stranded RNA genome • 50–70 nm in diameter	• Dengue virus • Rubella virus	• Dengue fever • Rubella (German measles) • Congenital rubella	• By bite of infected *Aedes aegypti* mosquito • By inhalation • Through placenta	• Demonstration of IgM antibody in serum by ELISA • Demonstration of NS antigen in serum • Isolation of virus Serology (ELISA for antibody detection)
5.	Reovirus	• Non-enveloped • Double stranded RNA genome (segmented) • 55–75 nm in diameter	• Rotavirus	• Diarrhea in children	• Feco-oral	• Demonstration of virus in the feces by ELISA • Detection of antibody in blood by ELISA
6.	Retroviruses	• Enveloped • Single stranded RNA genome • 0–120 nm in diameter • Contains reverse transcriptase enzyme	• Human immunodeficiency virus (HIV)	• Acquired immunodeficiency syndrome (AIDS)	• Sexual contract • Blood transfusion • Needle stick injury • Mother to newborn either transplacentally or perinatally • Feco-oral	• Detection of antibody in serum by ELISA

HEPATITIS VIRUSES

Viral hepatitis is a systemic disease with primary inflammation in the liver. Till now, there are six hepatitis viruses, i.e. hepatitis A, B, C, D, E, and G. Hepatitis B is DNA virus while others (A, C, D, E, G) contain RNA genome. Characteristics of major hepatitis virus are given in **Table 3.12**.

1. HEPATITIS A VIRUS (HAV—INFECTIOUS HEPATITIS)

Hepatitis A virus enters the body by oral route. The large majority of infections are asymptomatic. Symptoms include fever, malaise, anorexia, nausea, and vomiting and liver tenderness. These usually subside with the onset of jaundice. Recovery occurs over a period of 4–6 weeks.

HAV is 27 nm non-enveloped single stranded RNA viruses with an icosahedral symmetry. It belongs to the Picornavirus family.

A. Laboratory Diagnosis

Laboratory diagnosis can be made by:
1. Demonstration of virus
2. Detection of antibody

- **Demonstration of virus:**
  - *Immunoelectron microscopy (IEM):* The virus can be visualized by IEM in feces.
  - *Enzyme-linked immunosorbent assay (ELISA):* HAV antigen can be detected in feces by ELISA using monoclonal antibodies.
  - *Isolation:* The virus has been grown in human and simian cell cultures but it is not possible to grow them routinely from faeces of patients.
- **Detection of antibody:** Demonstration of specific antibody to HAV in the blood. ELISA kits for detecting IgM and IgG antibodies are available.

B. Prophylaxis

- General prophylaxis includes improved sanitation and prevention of fecal contamination of food and water.
- Passive prophylaxis with normal pooled human immunoglobulin before exposure to the virus or in the early incubation period may prevent or attenuate a clinical illness, while not necessarily prevent virus excretion.
- A formalin inactivated, alum conjugated vaccine containing HAV grown in human diploid cell culture is available. It is safe and effective A full course consists of two intramuscular injections of the vaccine. Second dose is administered 6 months after first dose. Protection lasts for 10–20 years.
- One attack of the disease gives life-long protection.

2. HEPATITIS B VIRUS (HBV—SERUM HEPATITIS)

Hepatitis B virus (HBV) belongs to the family Hepadnaviridae. It differs from hepatitis A in various aspects.

A. Morphology

HBV is a complex 42 nm double shelled particle. The outer surface or envelope of virus contains hepatitis B surface antigen (HBsAg). It encloses an inner icosahedral 27 nm nucleocapsid (core), which contains diploid cell hepatitis B core antigen (HBcAg). Inside the core is the genome, a circular double stranded DNA and a DNA polymerase. *Blumberg* and coworkers (1965) described a protein antigen in serum of an Australian aborigine, which gave protection a positive precipitation reaction with sera from two hemophiliacs who had received multiple transfusions.

TABLE 3.12: Characteristic features of major hepatitis virus.

Feature	HAV	HBV	HCV	HDV	HEV
Genome	RNA	DNA	RNA	RNA	RNA
Nomenclature	Picornaviridae	Hepadnaviridae	Flaviviridae	Deltavirus	Hepadnaviridae
Mode of transmission	Enteric	Parenteral, sexual, perinatal	Parenteral, sexual	Parenteral	Enteric
Antigen in blood	HAV	HBsAg, HBeAg	HCV	HDAg	HEV
Antibodies in blood	Anti-HAV	Anti-HBs, Anti-HBc, Anti-HBc	Anti-HCV	Anti-HDV	Anti-HEV
Chronic carrier state	No	Yes	Yes	Yes	No
Hepatic carcinoma	No	Yes	Yes	No	No

This antigen was named Australia antigen. It was subsequently established to be the surface component of hepatitis B virus (HBsAg). Electron microscopy of sera of hepatitis B patients shows three types of particles. The most abundant form is a spherical particle (22 nm in diameter) and the second type is tabular (22 nm in diameter) particle of varying length. These two types are antigenically identical and are the surface subunits of hepatitis B virus (HBsAg). The third double shelled spherical structure (42 nm in diameter). This particle is the complete hepatitis B virus and is called as **Dane particle.**

B. Antigenic Structure

- **HBsAg:** Surface antigens (envelope protein)
- **HBcAg:** It is the core (nucleocapsid) antigen of the virus. It is not detectable in patient's blood.
- **HBeAg:** It is the hidden antigenic component of core.
- **Viral genes and antigens:** The viral genome consists of two linear strands of DNA held in a circular configuration. Associated with one strand of DNA is a viral DNA polymerase.

C. Modes of Transmission

There are three important modes of transmission of HBV infection:
1. **Parenteral transmission:** Transmission of infection may result from accidental inoculation of minute amounts of blood, blood products or fluid containing HBV during medical, surgical or dental procedures.
2. **Perinatal transmission:** Transmission probably occurs when carrier mother's blood contaminates the mucous membranes of the newborn during birth.
3. **Sexual transmission:** HBV is present in body fluids such as semen and vaginal secretions, hence, it can be transmitted by sexual contact.

D. Clinical Features

Onset is slow, usually insidious but more severe. The incubation period varies from 6 weeks to 6 months. The course of acute HBV infection can be divided into three phases—preicteric, icteric and convalescent.

E. Hepatitis B Carriers

There are two types of hepatitis B carriers—super carriers and simple carriers.
1. **Super carriers:** They have HBeAg in blood and are highly infectious. Very minute amount of serum or blood can transmit the infection. These are called super carriers.
2. **Simple carriers:** They are more common type of carriers who have no HBeAg and a low level of HBsAg in blood. They transmit the infection only when large volumes of blood or serum are transferred, as in blood transfusion. These are named simple carriers.

F. Laboratory Diagnosis

Laboratory diagnosis of HBV infections can be carried out by detection of hepatitis B antigens and antibodies. These can be detected by sensitive and specific tests like ELISA and RIA.

Detection of Viral Markers

- **HBsAg:** HBsAg is recognized as a specific marker for HBV infection. It is the first marker to appear in blood after infection HBsAg disappears with recovery from clinical disease in most patients, however, it persists for years in carriers. Antibody to HBsAg appears within weeks after the disappearance of HBsAg and persists for very long periods. Anti-HBs are the protective antibody.
- **HBeAg:** Sera containing HBeAg are believed to be highly infectious and those with anti-HBe of little infectivity. The disappearance of HBeAg is followed by appearance of anti-HBe.
- **HBcAg:** It is not detectable in the serum but can be demonstrated in liver cells by immunofluorescence. Anti-HBc antibody usually appears in serum a week or two after the appearance of HBsAg. It remains lifelong and thus serves as a useful indicator of prior infection with HBV, even after all the other markers become undetectable.
- **Viral DNA polymerase:** It appears transiently in serum during pre-icteric phase.
- **Polymerase chain reaction (PCR):** HBV DNA level can be detected in serum by PCR. It is a highly sensitive test.

G. Prophylaxis

General Preventive Measures

These include health education, improvement of personal hygiene and strict attention to sterility. An important preventive measure is the screening for HBsAg and HBeAg in blood donors. Use of unsterile needles, syringes and other material must be avoided to prevent hepatitis B infection.

Immunization

- **Passive immunization:** Passive immunization may be employed following any accidental exposure to hepatitis B infection. Hepatitis B immunoglobulin (HBIG) is prepared from donors with high titres of anti-HBs. It can be given in doses of 300–500 IU intramuscularly.
- **Active immunization:** Following vaccines are available.
    - *Plasma derived vaccine:* Vaccine is prepared by purifying 22 nm particle of HBsAg from the plasma of healthy carriers. The particles are inactivated with formaldehyde. The vaccine is immunogenic and safe.
    - *Recombinant yeast hepatitis B vaccine:* It is produced plasmid by a recombinant DNA in yeasts in which a containing the gene of HBsAg has been incorporated. HBsAg particles produced are extracted and purified for use as vaccine. The vaccine is as immunogenic as plasma-derived vaccine. It is safe and free from side effects.
    Both vaccines are adsorbed with aluminum hydroxide as adjuvant, stored in cold but not frozen. Three doses at 0, 1 and 6 months are administered intramuscularly into deltoid muscle.

3. HEPATITIS C VIRUS (HCV)

Hepatitis C virus (HCV) belongs to the family Flaviviridae. It is a 50–60 nm virus with a linear single stranded RNA. It is transmitted by needle stick injuries, use of contaminated needles and syringes, transfusion of infected blood and blood products, and sexual intercourse. Maternal-neonatal transmission has also been reported. Clinical infection with hepatitis C is generally less severe with milder symptoms, absent or less marked jaundice.

Laboratory Diagnosis

It can be established by detection of anti-HC (antibody) by ELISA. Viral genome (HCV RNA) ca be detected by polymerase chain reaction (PCR) and by immunofluorescence.

Prophylaxis

Only general prophylaxis, such as blood or blood products screening, is possible.

4. HEPATITIS D VIRUS (HDV—DELTA ANTIGEN)

The HDV is a defective virus as it is dependent on the helper function of HBV for its replication and expression. It belongs to genus Deltavirus. It is spherical, 36–38 nm diameter, RNA particle surrounded by HBsAg envelope. The genome is a single stranded small circular molecule of RNA. It encodes its own nucleoprotein, the delta antigen or HDAg, but the outer envelope (HBsAg) of HDV is encoded by the genome of HBV coinfecting the same cell. HBV is necessary for the production of HDV virions.

Clinical Features

HDV infection can occur in presence of HBV under two situations:
1. Simultaneous infection with both HDV and HBV *(coinfection)*
2. Superinfection of an HBsAg carrier by HDV. Transmission occurs parenterally.

Laboratory Diagnosis

Diagnosis can be made by detecting the IgM anti-delta antibody in serum. ELISA and RIA kit are commercially available for detection of antibodies to HDV. HDAg (Delta antigen) is primarily expressed in liver cell nuclei, where it can be detected by immunofluorescence. It is occasionally present in serum.

Prophylaxis

No specific prophylaxis exists, but immunization with the hepatitis B vaccine is effective because delta antigen cannot infect person's immune to HBV. Screening of blood donors for HBsAg will also limit blood borne HDV infection.

5. HEPATITIS E VIRUS (HEV)

Hepatitis E virus belongs to family Hepevirida. They are spherical, non-enveloped and 27–38 nm in diameter. They possess single stranded RNA genome, which is surrounded by icosahedral capsid. It is primarily associated with ingestion of faecally contaminated drinking water. Clinically the disease resembles that of hepatitis A. The disease is generally mild and self limited.

Laboratory Diagnosis

- **Exclusion of hepatitis A and hepatitis B:** Hepatitis A can be excluded by IgM serology and hepatitis B by absence of HBsAg and anti HBc-IgM.
- **Immunoelectron microscopy:** Feces is examined by electron microscopy of aggregated hepevirus particles using monoclonal antibodies.
- **ELISA test and western blot assay:** These are used for detection of IgM and IgG antibodies.
- **Polymerase chain reaction (PCR):** HEV RNA can be detected in faeces or acute phase sera of patients by RT-PCR. It is gold standard test for diagnosis of acute HEV infection.
- **Prophylaxis:** Hepatitis E can be prevented by improved standards of sanitation and chlorinated water.

RETROVIRUSES

These are RNA viruses that belong to family Retroviridae. Members of this family possess reverse transcriptase (RNA directed DNA polymerase) enzyme which prepares a DNA copy of the RNA genome in host cell. The presence of enzyme reverse transcriptase is a characteristic feature.

HUMAN IMMUNODEFICIENCY VIRUS (HIV)

HIV occurs in two main types—HIV-1 and HIV-2.

A. Morphology

HIV is a spherical enveloped virus, about 90–120 nm in diameter. It contains two identical copies of single stranded RNA genome, in association with viral RNA is the reverse transcriptase enzyme. The virus core is surrounded by a nucleocapsid composed of protein. The virus contains a lipoprotein envelope. The major virus coded envelope glycoproteins are the projecting spikes on the surface and the anchoring transmembrane pedicles.

B. Modes of Transmission

There are three modes of transmission—sexual contact, parenteral and perinatal.
1. **Sexual contact:** This is the most important mode of transmission. Sexual transmission occurs among both homosexual as well as heterosexual individuals.
2. **Parenteral transmission:** It may occur through blood after receiving infected blood transfusions, blood products, sharing contaminated syringes and needles as in intravenous drug abusers or accidental inoculation.
3. **Perinatal transmission:** Infection may be transmitted from an infected mother to her child either transplacentally or perinatally.

C. Clinical Features

HIV infects all cells expressing at their surface the CD4 antigen, which is the receptor for the virus. It infects primarily the CD4+ lymphocytes. The clinical course of HIV infection can present as follows:
1. Acute HIV infection
2. Asymptomatic infection
3. Persistent generalized lymphadenopathy (PGL)
4. Symptomatic HIV infection

   When CD4+ cells fall below 200 per mm the titre of virus increases markedly and there is irreversible breakdown of immune defense mechanisms, it is defined as AIDS. Most of the patients with HIV disease die of infections other than HIV, e.g., opportunistic infections and malignancies as tabulated in **Table 3.13**. AIDS is the end stage of HIV infection. Acquired immunodeficiency syndrome (AIDS).

   By damaging your immune system, HIV interferes with your body's ability to fight infection and disease.

TABLE 3.13: Opportunistic infections and malignancies commonly associated with HIV infection.

I.	**Bacterial**
	Mycobacterial infections—tuberculosis and non-tuberculous infections
	M. avium complex
	Salmonellosis
II.	**Viral**
	CMV
	Herpes simplex
	Varicella-zoster
	Epstem-Barr (EB) virus
III.	**Mycotic**
	Pneumocystis jiroveci pneumonia
	Candidiasis
	Cryptococcosis
	Aspergillosis
	Histoplasmosis
	Coccidioidomycosis
IV.	**Parasitic**
	Toxoplasmosis
	Cryptosporidiosis
	Isosporiasis
	Generalized strongylodiasis
V.	**Malignancies**
	Kaposi's sarcoma
	B-cell lymphoma or non-Hodgkin's lymphoma

D. Laboratory Diagnosis

Specific Tests for HIV Infections

1. **Antigen detection:** The p24 antigen is the earliest virus marker to appear be a in the blood ELISA can be used for detection of this antigen. Virus isolation is an important test for diagnosis in window period when antibodies are absent in serum of patient.
2. **Virus isolation:** For diagnosis, virus is not routinely isolated. It can be isolated from CD4 lymphocytes of peripheral blood, bone-marrow and serum. Virus isolation is an important test for diagnosis in window period when antibodies are absent in serum of patient.
3. **Detection of viral nucleic acid:** Viral nucleic acid can be detected by polymerase chain reaction (PCR). The test is highly sensitive and specific. It is also useful for diagnosis in window period.
4. **Antibody detection:** Demonstration of antibodies is the simplest and most commonly employed technique for diagnosis. It may take several weeks to months for antibodies to appear after infection. HIV infected persons remain negative for antibodies during window period, when initial viral replication takes place for about 2–3 weeks.

There are two types of serological tests—screening and supplemental.
1. **Screening tests:**
   – *ELISA test:* ELISA is the method most commonly used. It is highly sensitive and specific test. It is an extremely good screening test and most laboratories use a commercial ELISA kit that contains both HIV-1 and HIV-2.
   – Saliva is an acceptable alternative to serum for antibody testing by ELISA.
   – *Rapid tests:* These tests take less than 30 minutes and do not require expensive equipment. The rapid tests include dot-blot assay, particle agglutination, HIV spot and comb tests.
   – *Simple tests:* They take 1–2 hours and do not require expensive equipment.

– *Supplemental test:*
  - Western blot test: In this test, HIV proteins are separated and these proteins are blotted on to strips of nitrocellulose paper. These strips are reacted with test sera. Antibodies to HIV proteins, if present in test serum, combine with different fragments of HIV. The position of the color band on the strip indicates the fragment of antigen with which antibodies have reacted.
  - A positive result in any one screening test may not be accepted without confirmation. As the test is cumbersome, costly and not readily available, different strategies are followed for confirmation. The practice now is to perform either two different types of ELISA or an ELISA with any of the rapid tests. A serum positive in both tests is considered positive.
2. **Non-specific tests:**
   – *Total and differential leukocyte count:* In AIDS, there is leukopenia with a lymphocyte count less than 400 per mm^3.
   – *T-lymphocyte subset assays:* The normal CD4: CD8 T-cell ratio of 2: 1, is reversed to 0.5:1 in cases of AIDS. The count of CD4 lymphocytes falls below 200 per mm^3.

E. Prevention

The following preventive measures are recommended.
- **Sexual contact:** The use of condoms can prevent transmission of the virus.
- **Sharing needles:** Contaminated syringes or needles should not be shared.
- **Blood:** All blood and blood products are to be screened for HIV. This also applies to donation of cornea, semen, marrow, kidney and other organs.
- Isolation of AIDS patient and initiation of treatment.
- **Control of infection:** Screening of individuals within risk groups helps to identify the HIV infected persons.

F. Prophylaxis

No effective vaccine has yet been found out.

G. Antiretroviral Therapy (ART)

Specific treatment with antiretroviral drugs is the mainstay in the management of HIV infection. Highly active antiretroviral therapy (HAART) is effective in inhibition of HIV replication in most of the HIV-infected individuals but major drawback with this therapy is the selection of resistant mutants. Antiretroviral drugs include both nucleoside and non-nucleoside inhibitors of enzyme reverse transcriptase, viral pretease inhibitors, fusion inhibitor, integrase inhibitor and entry inhibitor **(Table 13.14)**. These drugs have been used as monotherapy or in various combinations. Adverse reactions and high cost restrict their wide use in developing countries.

H. Postexposure Prophylaxis (PEP)

Exposure to blood, body fluid, other potentially infected material or an instrument contaminated with one of these materials may lead to risk of acquiring HIV infection. The risk of infection varies with the type of exposure and other factors. Most exposures do not result in infection. Following exposure, postexposure prophylaxis (PEP) may be required depending up or the category of exposure and HIV status of exposure source. Zidovudine 300 mg BD and Lamivudine 150 mg BD are used in combination for a period of 4 weeks. In selected cases, Indinavir 800 mg TDS is added to this combination of drugs according to PEP guidelines. To be effective these drugs must be started within the first 72 hours and ideally within 2 hours. Both risk of infection and possible side-effects of antiretroviral drugs should be carefully considered when deciding to start PEP.

TABLE 13.14: Antiretroviral drugs.

Nucleoside reverse transcriptase inhibitors (NRTIs)	Non-nucleoside reverse transcripase inhibitors (NNRTIs)	Protease inhibitors	Fusion inhibitos	Integrase inhibitor	Entery inhibitor (CCR5-co-recetor antagonist)
Zidovudine (AZT, azidothymidine)	Nevirapine (NVP) Delaviridine (DLV)	Saquinavir (SQT) Ritonavir (RTV)	Enfuvirtide (T20)	Raltegravir (RAL)	Maraviroc (MVC)
Didanosine (ddI)	Efavirnez (EFV)	Indinavir (IDV)			
Zalcitabine (ddc)	Etravirine (ETR)	Nelfinavir (NFV)			
Stavudine (d4T)		Lopinavir (LPV)			
Lamivudine (d4T)		Amprenavir			
Abacavir (ABC)		Tipranavir (TPV)			
Tenofovir		Atazanavir (ATV)			
Emitricitabine (FTC)		Fosamprenavir (FPV)			

Chapter 3: Pathogenic Organisms

MEDICAL MYCOLOGY

Study of fungus is called Mycology. All fungi are eukaryotic. Water, soil and decaying organic debris are natural habitat. Fungi are obligate aerobes.

Fungal Diseases

A. Superficial mycoses
B. Subcutaneous mycoses
C. Systemic mycoses
D. Opportunistic mycoses

A. Superficial Mycoses

Further divided into surface infections (*Tinea versicolor* and *Tinea nigra*) and cutaneous infections (dermatophytes).

Dermatophytes

Dermatophytes are group of fungi that infect only superficial keratinized tissue (skin, hair, nails) without involving the living tissue.
- They break down and utilize keratin
- They are incapable of penetrating subcutaneous tissue
- They cause dermatophytoses also called as ringworm infection.

Classification of dermatophytes:
Trichophyton: Hair, skin, nails
Microsporum: Hair, skin
Epidermophyton: Skin, nails

	Features	Trichophyton	Microsporum	Epidermophyton
Macroconidia	Shape	Clavate or cigar shaped	Fusiform or spindle shaped	Club shaped
	Size	(8–50 µm × 4–8 µm)	(7–20 × 35–125 µm, up to 160 µm long)	(6–10 × 8–15 µm)
	Nature of wall	Smooth walled	Thick walled	Thin walled
	Septation	0–4 septate	5–15 septate	Less than 5 septate
Microconidia	Shape	Spherical or clavate	Clavate	Absent
	Size	(2.5–4 µm) (2–3 × 3–4 µm)	(2.5–3.5 × 4–7 µm)	—
Part of the body infected		Ringworm of scalp, body, beard and nails, Athlete's foot	Ringworm of scalp and skin	Ringworm of groin and nails
Principal targets Transmission		Hair, skin, nails Human to human, animal to human	Scalp hair, skin Animal to human, soil to human, human to human	Skin, nails Strictly human to human

B. Subcutaneous Mycoses

- **Mycetoma:**
  - It is a chronic granulomatous infection of the subcutaneous tissue, usually infecting the foot and rarely the other parts of the body
  - The disease was first described in Madurai, South India, so referred as Madura foot or Maduramycosis.
  - It is caused by a number of actinomycetes and filamentous fungi.
  - Causative agent enters the body, thus the disease begins as subcutaneous swelling of foot, which enlarges and burrows into the deeper tissues producing characteristic abscess. Abscess bursts with the formation of chronic multiple sinuses discharging viscid, seropurulent fluid containing granules.
  - Diagnosis is made by examination of granules
  - Actinomycotic mycetoma responds to sulfonamides and antibiotics.
- **Sporotrichosis:**
  - Sporotrichosis is a nodular, ulcerating disease of skin and subcutaneous tissue
  - Fungus gains access through thorn pricks or some injuries

- Causative agent—*Sporothrix schenkii*
- *S. schenkii* occurs in yeast phase in the tissues and in cultures at 37°C, in mycelial phase in 22–25°C.
- Yeast phase appears as cigar shaped cells and mould forms contain hyphae carrying flower like clusters of small conidia borne on delicate sterigmata.

- **Rhinosporidiosis:**
    - It is a chronic granulomatous disease characterized by formation of friable polyps, usually confined to nose, mouth and eye.
    - Causative agent—*Rhinosporidium seeberi*
    - Mode of infection is frequent contact with stagnant water or aquatic life
    - Diagnosis is made on basis of Sporangia. On H&E stain—shows large number of endospores with the sporangia embedded in a stroma of connective tissue and capillaries. Each sporangium (10–200 µm) contains thousands of endospores (6–7 µm in diameter).

C. Systemic Mycoses

- **Histoplasmosis:**
    - Causative agent is *Histoplasma capsulatum*. It is an intercellular parasite.
    - Primarily the disease of reticuloendothelial system.
    - Fungus is mainly present in soil enriched with the excreta of birds or bats
    - Human infection is by inhalation of spores
    - Disseminate histoplasmosis develops in minority of infected individuals.
    - Granulomatous and ulcerative lesions may develop on skin or mucosa.
    - Microscopically-appears as small oval yeast cell (2–4 µm in diameter), packed within the cytoplasm of macrophages and monocytes. Yeast phase is formed in culture at 37°C. White cottony mycelial growth containing large (8–20 µm) thick walled, spherical spores with tubercles or finger like projections appear at 25°C.
- **Blastomycosis:**
    - *Causative agent: Blastomyces dermatitidis*, a dimorphic fungus
    - It is a chronic infection of lungs which may spread to tissues, particularly skin, bone and genitourinary tract.
    - *Microscopically:* In tissues and cultures at 37°C, fungus appears as spherical or oval budding yeast cells with thick, double contoured walls. Each cell has only a single broad based bud. At 25°C the culture is filamentous with septate hyphae and many round or oval conidia.
    - Inhalation of conidia of fungus growing as saprophytes in the soil.
    - Disseminated lesions are found in immunocompromised patients including AIDS cutaneous blastomycosis.
- **Paracoccidioidomycosis:**
    - *Causative agent: Paracoccidioides brasiliensis*, a dimorphic fungus.
    - Infected by inhalation of spores from environmental sources
    - Primary pulmonary infection that spreads by hematogenous route to mucous membranes of mouth, nose, lymph node, skin producing granulomatous lesions. Ulcerative granulomas of buccal and nasal mucosa are prominent feature.
    - *Microscopically:* Grows as yeast cells with multiple buds at 37°C and mycelia at 25°C.

D. Opportunistic Mycoses

- **Candidiasis:**
    - *Causative agent: Candida albicans.*
    - It is an infection of skin, mucosa and internal organs caused by yeast like fungus *Candida albicans*, normally an inhabitant of skin, GIT, oral and vaginal cavities.
    - *Morphology:* Ovoid, spherical budding yeast cells 3–5 µm in diameter.
    - Its is an opportunistic fungus. Predisposing factors are diabetes, immunodeficiency, malignancy, prolonged administration of antibiotics, patients on immunosuppressive drugs and intravenous catheters.
    - Lesions caused are mucocutaneous lesions, such as oral thrush, vulvovaginitis, balanitis, conjunctivitis, keratitis
    - *Skin and nail infections:* Infections of axillae, groin, perineum, infection of finger webs, nail folds and nails.
    - *Systemic candidiasis:* UTI, intestinal candidiasis, pulmonary candidiasis, endocarditis, meningitis, septicemia.
    - *Microscopically on KOH mount* (**Fig. 3.20A**)*:* Budding yeast cells with pseudohyphae are seen. On SDA—creamy, pasty colonies appear. Germ tube test can also be done to differentiate *C. albicans* from non-albicans *Candida* (**Fig. 3.20B**).

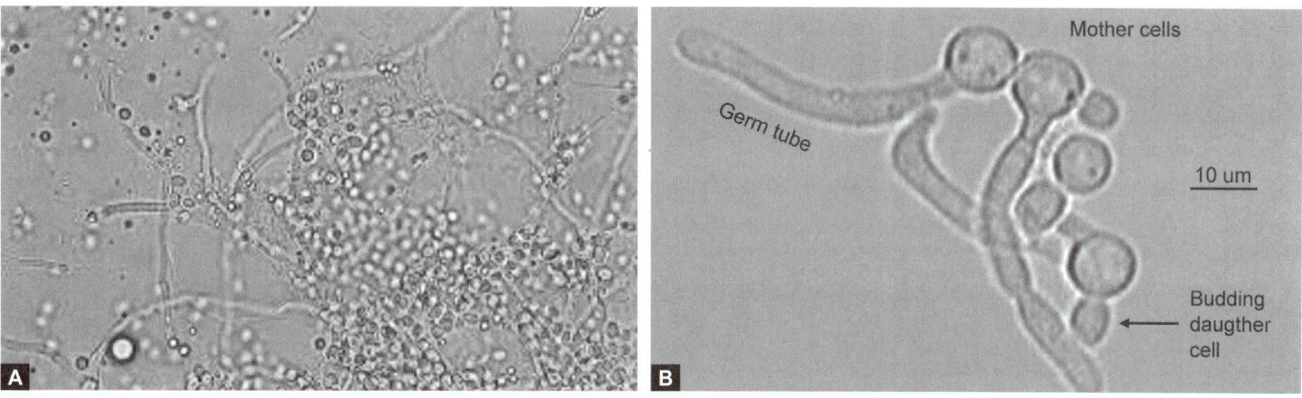

Figs. 3.20A and B: KOH mount: (A) Oval budding yeast cells; (B) Germ tube test.

- ***Cryptococcus:***
    - *Causative agent is:* Cryptococcus neoformans.
    - It is a soil saprophyte and is particularly abundant in feces of pigeons. Source of infection is usually acquired by inhalation of dust containing yeast cells.
    - It is pathogenic and is mainly seen in immunocompromised host. Pulmonary cryptococcosis leads to mild pneumonitis.
    - Cryptococcal meningitis occurs by hematogenous spread.
    - *Specimens to be collected are:* CSF, sputum, pus, brain tissue
    - On India ink **(Figs. 3.21A and B)***:* Capsule appears as clear halo around the yeast cells.
    - *On SDA:* Smooth, mucoid, cream colored colonies and LPCB mount shows round budding yeast cells are seen.

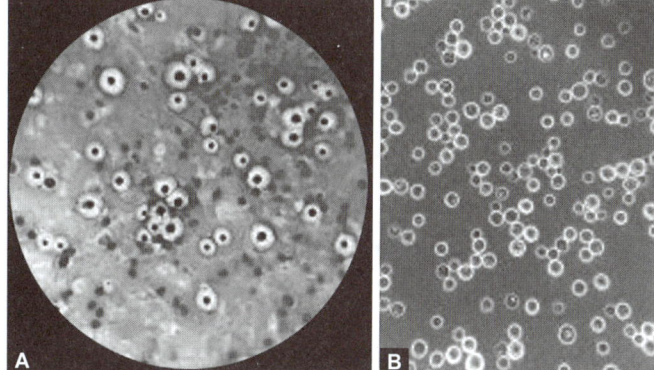

Figs. 3.21A and B: (A) Round yeast cells India ink; (B) Capsule of *Cryptococcus.* (For color version, see Plate 5)

    - Latex agglutination test for cryptococcal capsular polysaccharide antigen can be detected in CSF, serum or urine.
- **Aspergillosis:**
    - Caused by *Aspergillus fumigatus*. Other important species are *A. flavus* and *A. niger*
    - Mainly caused by inhalation of *Aspergillus* conidia or mycelia fragments which are present on the decaying matter, soil or air.
    - Three clinical forms generally occur as:
        1. Respiratory disease—*Aspergillus* asthma, bronchopulmonary aspergillosis, aspergilloma
        2. Invasive aspergillosis
        3. Superficial infections, such as mycotic keratitis and otomycosis.
    - *Microscopically:* On KOH mount—thin septate hyphae are seen with characteristic dichotomous branching (at acute angle of 45°C).
    - *On SDA:* Colonies appear as **(Figs. 3.22A to C)**:
        - *A. fumigatus*—green colored
        - *A. flavus*—golden yellow colored
        - *A. niger*—black colored
    - On LPCB mount-branching thin septate hyphae. Asexual conidia are arranged in chains, with sterigmata on the expanded ends of conidiophores

ZYGOMYCETES

Zygomycetes are a group of fungi whose members generally produce nonseptate or aseptate or rarely septate hyphae which branch irregularly and have irregular diameter. Mucormycosis is a general term for infections caused by a group of filamentous fungi belonging to the class *Glomeromycetes*, which because of recent taxonomic reclassification has replaced the former class name *Zygomycetes*. Some zygomycetes have vegetative hyphae in form of stolons. It is divided into three parts—*Mucor, Rhizopus* and *Absidia*. Mucorales characteristically produce large, ribbon-like aseptate hyphae with irregular diameter hence, their frequent characterization in tissue as aseptate fungi.

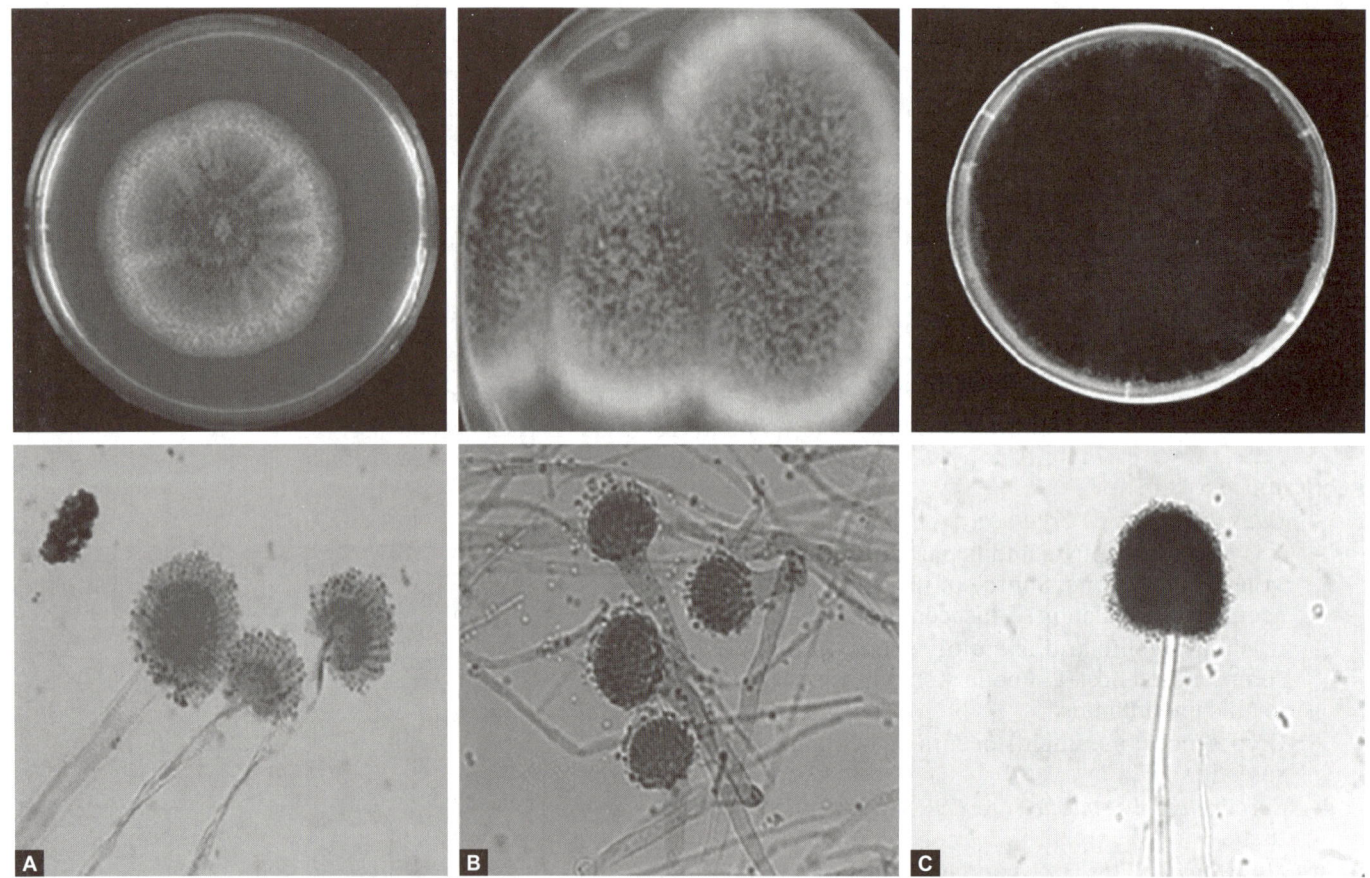

Figs. 3.22A to C: (A) *A. flavus*; (B) *A. fumigatus*; (C) *A. niger*. (For color version, see Plate 5)

Mucor

- On SDA-colonies are fast growing color varying from brownish gray to blackish.
- Microscopy on LPCB mount, sporangiospores are of two types—elongated sporangiosphore comprising of 20–50 sporangia, columella spherical to ellippsoidal. Sporangiospores (4–7 um) smooth walled, ellipsoidal.

Rhizopus

- On SDA-colonies are rapidly growing, woollt, tall colonies, whitish to gray brown.
- Microscopy on LPCB mount—hyaline stolon slightly brown at the nodes where rhizoids and sporangiospores are produced. Sporangiospores are in tufts, unbranched with sporangia which are spherical, brownish gray to black, columella 50–70% of sporangium.

Absidia

- On SDA—colonies are floccose, light olive gray colony, mycelium profusely branched with stolons and rhizoids.
- Microscopy on LPCB mount—sporangiospores are solitary or in groups branch repeatedly to form corymbs. Sporangia are pyriform to spherical, columella is hemispherical to ovoid having 1–2 nipple like projections and a long conical apophysis.

MEDICAL PARASITOLOGY

- Medical parasitology deals with parasites which infect and produce disease in humans.
- Classification of medically important parasites are:

Group	Examples
Parasites	
Amoebae	Entamoeba histolytica E. gingivalis
Flagellates	Giardia lamblia Trichomonas vaginalis Leishmania species
Sporozoa	Plasmodium falciparum Plasmodium vivax Toxoplasma
Ciliates	Balantidium coli
Helminths	
Trematodes	Fasciola species Schistosoma species
Cestodes	Taenia spp. Echinococcus species
Nematodes	Roundworm Hookworm Threadworm

Stool Examination (Fig. 3.23)

Procedure

- A drop of normal saline is placed on the center of a clean slide.
- About 2 mg of the given sample of stool is emulsified in the saline.
- A cover slip is then placed on the emulsion avoiding air bubbles.
- After reducing the light by lowering the condenser and using the concave mirror, the preparations first screened under low power.
- When a cyst or an ovum is seen the details are observed by focusing under high power.
- If cysts are seen, another preparation is made by emulsifying about 3 mg of stool sample in Lugol's Iodine. This helps to stain the nuclei.

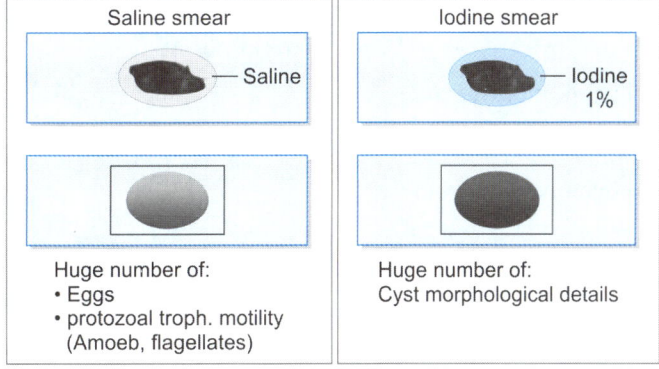

Fig. 3.23: Stool examination.

Advantages of Iodine

- Lugol's iodine stain is intended to be used with wet mount preparations and concentration techniques for the detection of intestinal protozoa.
- Lugol's iodine is a rapid, non-specific contrast dye that is added to direct wet mounts of fecal material to aid in differentiating parasitic cysts from host white blood cells.

- Iodine stains protozoan nuclei and intracytoplasmic organelles as brown, making them easier to identify. It paralyzes the motility of organisms and may hinder some parasitic structures.

- ***Entamoeba histolytica:***
  - Quadrinucleate cyst, measures 18–40 μm in size
  - Surrounded by thick chitinous wall. 1–4 chromatoid bars are present.
  - Cysts are present in lumen of colon and formed feces.
  - Causes intestinal amoebiasis and extraintestinal amoebiasis
  - *Laboratory diagnosis:*
    - Stool examination: Normal saline preparation is useful for demonstration of actively motile trophozoites. Charcot-Leyden crystals may appear in saline preparation.
    - Stool ELISA to detect antigens of *E. histolytica* in feces
    - Indirect hemagglutination test and ELISA to detect later stages of invasive intestinal amoebiasis
    - DNA probes and PCR can be done

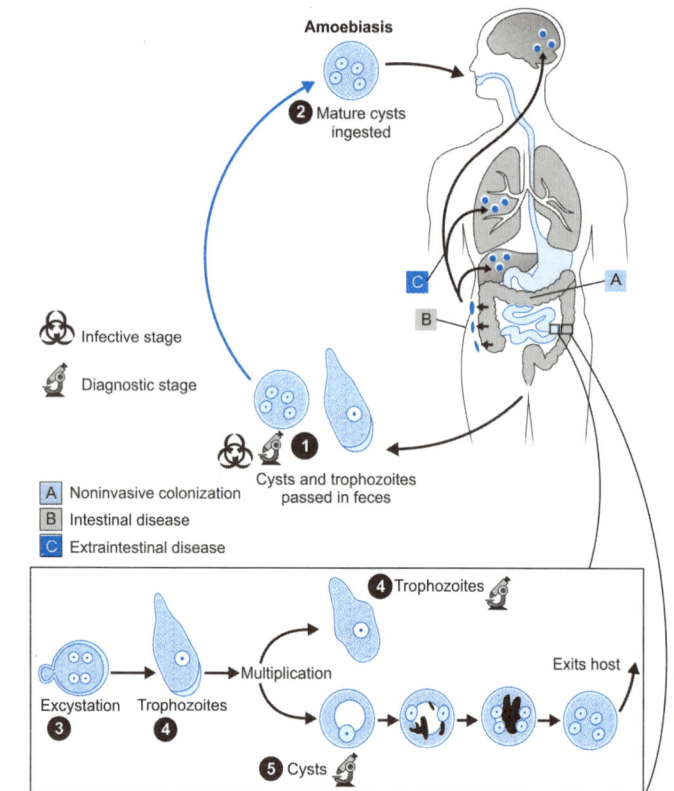

- ***Giardia lamblia:***
  - Lives in duodenum and upper jejunum
  - Cysts are oval ellipsoidal in shape with thick cyst wall
  - Bilaterally symmetrical with two axostyles placed diagonally
  - Two pairs of nuclei are also present
  - Demonstration by Entero-test.
  - Patient may complain of persistent loose stools and mild steatorrhea
  - *Laboratory diagnosis:*
    - On microscopy: Demonstration of *Giardia trophozoites* and cysts in freshly passed stool by saline and iodine mount.
    - Trophozoites can also be demonstrated from bile fluid

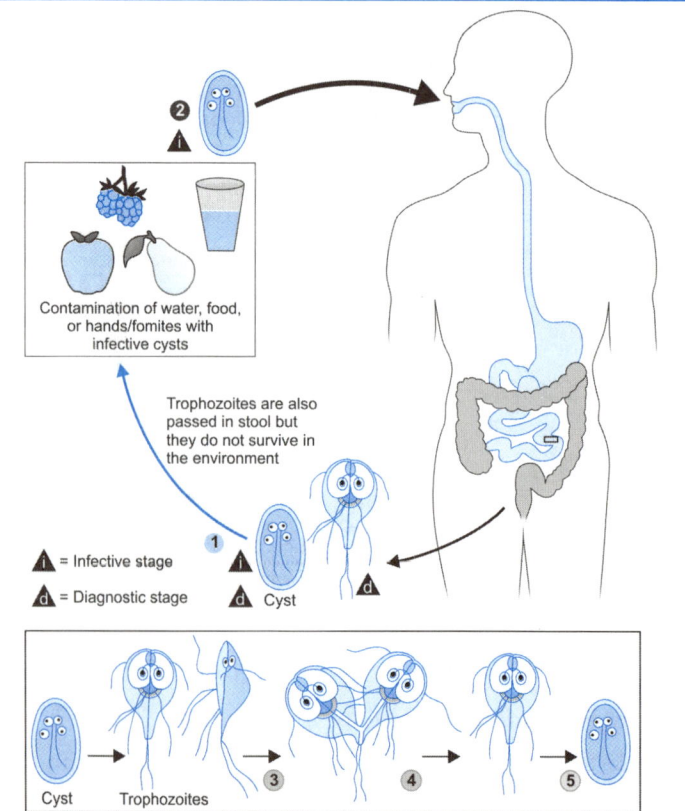

- **Beef-containing Cysticercus bovis (Taenia saginata):**
  – Large, 5–10 meters in length
  – Scolex is rhomboidal
  – 2 mm in diameter
  – Four suckers are present, pigmented
  – Lacks rostellum and hooklets
  – Bile-stained ova seen.
  – Stool examination on wet mount shows eggs can be seen.
  – Naked eye examination of stool shoes segments of *Taenia* spp. Head and the gravid segment are helpful in species identification
  – *Diagnosis of cysticercosis:*
    ♦ Biopsy examination of subcutaneous nodules for cysticerci
    ♦ Eosinophilia
    ♦ CT scan of brain show lesions

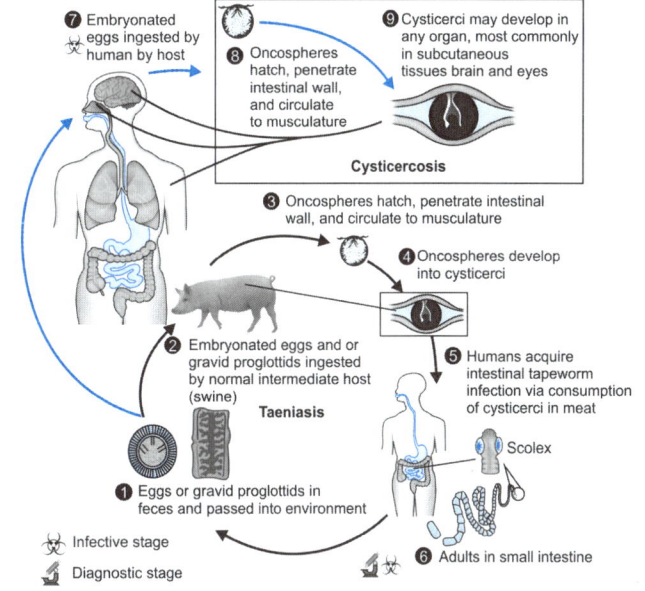

- **Pork-containing Cysticercus cellulosae (Taenia solium):**
  – Small, 2–3 meters in length, globular
  – Possess rostellum and hooklets
  – Suckers are not pigmented
  – *Cysticercus cellulosae:* Larval stage of *T. solium* developing in the muscles of intermediate host, i.e., pig.
  – A mature cyst is an ellipsoidal body and the long axis of the cyst is parallel to muscle fiber.
  – This cyst develops further when ingested by man, its definitive host.

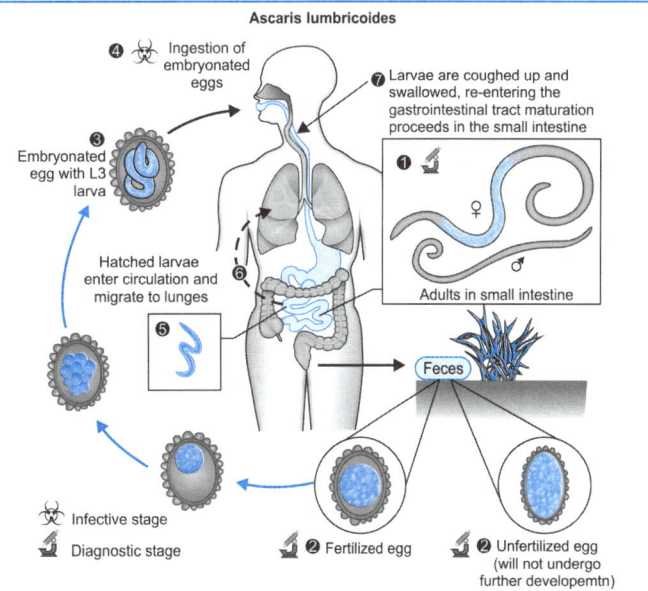

- **Ascaris lumbricoides:**
  – Infection of *Ascaris lumbricoides* is due to migrating larva or adult worms. Presence of larva in the lung may lead to pneumonia.
  – *Laboratory diagnosis:*
    ♦ On stool microscopy—adult worm or eggs can be demonstrated.
    ♦ Barium meal—demonstrate the presence of adult worn in small intestine
    ♦ Antibodies of A. lumbricoides can be demonstrated. It is useful for extraintestinal ascariasis
    ♦ Round to oval in shape, 60–75 µm in size
    ♦ Bile stained
    ♦ Surrounded by thick, transparent shell, consisting of vitelline membrane
    ♦ Outermost layer is coarsely, regular, albuminoid.

- **Unfertilized egg of *Ascaris lumbricoides*:**
  - Narrower and longer, 90 × 55 µm in size
  - Bile stained
  - Egg contains small atrophied ovum with thin shell within an irregular coating of albumin
  - Heaviest of helminthic egg, do not float in saturated solution of common salt.

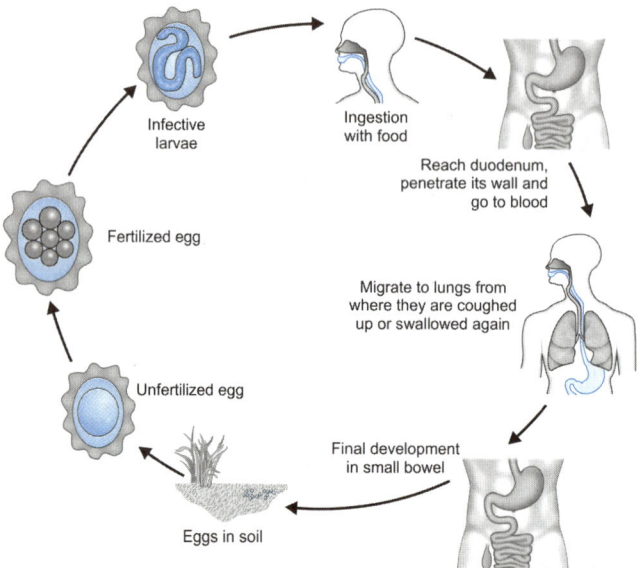

- ***Ancylostoma duodenale:***
  - *Infective:* Filariform larva
  - *Portal of entry:* Skin
  - *Cutaneous larva migrans:* Filariform larva wander about the skin and produce a reddish itchy papule along the path traversed by them.
  - *Lesions in the lungs:* Bronchitis and brochopneumonia occurs
  - *Laboratory diagnosis:*
    - On direct microscopy of stool—egg of *A. duodenale*
    - Duodenal contents may reveal eggs or adult worms.
    - Blood examination reveals microcytic, hypochromic anemia and eosinophilia
    - Eggs are oval and elliptical, 60 × 40 µm in size
    - Non-bile stained
    - Possess a segmented ovum with four blastomeres
    - Clear space between the segmented ovum and egg shell.

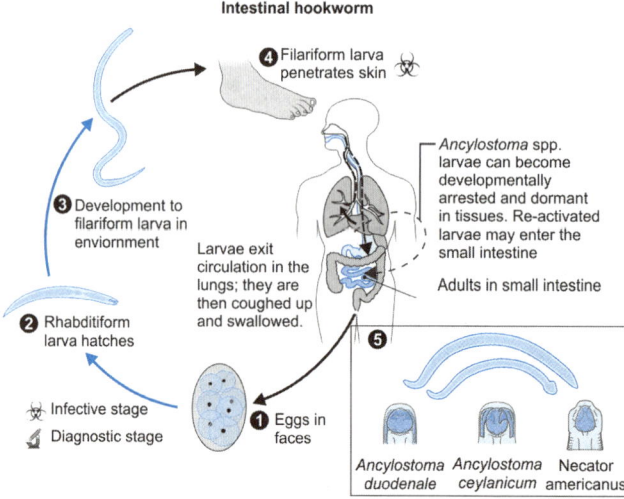

- ***Enterobius vermicularis*:**
    - *E. vermicularis* can cause pruritus ani and an eczematous condition around the anus and perineum
    - Laboratory diagnosis:
        - Eggs of *Enterobius vermicularis* are demonstrated in the scrapings from perianal swab by a National Institute of Health (NIH) swab.
        - Non-bile stained
        - Embryonated egg is the infective stage
        - Egg shell is thin, hyaline, transparent, encloses larva.

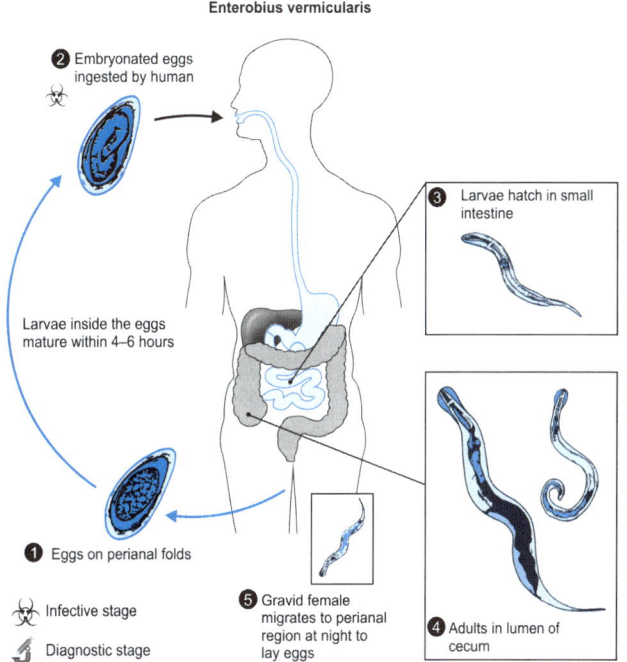

- **Trypanosomes:**
    - Morphological forms—trypomastigote and amastigote
    - Trypomastigote is infective form found in peripheral blood, C-shaped 20 μm in size
    - Kinetoplast is situated in the posterior end
    - Stained by Giemsa and Wright stains
    - Undulating membrane is present.

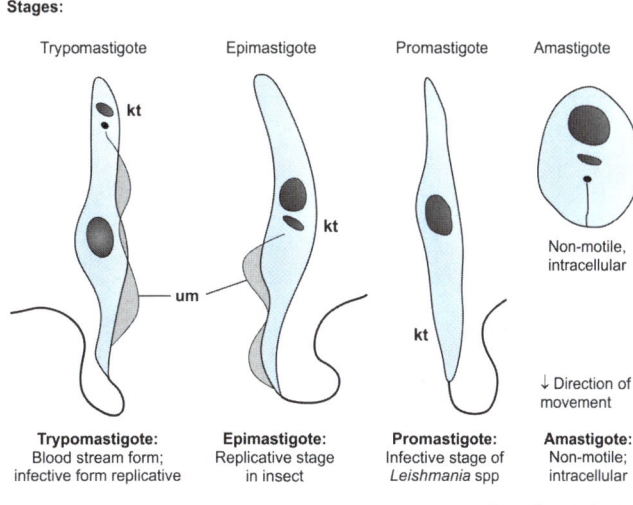

- ***Leishmania donovani:***
  - *Morphological forms:* LD bodies and promastigotes
  - *Promastigote:* Cells are elongated, posterior end is pointed
  - Long flagellum projects from posterior end
  - *Amastigote form:* Resides in reticuloendothelial system, is oval body measuring 2–4 µm in size. Can be stained by Wright and Giemsa stain.

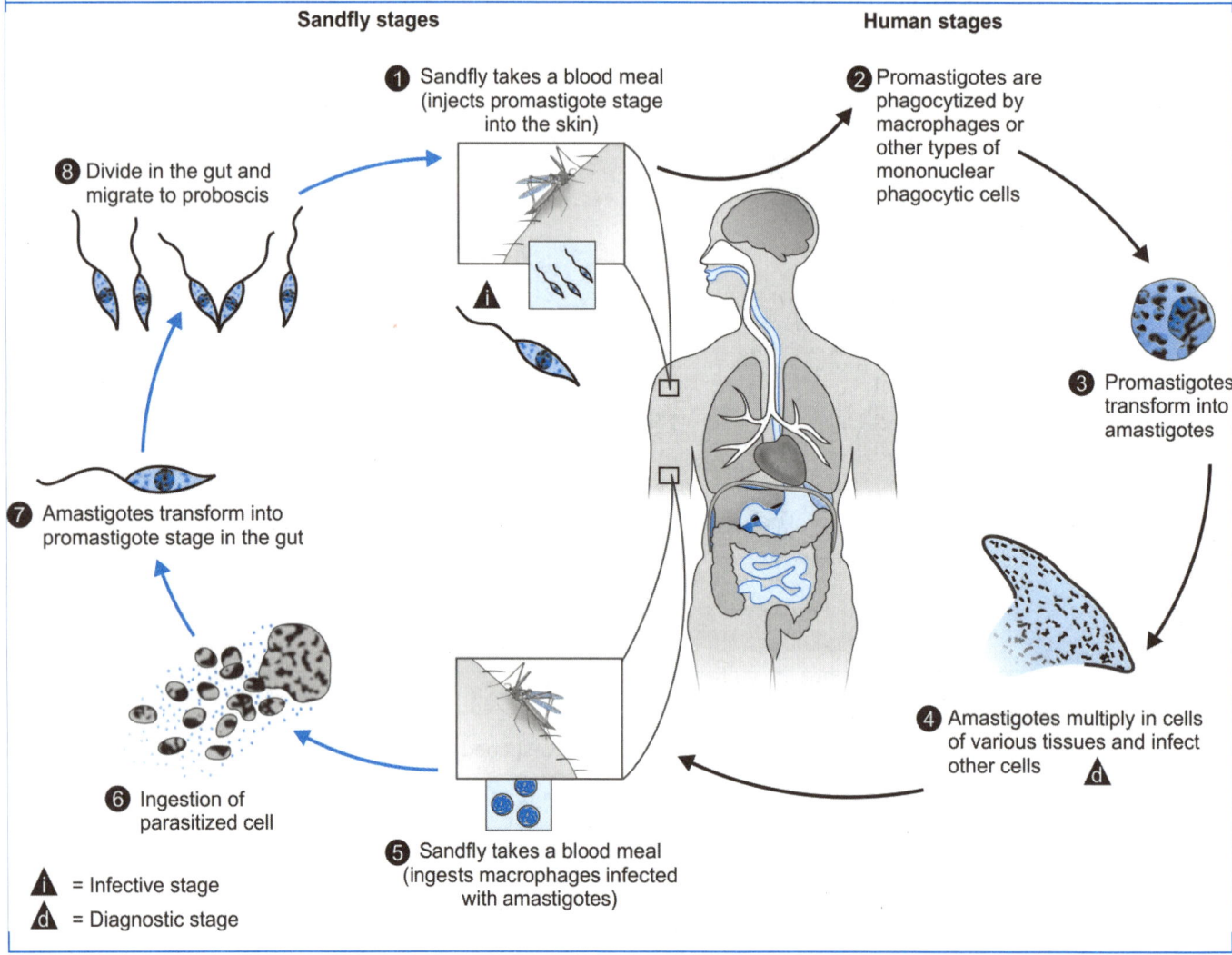

CAUSATIVE ORGANISM FOR MALARIA—*PLASMODIUM FALCIPARUM*

Different stains used are: Giemsa, Leishman, Romanowsky, Wright's and Jaswant Singh Bhattacharya stain
- **Thick smear:** For Identification of malaria
- **Thin smear:** For species identification.
- **Occurrence of multiple rings with accole formation:** Diagnostic of *P. falciparum*.

Malarial Smear

See **Figures 3.24 and 3.25**.

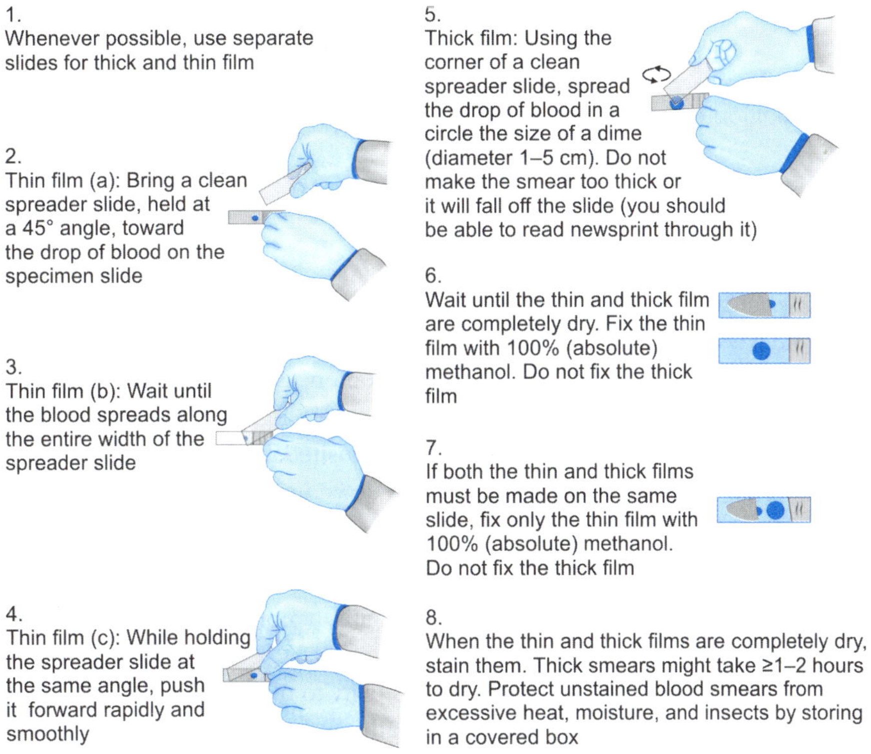

1. Whenever possible, use separate slides for thick and thin film

2. Thin film (a): Bring a clean spreader slide, held at a 45° angle, toward the drop of blood on the specimen slide

3. Thin film (b): Wait until the blood spreads along the entire width of the spreader slide

4. Thin film (c): While holding the spreader slide at the same angle, push it forward rapidly and smoothly

5. Thick film: Using the corner of a clean spreader slide, spread the drop of blood in a circle the size of a dime (diameter 1–5 cm). Do not make the smear too thick or it will fall off the slide (you should be able to read newsprint through it)

6. Wait until the thin and thick film are completely dry. Fix the thin film with 100% (absolute) methanol. Do not fix the thick film

7. If both the thin and thick films must be made on the same slide, fix only the thin film with 100% (absolute) methanol. Do not fix the thick film

8. When the thin and thick films are completely dry, stain them. Thick smears might take ≥1–2 hours to dry. Protect unstained blood smears from excessive heat, moisture, and insects by storing in a covered box

Fig. 3.24: Steps of malarial smear.

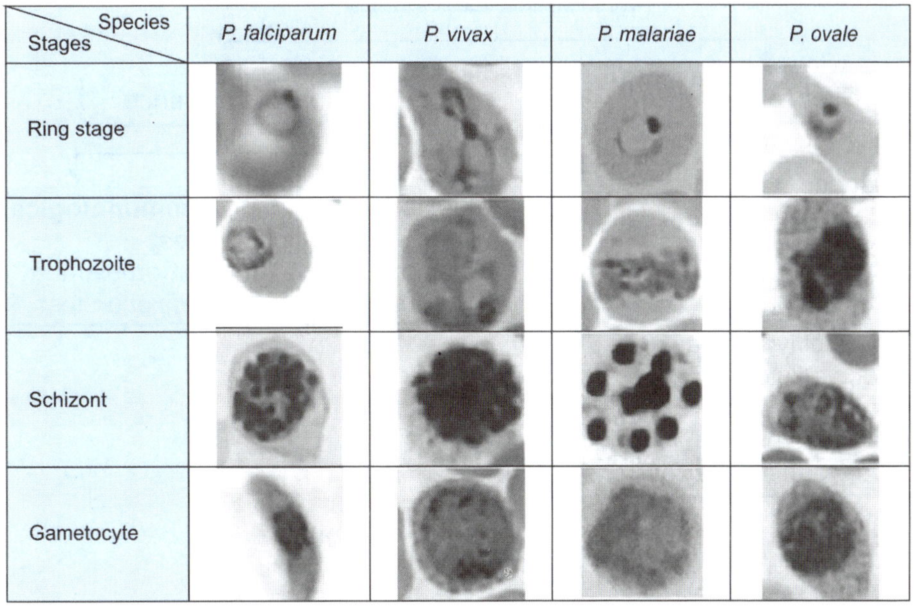

Stages \ Species	P. falciparum	P. vivax	P. malariae	P. ovale
Ring stage				
Trophozoite				
Schizont				
Gametocyte				

Fig. 3.25: Draw malarial smear. *(For color version, see Plate 6)*

Quantitative Buffy Coat

Acridine orange (AO) binds deoxyribonucleic acids and ribonucleic acids. The malaria parasite binds acridine orange in the nucleus and the cytoplasm and emits green and red fluorescence when excited at 480 nm allowing the detection and examination of parasite morphology by fluorescent microscopy.

Rapid diagnostic tests: RDTs for detection of antigen. Antigens targeted by RDTs are:
- Histidine rich protein-II (HRP-II)
- Parasite lactate dehydrogenase (pLDH)
- Aldolase.

Complications

Anemia, hemoglobinuria, hemoglobinemia, black water fever, acute renal failure, tropical splenomegaly, cerebral malaria, hypoglycemia.

FILARIA

Causative agent for filariasis: *Wuchereria bancrofti*

Wuchereria bancrofti is mainly confined to tropics. In India it is distributed along the sea coasts and also along the banks of big rivers. Wuchereria bancrofti passes its life cycle in two hosts i.e. Man (definitive host) and mosquito (intermediate host). Adult worms are harboured in lymphatic system of man. After fertilization, Microfilariae (embryos) are discharged by gravid female and reach the blood stream. Microfilariae undergo further development in mosquito and become infective for man. When the infected mosquito bites a human being, the larvae are deposited on the skin near the site of puncture. Infective larvae penetrate the skin and reach lymphatic channels and settle down usually in inguinal, scrotal and abdominal lymph nodes, where they develop into adult worms.

Wuchereria bancrofti mainly causes Filariasis, which is of two types:
1. **Classical filariasis (caused by adult worm):** Leads to lymphangitis, lymphadenitis, lymphoedema with hypertrophy of affected part (elephantiasis), lymphangiovarix, hydrocele and chyluria
2. **Occult filariasis (caused by embryos):** It is due to hypersensitivity to microfilarial antigens. Patient develops massive eosinophilia, hepatosplenomegaly, generalized lymphadenopathy and pulmonary symptoms, microfilariae

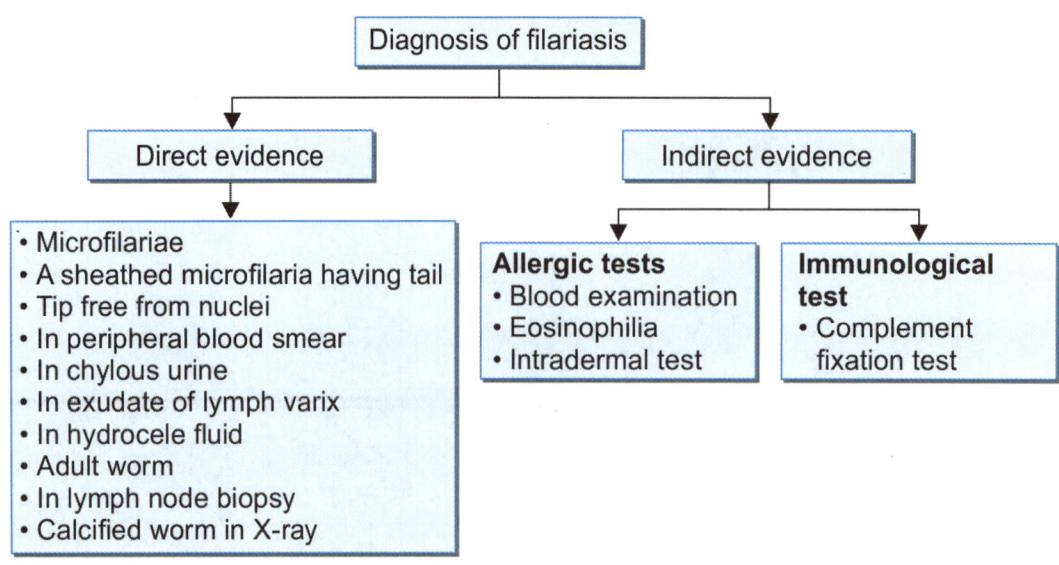

Mention the Infective Forms of the Following Protozoans (Table 3.15)

TABLE 3.15: Infective forms of the following protozoans.

Protozoan	Infective forms
Entamoeba histolytica	Tetranucleate cyst
Naegleria fowleri	Trophozoite
Acanthamoeba nigricans	Trophozoite and cyst
Giardia lamblia	Cyst
Trichomonas vaginalis	Trophozoite
Leishmania	Promastigote
Balantidium coli	Cyst
Plasmodium	Sporozoite
Toxoplasma gondii	Oocyst
Cryptosporidium	Oocyst and tissue cyst

Mention the Infective Forms of the Following Helminths (Table 3.16)

TABLE 3.16: Infective forms of the following helminths.

Helminth	Infective form
Taenia	Cysticercus bovis (T. saginata) and Cysticercus cellulosae (T. solium)
Diphyllobothrium latum	Plerocercoid larvae
Echinococcus granulosus	Egg
Hymenolepis nana	Egg
Fasciola	Metacercaria larva
Paragonimus westermani	Metacercaria larva
Schistosoma	Cercaria larva
Ascaris lumbricoides	Egg
Ancylostoma duodenale	Filariform larva
Trichinella spiralis	Encysted larva
Strongyloides stercoralis	Filariform larva
Trichuris trichiura	Egg
Enterobius vermicularis	Egg
Filarial worms	3rd stage larva
Dracunculus medinensis	3rd stage larva

CHAPTER 4

Immunity

Chapter Outline

- Immunity Definition and Types, Classification
- Antigen and Antibody Reactions
- Serological Tests
- Hypersensitivity Reactions
- Structure of Immunoglobulins: Types and Properties
- Vaccines: Types and Properties, Classification
- Immunization Schedule

Immunity is defined as the resistance offered by the body against any foreign agent including microorganisms. The immune system is evolved as a defense against infectious diseases. An immune response consists of five parts:

1. Recognition of material recognized as foreign and dangerous.
2. An early innate (non-specific) response to this recognition.
3. A slower specific response to a particular antigen, known as adaptive responses.
4. Non-specific augmentation of this response.
5. Memory of specific immune responses, providing a quicker and larger response when that particular antigen is encountered the second time **(Flowchart 4.1)**.

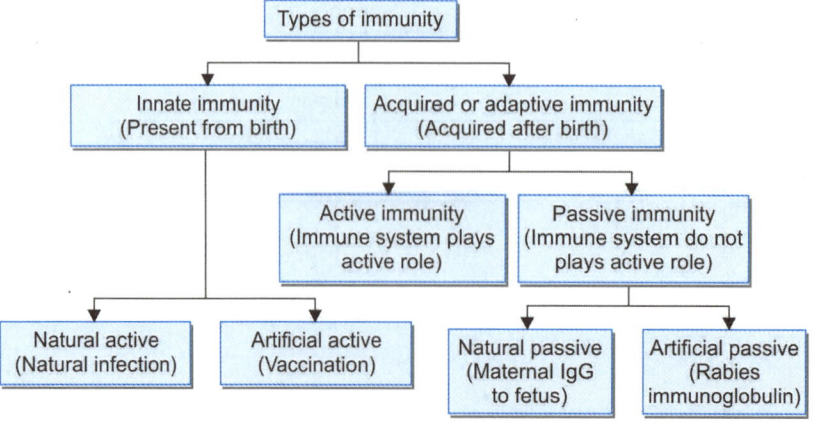

Flowchart 4.1: Classification of immunity.

Chapter 4: Immunity

TYPES OF IMMUNITY

Innate Immunity (Table 4.1)

Innate immunity represents the first line of defense to an intruding pathogen. It is also known as inborn immunity or resistance against infection which a person is having from birth.

Properties of Innate Immunity

- It is the first line of defense of body and acts in minutes.
- It is an antigen-independent (non-specific) defense mechanism that is used by the host immediately or within hours of encountering an antigen.
- The innate immune response has no immunologic memory, therefore, it is unable to recognize or "memorize" the same pathogen should the body be exposed to it in the future.
- It is non-specific. It cannot fight with all infections, i.e., its diversity is limited.

Mechanisms of Innate Immunity

Epithelial Surfaces

Skin: It not only acts as a mechanical barrier to microorganisms but also provides bactericidal secretions. The high concentration of salt in drying sweat, the sebaceous secretions and long chain fatty acids contribute to bactericidal activity.
Respiratory secretions: The inhaled particles are arrested in the nasal passages on the moist mucous membrane surfaces. The mucous secretions of respiratory tract act as a trapping mechanism and hair like cilia propels the particles towards the pharynx where it is swallowed or coughed out. The cough reflex is important defense mechanism.
Intestinal tract: The mouth possesses saliva which has an inhibitory effect on many microorganisms. Some bacteria may be swallowed and are destroyed by acidic pH of gastric juices.
Conjunctiva: Tears have a major role by flushing away bacteria and other dust particles. In addition, lysozyme present in tears has a bactericidal effect.
Genitourinary tract: The flushing action of urine eliminates bacteria from the urethra. The acidic pH of vaginal secretions in female, due to fermentation of glycogen of *Lactobacillus* (normal flora), renders vagina free of many pathogens.

Antibacterial Surfaces

There are number of non-specific antibacterial substances present in blood and tissues. These substances are properdin, complement, and lysozyme.

Cellular Factors

When the infective agent crosses the barrier of epithelial surfaces, tissue factors come into play for defense. When an infective agent invades tissue, an exudative inflammatory reaction occurs by accumulation of phagocytes at the site of infection.

Acquired or Adaptive Immunity (Table 4.2)

It is defined as a resistance that an individual acquired by an individual during life against any foreign substance (microbes, etc.).

TABLE 4.1: Types of innate immunity.

Types of innate immunity based on genetic makeup		
Species specific	**Racial specific**	**Individual immunity**
This is a type of innate immunity at species level in which all the members of species are immune against a particular pathogen, e.g., *Bacillus anthrax* infects humans but not chickens	This is a type of innate immunity present in a particular race against a particular pathogen, e.g., Negroes of America are susceptible to tuberculosis then whites	This is a type of innate immunity present confined to a particular person
Factors determining the degree of innate immunity: • Age • Hormone disorder • Sex		

TABLE 4.2: Difference between innate and acquired immunity.

Innate immunity	Acquired immunity
It is the resistance towards infection that a person possesses by birth	It is the resistance towards infection that a person possesses after birth during his life time
Immune response occurs in minutes	Immune response occurs in days
Prior exposure with microbe (or antigen) is not required	Prior exposure with microbe (or antigen) is required as it develops after antigenic exposure
Diversity is limited, it acts via restricted set of reactions	Diversity is wide; it acts via more varied and specialized responses
Immunological memory response is absent	Immunological memory response is present
It is not specific	It is specific
Host cell receptors are non-specific, e.g., Toll-like receptors	Host cell receptors are specific, e.g., T cell receptors and B cell receptors
Components	
Anatomical barrier, such as skin and mucosa	T cells B cells Classical complement pathway Cytokines: IL-2, IL-4, IL-5 and INF-α
Physiological barrier, such as temperature, low pH	
Phagocytes (neutrophils, monocytes and macrophages)	
Natural killer cells	
Mast cells, macrophages and dendritic cells	
Complement pathways (alternate and mannose binding pathway)	
Fever and inflammatory responses	
Normal resident flora	
Acute phase reactant proteins (APRs)	
Cytokines: IL-1, IL-6, IL-8, IL-12, IL-16, IL-18 and INF-α, IFN-α, β, TGF-β	

The primary functions of the adaptive immune response are: The recognition of specific "non-self" antigens, distinguishing them from "self" antigens; the generation of pathogen-specific immunologic effector pathways that eliminate-specific pathogens or pathogen-infected cells; and the development of an immunologic memory that can quickly eliminate a specific pathogen resulting in infections.

Properties of Acquired Immunity

- It is mainly mediated by T and B cells.
- Response occurs on days as it requires activation of T and B cells following microbial entry which takes many days.
- Prior microbial exposure is required.
- It is highly specific. Memory component is present, a portion of T and B cells become memory cells after contact with microbe.

Types of Acquired Immunity

A. Active Immunity

Further divided into two types:
1. **Natural:** Through clinical or subclinical infection
2. **Artificial:** Induced by vaccination

Mechanism: Active immune response stimulates both humoral and cell mediated immunity.

- **Humoral immunity:** Antibody mediated—it depends on the synthesis of antibodies by plasma cells. These cells produce specific circulating antibody which combines specifically with the antigens and modify their activity.
- **Cell mediated immunity (CMI):** It depends on T-lymphocytes developed against certain antigens. The cell mediated immunity by sensitized T-lymphocytes is important in resistance to chronic bacterial infections.

Chapter 4: Immunity

Types of active immunity:
- *Natural active immunity:* It is acquired by natural subclinical or clinical infections.
- *Artificial active immunity:* It is produced by vaccination. Vaccines are prepared from live, attenuated or killed microorganisms, antigens or toxoids.

B. Passive Immunity

Subdivided into two types:
1. **Natural:** Through transplacentally maternal IgG antibodies—transferred from mother to fetus or infant. Transfer of maternal antibodies to fetus transplacentally and to infant through milk (colostrum) protects them till their own immune system matures to function.
2. **Artificial:** Induced by antiserum injection. It is through parenteral administration of antibodies. The agents used for artificial passive immunity are hyperimmune sera of animal or human origin, convalescent sera and pooled human gamma globulin.

Uses of passive immunization:
- To provide immediate short-term protection in a nonimmune host, faced with the threat of a serious infection.
- For suspension of active immunity which may be injurious. Example is to use Rh immunoglobulin during delivery to prevent immune response to Rh factor in Rh negative mother with Rh positive babies.
- For treatment of serious infections.

Herd Immunity

It refers to the overall resistance in a community. When herd immunity is low, chances of epidemics increase on introduction of a suitable pathogen. Eradication of any communicable disease depends on development of high level of herd immunity rather than of immunity in individual.

ANTIGEN-ANTIBODY REACTIONS

Antigen

An antigen is a substance which when introduced into a body evokes immune response to produce a specific antibody with which it reacts in an observable manner.

Types of Antigen

Complete antigen: These are substances which can induce antibody formation by themselves and can react specifically with antibodies.

Haptens: These are substances which are unable to induce antibody formation on its own but can become immunogenic (capable of inducing antibodies) when covalently linked to proteins called carrier proteins. Epitope is a smallest unit of antigenicity.

Factors of antigenicity are:
- Foreignness
- Size
- Chemical nature
- Species specificity
- Isospecificity
- Autospecificity
- Organ specificity
- Heterophile specificity

Antibody (Immunoglobulins)

Antibodies are substances which are formed in the serum and tissue fluids in response to an antigen and react with that antigen specifically and in some observable manner. Chemical nature of antibodies is globulin and they are named as immunoglobulins. They are mainly synthesized by plasma cells.

Immunoglobulins can be divided into five different classes, based on differences in the amino acid sequences in the constant region of the heavy chains. All immunoglobulins within a given class will have very similar heavy chain constant regions.
1. **IgG:** Gamma heavy chains
2. **IgM:** Mu heavy chains
3. **IgA:** Alpha heavy chains
4. **IgD:** Delta heavy chains
5. **IgE:** Epsilon heavy chains

STRUCTURE AND SOME PROPERTIES OF IMMUNOGLOBULIN CLASSES AND SUBCLASSES

A. Immunoglobulin G (IgG) (Fig. 4.1)

Structure

- IgG is the most versatile immunoglobulin because it is capable of carrying out all of the functions of immunoglobulin molecules.
- IgG is the major Ig in serum—75% of serum IgG.
- IgG is the major Ig in extravascular spaces.
- **Placental transfer:** IgG is the only class of Ig that crosses the placenta. Transfer is mediated by a receptor on placental cells for the Fc region of IgG. Not all subclasses cross equally well; IgG2 does not cross well.
- **Fixes complement:** Not all subclasses fix equally well binding to cells—macrophages, monocytes, PMNs and some lymphocytes have Fc receptors for the Fc region of IgG.

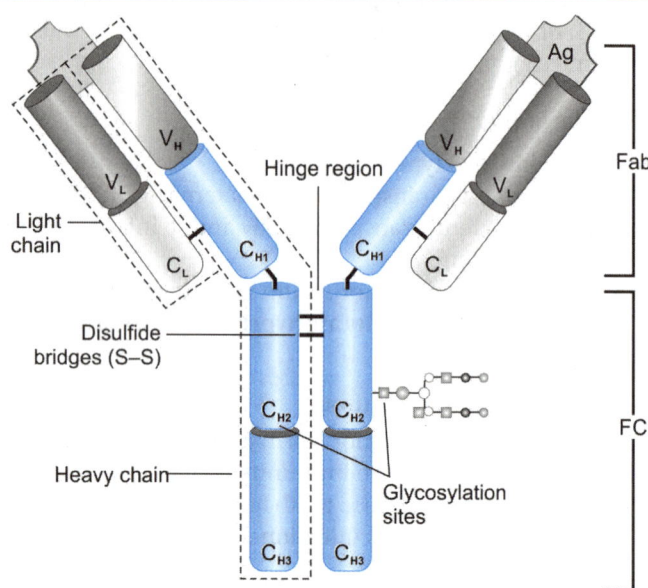

Fig. 4.1: Diagrammatic representation of IgG molecule.

B. Immunoglobulin M (IgM) (Fig. 4.2)

Structure

- The structure of IgM is a pentamer consisting of 5 immunoglobulin subunits and one molecule of J chain, which joins the Fc region of basic subunit. In the pentameric form, all heavy chains are identical and all light chains are identical.
- IgM is the third most common serum Ig.
- IgM is the first Ig to be made by the fetus and the first Ig to be made by B cells when it is stimulated by antigen.
- As a consequence of its pentameric structure, IgM is a good complement fixing Ig. Thus, IgM antibodies are very efficient in leading to the lysis of microorganisms.
- IgM binds to some cells via Fc receptors.

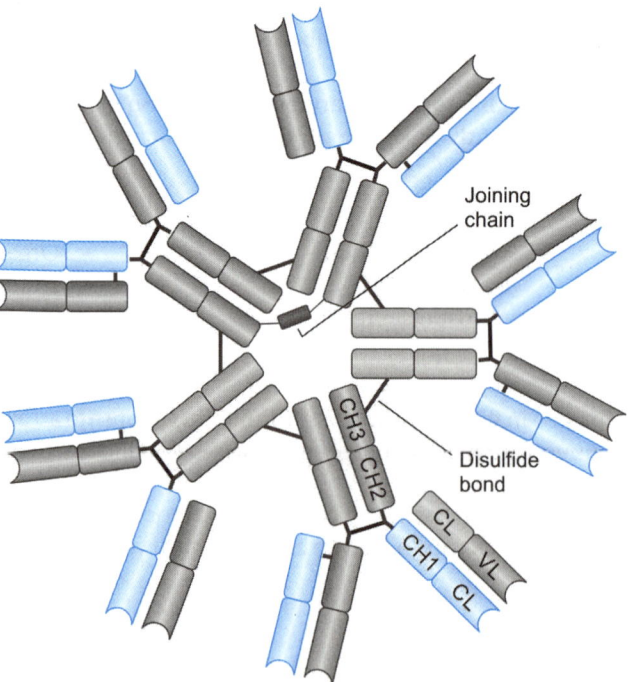

Fig. 4.2: Diagrammatic representation of IgM molecule.

C. Immunoglobulin A (IgA) (Fig. 4.3)

Structure

- IgA is found in secretions, it also has another protein associated with it called the secretory piece or T piece.
- IgA is the 2nd most common serum Ig.
- IgA is the major class of Ig in secretions—tears, saliva, colostrum, mucus. Since, it is found in secretions secretory IgA is important in local (mucosal) immunity.
- Normally, IgA does not fix complement, unless aggregated. IgA can binding to some cells—PMN's and some lymphocytes.

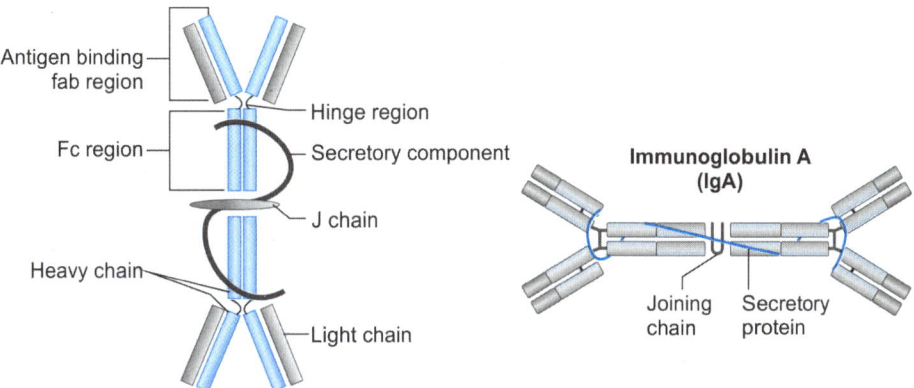

Fig. 4.3: Diagrammatic representation of IgA molecule.

D. Immunoglobulin D (IgD)

Structure

- IgD exists only as a monomer. Resembles IgD structurally.
- IgD is found in low levels in serum; its role in serum is uncertain.
- IgD is primarily found on B cell surfaces where it functions as a receptor for antigen. IgD on the surface of B cells has extra amino acids at C-terminal end for anchoring to the membrane.
- It also associates with the Ig-alpha and Ig-beta chains.

E. Immunoglobulin E (IgE) (Fig. 4.4)

Structure

- IgE exists as a monomer and has an extra domain in the constant region. Mainly produces in the linings of respiratory and intestinal tracts.
- IgE is the least common serum Ig since it binds very tightly to Fc receptors on basophils and mast cells even before interacting with antigen.
- Involved in allergic reactions—as a consequence of its binding to basophils an mast cells, IgE is involved in allergic reactions. Binding of the allergen to the IgE on the cells results in the release of various chemical mediators that result in allergic symptoms.
- IgE also plays a role in parasitic helminth diseases. Since serum IgE levels rise in parasitic diseases, measuring IgE levels is helpful in diagnosing parasitic infections. Eosinophils have Fc receptors for IgE and binding of eosinophils to IgE-coated helminths results in killing of the parasite.
- IgE does not fix complement.

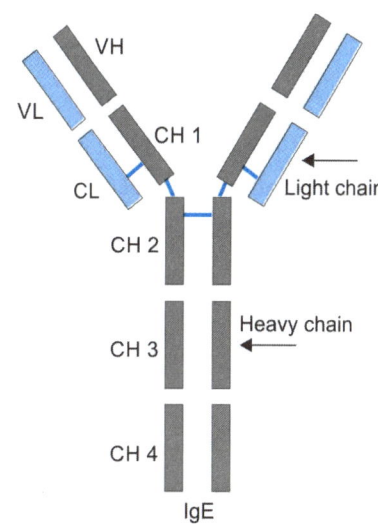

Fig. 4.4: Diagrammatic representation of IgE molecule.

ANTIGEN-ANTIBODY REACTIONS

Antigen combines with its specific antibody in an observable manner and the reaction between antigen and antibody is specific.

Characteristics of antigen-antibody reactions are:
- Reaction is specific, an antigen combines only with its homologous antibody and vice-versa. However, cross-reactions may occur due to antigenic similarity.
- Entire molecules of antigen and antibody can react and not the fragments.
- Reaction is firm, but reversible.

Types of Antigen–Antibody Reactions

Conventional Techniques
- Precipitation reaction
- Agglutination reaction
- Complement fixation test
- Neutralization test

Newer Techniques (Labeled Assays)
- Enzyme-linked immunosorbent assay (ELISA)
- Immunofluorescence assay (IFA)
- Radioimmunoassay (RIA)
- Chemiluminescence-linked immunoassay (CLIA)
- **Rapid test:** Cassette ELISA, lateral flow test (Immunochromatographic test), flow through assay.

A. Precipitation Reactions

Definition

When a soluble antigen reacts with its specific antibody in the presence electrolyte at optimal temperature and pH, it leads to formation of antigen-antibody complex in the form of insoluble precipitate band when gel containing medium is used or insoluble floccules or precipitate ring when liquid medium is used.

- **Precipitation in liquid medium:**
    - *Ring test:* Ascoli's Thermoprecipitation test, streptococcal grouping by Lancefield's technique
    - *Slide test:* Flocculation test—VDRL test for syphilis
    - *Tube test:* Kahn's test for syphilis
- **Precipitation in gel (immunodiffusion):**
    - Single diffusion in one dimension (Oudin procedure)
    - Double diffusion in one dimension (Oakley Fulthrope procedure)
    - Single diffusion in two dimensions (Radial immunodiffusion)
    - Double diffusion in two dimensions (Ouchterlony procedure)
- Immunoelectrophoresis
- **Electroimmunodiffusion:**
    - Countercurrent immunoelectrophoresis (CIEP)
    - Rocket electrophoresis

B. Agglutination Reactions

Definition

When a particulate or insoluble antigen is mixed with its specific antibody in the presence of electrolytes at a suitable temperature and pH, particles are clumped or agglutinated.

- **Direct agglutination test:**
  - *Slide agglutination test:* For blood grouping and cross matching
  - *Tube agglutination test:* Widal test for enteric fever
  - *Heterophile agglutination test:* Weil felix for typhus fever, Paul Bunnell test for infectious mononucleosis
  - *Microscopic agglutination:* For leptospirosis
- **Passive agglutination test (for antibody detection):** A precipitation reaction can be converted into agglutination test by attaching soluble antigens to the surface of carrier, such as latex particles, bentonite and red blood cells.
  - *Latex agglutination test (LAT)* **(Fig. 4.5)**: For detection of ASO (antistreptolysin antibody), CRP, RA
  - Indirect hemagglutination test

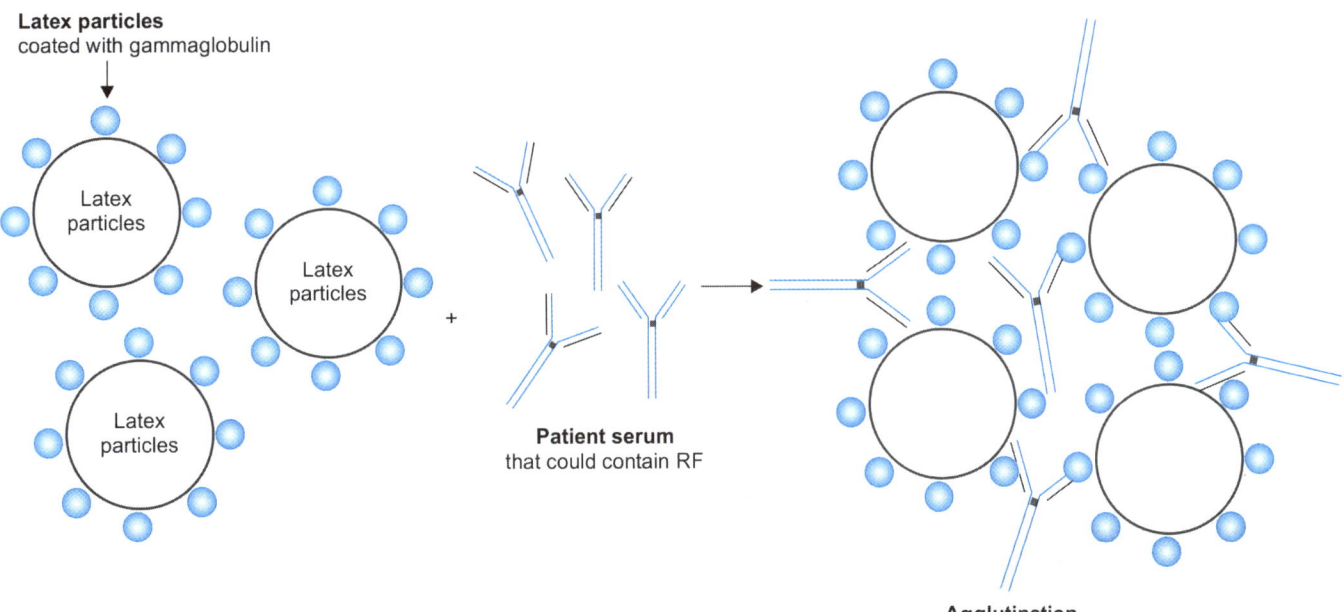

Fig. 4.5: Latex agglutination test.

- **Reverse passive agglutination reaction:** When instead of antigen, antibody is absorbed on the carrier particles for estimation of antigens.
  - *Coagglutination test: Staphylococcus aureus* (protein A) acts as a carrier molecule. Specific antibody binds with Fc portion and Fab site remain free. Such sensitized cells are used for detection of antigen. For example, *Salmonella typhi* antigen in serum
  - For detection of hepatitis B surface antigen (HBsAg)

PRINCIPLE AND APPLICATIONS OF COOMBS TEST

It is performed to diagnose Rh incompatibility by detecting Rh antibody from mother's and baby's serum. It is used to test for autoimmune hemolytic anemia.

A. Direct Coombs Test

Direct Coombs test (also known as the direct antiglobulin test or DAT) is used to detect if antibodies have bound to RBC surface antigens **in vivo**. A blood sample is taken, and the RBCs are washed and then incubated with antihuman globulin. If this produces agglutination of RBCs, the direct Coombs test is positive, e.g., erythroblastosis fetalis.

B. Indirect Coombs Test

Indirect Coombs test (also known as the indirect antiglobulin test or IAT) is used to detect in vitro antibody-antigen reactions. It is used to detect very low concentrations of antibodies present in a patient's plasma/serum prior to a blood transfusion. In antenatal care, this test is used to screen pregnant women for antibodies that may cause hemolytic disease of the newborn. The IAT can also be used for compatibility testing, antibody identification **(Fig. 4.6)**.

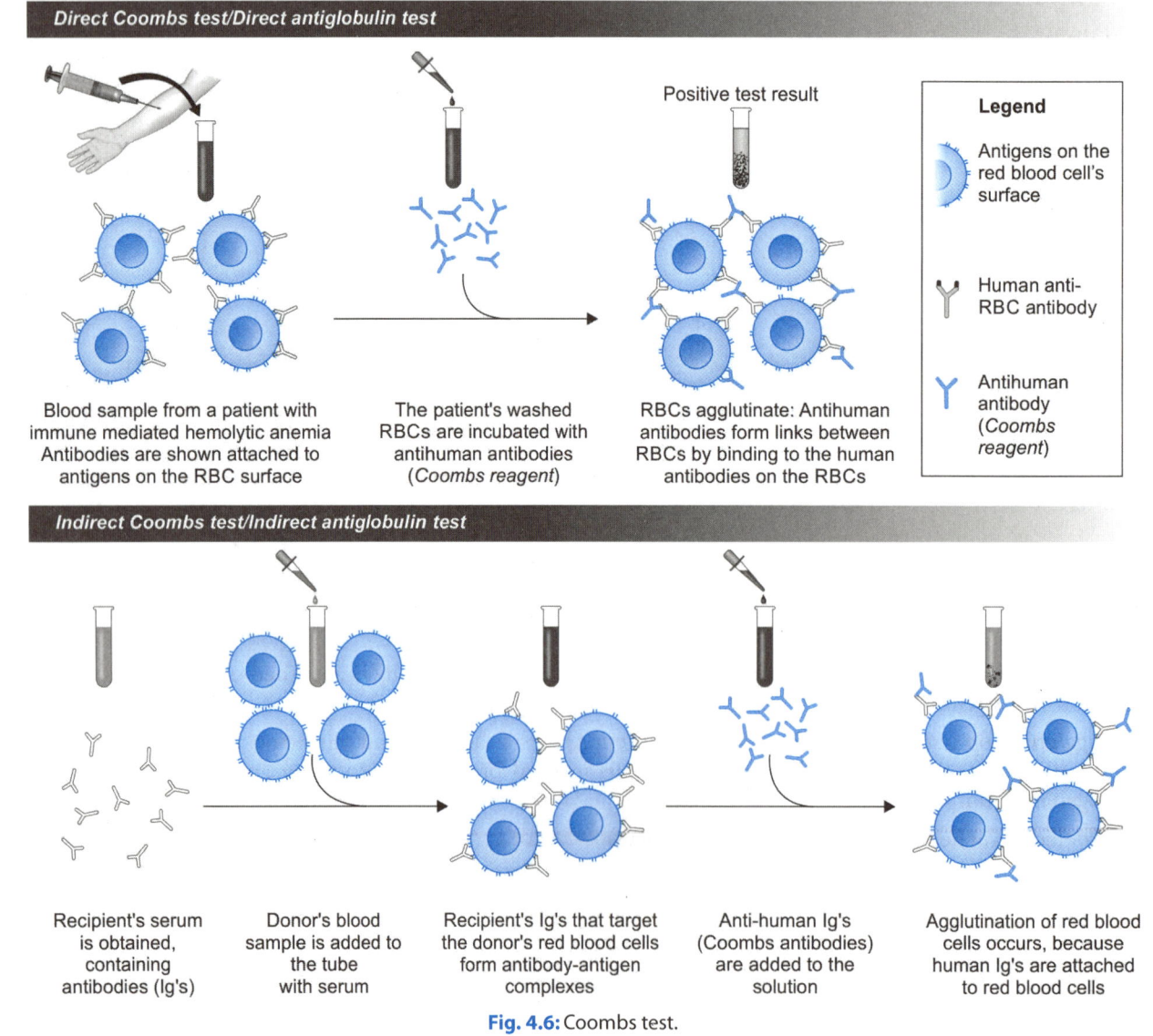

Fig. 4.6: Coombs test.

C. Complement Fixation Test (Fig. 4.7)

Principle
It is a two-way step. When antigen and antibodies are mixed, complement is fixed to the antigen-antibody complex. It can be detected by adding ambo receptors (Sheep RBCs coated with anti-sheep RBC antibody).

First Step
Antigen (soluble or particulate) + test serum + guinea pig complement are all added together.
- **If the test serum is positive for antibody** → Ag-Ab complex is formed. Complement gets fixed to the complex, so there will be no free complements in the serum.
- **If the test serum is negative for antibody** → there is no Ag-Ab complex. Complements are not fixed, hence remain free in the serum.

Second Step
A hemolysis indicator system is added. It consists of sheep RBCs coated with its antibodies called ambo receptors.
- If the test serum is positive for antibody → no free complement in serum for binding to ambo receptors → No hemolysis.
- If the test serum is negative for antibody → free complement attached to ambo receptors bound on sheep RBCs → Hemolysis.

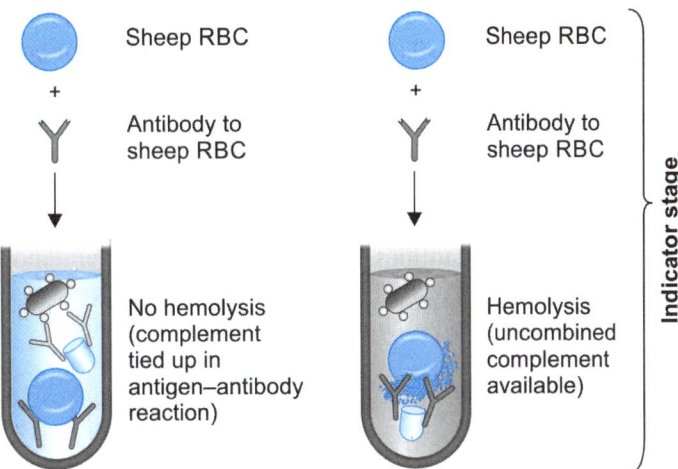

Fig. 4.7: Complement fixation test.

D. Immunofluorescence

Principle
Fluorescence refers to absorbing high energy-shorter wavelength ultraviolet light rays by the fluorescent compounds and in turn emitting visible light rays with a low energy-longer wavelength. Commonly used fluorescent dyes are fluorescein isothiocyanate, rhodamine.

Types of Immunofluorescence Tests are (Fig. 4.8)
- **Direct immunofluorescence test:** Specific antibodies tagged with fluorescent dye are used for detection of unknown antigen. If antigen is present, it reacts with labeled antibodies and fluorescence can be observed.
- **Indirect immunofluorescence assay:** A known antigen is fixed on slide and unknown antibody in patient's serum attaches to the known antigen on the slide. For detection of antigen-antibody reaction, fluorescein tagged antibody to human globulin is added, thus which is observed under fluorescent microscope.

Applications
- Detection of autoantibodies—(antinuclear antibody) in autoimmune diseases
- Detection of bacteria in blood, CSF, urine, feces, tissue and other specimens
- Detection of microbial antigens-rabies antigen in corneal smear
- Detection of viral antigens in cell lines inoculated with the specimens.

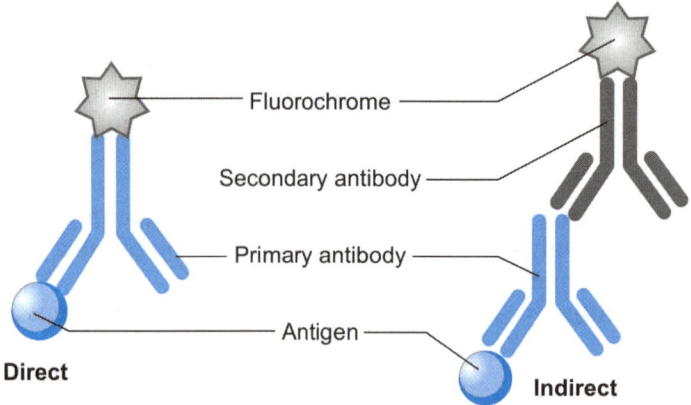

Fig. 4.8: Immunofluorescence.

E. Radioimmunoassay (RIA)

Radioimmunoassay (RIA) is an immunoassay that is based on competition for a fixed amounts of specific antibody between a known radiolabeled antigen and unknown unlabeled (test) antigen. After antigen-antibody reaction, antigen is separated into 'free' and 'bound' fractions and their radioactivity is measured **(Fig. 4.9)**.

It uses radiolabeled molecules in a stepwise formation of immune complexes. An RIA is a very sensitive in vitro assay technique used to measure concentrations of substances, usually measuring antigen concentrations.

Uses

- The test can be used to determine very small quantities (e.g., nanogram) of antigens and antibodies in the serum.
- The test is used for quantitation of hormones, drugs, HBsAg, and other viral antigens.
- Analyze nanomolar and picomolar concentrations of hormones in biological fluids.

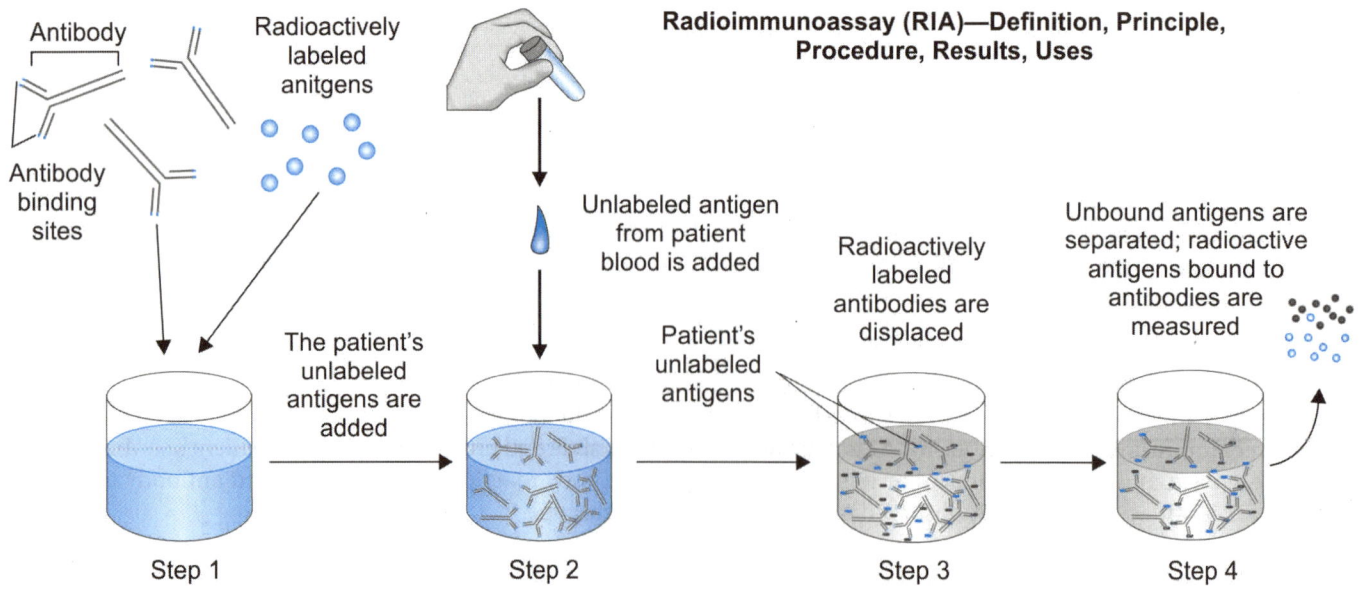

Fig. 4.9: Radioimmunoassay.

F. ELISA (Enzyme-linked Immunosorbent Assay)

Principle
ELISA can provide a useful measurement of antigen or antibody concentration. There are two components:
1. **Immunosorbent:** An absorbing material (polyvinyl, polystyrene) is used that specifically absorbs the known antigen or antibody present in serum.
2. **Enzyme:** Is used to label one of the components of immunoassay.

Following antigen-antibody reaction, chromogenic substrate specific to enzyme (o-phenylenediamine for peroxidase and p-nitrophenyl phosphate for alkaline phosphatase) is added. Reaction is detected by reading optical density.

(Ag + AB complex) – enzyme + substrate → activates the chromogen → color change → Detected by spectrophotometry

Types of ELISA (Figs. 4.10A to D)
- Direct ELISA—used for detection of antigen
- Indirect ELISA—used for detection of antibody/antigen
- Sandwich ELISA—used for detection of antigen-direct (single Ab) and indirect (double Ab) sandwich ELISA
- Competitive ELSA—used for detection of antigen/antibody
- Cassette ELISA (Cylinder ELISA)—used for detection of antibody

Applications
- **For antigen detection:** Hepatitis B surface antigen, hepatitis B inner core antigen, NS1 dengue antigen
- **For antibody detection:** Hepatitis B, C, HIV, dengue, Epstein-Barr virus, herpes simplex virus, toxoplasmosis, leishmaniasis

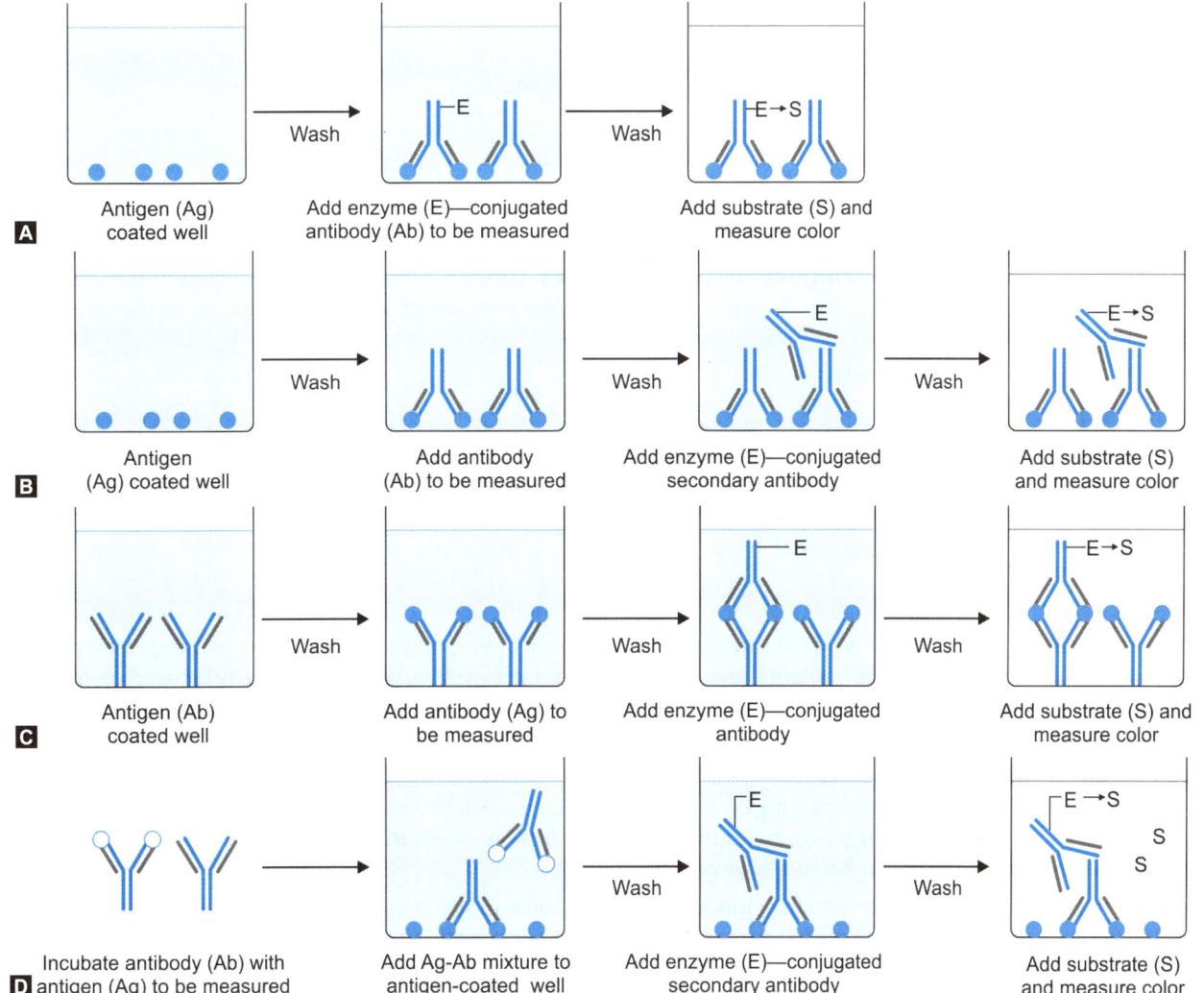

Figs. 4.10A to D: ELISA types: (A) Direct ELISA; (B) Indirect ELISA; (C) Sandwich ELISA; (D) Competitive ELISA.

VACCINES

A vaccine is a biological preparation that provides active acquired immunity to a particular infectious or malignant disease. It typically contains an agent that resembles a disease-causing microorganism and is often made from weakened or killed forms of the microbe, its toxins, or one of its surface proteins.

The agent stimulates the body's immune system to recognize the agent as a threat, destroy it, and to further recognize and destroy any of the microorganisms associated with that agent that it may encounter in the future. Vaccines can be prophylactic (to prevent or ameliorate the effects of a future infection by a natural or 'wild' pathogen), or therapeutic (to fight a disease that has already occurred).

The main types of vaccines that act in different ways are:

- **Live-attenuated vaccines:** Live-attenuated vaccines inject a live version of the germ or virus that causes a disease into the body. Although the germ is a live specimen, it is a weakened version that does not cause any symptoms of infection as it is unable to reproduce once it is in the body.
  - BCG for tuberculosis
  - Sabin vaccine for poliomyelitis
  - MMR vaccine for measles, mumps and rubella
  - Rotavirus
  - Smallpox
  - Chickenpox
  - Yellow fever
- **Inactivated vaccines:** An inactivated vaccine uses a strain of a bacteria or virus that has been killed with heat or chemicals. This dead version of the virus or bacteria is then injected into the body.
  - Hepatitis A
  - Flu
  - Polio
  - Rabies
- **Subunit, recombinant, conjugate, and polysaccharide vaccines:** Subunit, recombinant, conjugate, and polysaccharide vaccines use particular parts of the germ or virus. They can trigger very strong immune responses in the body because they use a specific part of the germ
  - Hib (*Hemophilus influenza* type b)
  - Hepatitis B
  - Human papillomavirus (HPV)
  - Whooping cough
  - Pneumococcal disease
  - Meningococcal disease
  - Shingles
- **Toxoid vaccines:** Toxoid vaccines use toxins created by the bacteria or virus to create immunity to the specific parts of the bacteria or virus that cause disease, and not the entire bacteria or virus. The immune response is focused on this specific toxin. Toxoid vaccines do not offer lifelong immunity and need to be topped up over time. Toxoid vaccines are used to create immunity against diphtheria and tetanus.
- **mRNA vaccines:** This technology has been in development for decades. mRNA vaccines have benefits, such as short manufacturing times and low manufacturing costs. However, they have to be kept at low temperatures due to the fragility of the mRNA. Vaccines work by triggering an immune response from proteins they synthesize. They induce both cellular and humoral immunity. The first mRNA vaccine is for COVID-19.
- **Viral vector vaccines**: Viral vector vaccines modify another virus and use it as a vector to deliver protection from the intended virus. Some of the viruses used as vectors include adenovirus, influenza, measles virus and vesicular stomatitis virus (VSV).

UNIVERSAL IMMUNIZATION SCHEDULE

India's Immunization Programme is one of the largest public health programs in the world. Launched as Expanded Programme on Immunization in 1978, it was renamed as Universal Immunization Programme in 1985 when it was expanded beyond urban areas **(Tables 4.3 and 4.4)**.

It targets 3.04 crore pregnant women and 2.7 crore newborns annually. More than 1.2 crore immunization sessions are being conducted annually. Under UIP, immunization is being provided free of cost against 12 vaccine preventable diseases:

Nationally against 11 diseases: *Diphtheria, pertussis, tetanus, polio, measles, rubella, severe form of childhood tuberculosis, rotavirus diarrhea, hepatitis b, meningitis and pneumonia caused by hemophilus influenza type b and pneumococcal pneumonia and sub-nationally against 1 disease—japanese encephalitis* (JE vaccine is provided only in endemic districts).

TABLE 4.3: National Immunization Schedule for infants, children and pregnant women.

Age	Vaccines given
Birth	Bacillus Calmette Guerin (BCG), oral polio vaccine (OPV)-0 dose, Hepatitis B birth dose
6 Weeks	OPV-1, pentavalent-1, rotavirus vaccine (RVV)-1, fractional-dose of inactivated polio vaccine (fIPV)-1, pneumococcal conjugate vaccine (PCV)-1
10 weeks	OPV-2, pentavalent-2, RVV-2
14 weeks	OPV-3, pentavalent-3, fIPV-2, RVV-3, PCV-2
9–12 months	Measles and rubella (MR)-1, JE-1*, PCV-booster
16–24 months	MR-2, JE-2*, diphtheria, pertussis and tetanus (DPT)-booster-1, OPV-booster
5–6 years	DPT-booster-2
10 years	Tetanus and adult diphtheria (Td)
16 years	Td
Pregnant mother	Td1, 2 or Td booster**

*One dose if previously vaccinated within 3 years
**JE vaccine is introduced in selected endemic districts after the campaign.

Cold Chain System, Vaccines and Logistics

- Cold chain is a system of storing and transporting vaccine at the recommended temperature range from the point of manufacture to point of use. India has built a vast cold chain infrastructure to ensure that only potent and effective vaccines reach millions of beneficiaries across the country.
- There are more than 29,000 Cold Chain Points (CCPs) across the country where the vaccines are stored and further delivered to the lower-level stores/immunization sessions attached to it.
- The vaccines are supplied by manufacturers directly to four Government Medical Store Depots (at Karnal, Mumbai, Chennai and Kolkata) which act as national buffer stores as well as to state and selected regional vaccine stores.
- Transportation of vaccines from the manufacturers to GMSDs/SVSs/RVSs and from the GMSDs to SVSs/RVs are normally done through air transportation except for the small distances which are done by road.
- Transportation from States/Regional stores to districts are done in cold boxes using insulated vaccine vans.
- National Cold Chain Management Information System (NCCMIS) is the repository for the CCEs under immunization program, which helps in tracking the CCP wise status and sickness rate of the CCEs.

TABLE 4.4: Immunization program of India.

	For infants			
Vaccine	*When to give*	*Dose*	*Route*	*Site*
Bacillus Calmette-Guerin (BCG)	At birth or as early as possible till one year of age	0.1 mL (0.05 mL until 1 month age)	Intradermal	Left upper arm
Hepatitis B—Birth dose	At birth or as early as possible within 24 hours	0.5 mL	Intramuscular	Anterolateral side of mid-thigh
Oral polio vaccine (OPV)-0	At birth or as early as possible within the first 15 days	2 drops	Oral	Oral
OPV 1, 2 and 3	At 6 weeks, 10 weeks and 14 weeks (OPV can be given till 5 years of age)	2 drops	Oral	Oral
Pentavalent 1, 2 and 3	At 6 weeks, 10 weeks and 14 weeks (can be given till one year of age)	0.5 mL	Intramuscular	Anterolateral side of mid-thigh
Pneumococcal conjugate vaccine (PCV)	Two primary doses at 6 and 14 weeks followed by booster dose at 9–12 months	0.5 mL	Intramuscular	Anterolateral side of mid-thigh
Rotavirus (RVV)	At 6 weeks, 10 weeks and 14 weeks (can be given till one year of age)	Rotaract: 5 drops (liquid vaccine) Retail lyophilized vaccine—2.5 mL Rotasiil liquid—2 mL	Oral	Oral
Inactivated polio vaccine (IPV)	Two fractional dose at 6 and 14 weeks of age	0.1 mL	Intradermal two fractional dose	Intradermal: Right upper arm
Measles rubella (MR) 1st dose	9 completed months–12 months. (Measles can be given till 5 years of age)	0.5 mL	Subcutaneous	Right upper arm
Japanese encephalitis (JE)-1	9 completed months–12 months	0.5 mL	Subcutaneous (Live attenuated vaccine) intramuscular (Killed vaccine)	Left upper arm (Live attenuated vaccine) Anterolateral aspect of mid thigh (Killed vaccine)
Vitamin A (1st dose)	At 9 completed months with measles—rubella	1 mL (1 lakh IU)	Oral	Oral
For children				
Diphtheria, pertussis and tetanus (DPT) booster-1	16–24 months	0.5 mL	Intramuscular	Anterolateral side of mid-thigh
MR 2nd dose	16–24 months	0.5 mL	Subcutaneous	Right upper arm
OPV booster	16–24 months	2 drops	Oral	Oral
JE-2	16–24 months	0.5 mL	Subcutaneous (Live attenuated vaccine) Intramuscular (Killed vaccine)	Left upper arm (Live attenuated vaccine) Anterolateral aspect of mid thigh (Killed vaccine)
Vitamin A (2nd to 9th dose)	16–18 months. Then subsequently one dose every 6 months up to the age of 5 years	2 mL (2 lakh IU)	Oral	Oral
DPT booster-2	5–6 years	0.5 mL	Intramuscular	Upper arm
Td	10 years and 16 years	0.5 mL	Intramuscular	Upper arm
For pregnant women				
Tetanus and adult diphtheria (Td)-1	Early in pregnancy	0.5 mL	Intramuscular	Upper arm
Td-2	4 weeks after Td-1	0.5 mL	Intramuscular	Upper arm
Td-booster	If received 2 Td doses in a pregnancy within the last 3 years	0.5 mL	Intramuscular	Upper arm

SECTION II

Infection Control and Safety

Chapter 5: Hospital Acquired Infections
Chapter 6: Isolation Precautions and Use of Personal Protective Equipments
Chapter 7: Hand Hygiene
Chapter 8: Disinfection and Sterilization
Chapter 9: Specimen Collection
Chapter 10: Biomedical Waste Management
Chapter 11: Antimicrobial Stewardship
Chapter 12: Patient Safety Indicators
Chapter 13: International Patient Safety Goals
Chapter 14: Safety Protocols
Chapter 15: Employee Safety Indicators

CHAPTER 5

Hospital Acquired Infections

Chapter Outline

- Hospital Acquired Infections
- Types of Hospital Acquired Infections
- Surveillance of HAI-Infection Control Team and Infection Control Committee
- Hospital Infection Control Committee and Infection Control Team

INTRODUCTION

Hospital acquired infections (HAI's) are also known as healthcare-associated infections (HCAIs) or nosocomial infections.

Healthcare-associated Infections (HAIs)

Definition

- Infections in hospitalized patients which were not present or incubating at the time of admission. An infection acquired in a medical setting in the course of medical treatment.
    - An infection is considered an HAI if all elements of a CDC/NHSN site-specific infection criterion were first present together on or after the 3rd calendar day of admission to the facility (the day of hospital admission is day 1).
    - HAIs may be caused by infectious agents from endogenous or exogenous sources:
        - Endogenous sources are body sites, such as the skin, nose, mouth, gastrointestinal (GI) tract, or vagina that are normally inhabited by microorganisms.
        - Exogenous sources are those external to the patient, such as patient care personnel, visitors, patient care equipment, medical devices, or the healthcare environment.
- HAIs can happen in any healthcare facility, including hospitals, ambulatory surgical centers, end-stage renal disease facilities, and long-term care facilities.
- Bacteria, fungi, viruses, or other less common pathogens can cause HAIs.
- Prevention of nosocomial infection is the responsibility of all individuals and services provided by healthcare setting.

This also includes the occupational infection among staff and also the infection which appears after the discharge from hospital. HAIs are a danger to patient wellbeing and safety and put a great burden in the treatment of patient as mainly the etiological agent responsible are drug resistant. Preventing HAIs is critical to patient safety and nursing staff is the one whose role is directly involved in the prevention of HAIs.

The Following Infections are not Considered Healthcare Associated

- Infections associated with complications or extensions of infections already present on admission, unless a change in pathogen or symptoms strongly suggests the acquisition of a new infection.
- Infections in infants that have been acquired transplacentally (e.g., herpes simplex, toxoplasmosis, rubella, cytomegalovirus, or syphilis) and become evident on the day of birth or the next day.
- Reactivation of a latent infection (e.g., herpes zoster, herpes simplex, syphilis, or TB)

Factors Affecting HAIs

The various risk factors which increase the chances of getting HAI to a patient are as following:

1. Extreme age: Premature babies and very old people are at high risk.
2. Underlying medical condition: People with disease, such as diabetes, Leukemia's, etc.
3. Low immune status: A person with low immune status can develop HAIs easily, such as HIV patients.
4. Prolonged stay or hospitalization
5. Inadequate knowledge about hand sanitization/hand washing
6. Any long and complicated surgery especially, such as neuro and ortho surgeries.
7. Overuse and under use of antibiotics
8. Instrumentation, such as catheters, IV sets, etc., applied in aseptic conditions increase the chances of HAIs. Patients admitted in intensive care units (ICUs) are at high risk to develop HAIs.
9. Transfusion of blood and other IV products if not screened can transmit various diseases.
10. Poor hospital infection control practices.

Sources of Healthcare-associated Infections

There can be two types of sources of HAIs:
1. **Endogenous source:** This includes the normal flora of an individual which when gets altered by the different medical procedures produces disease. Large number of HAIs are of endogenous sources.
2. **Exogenous sources:** They can of different types:
   a. *Healthcare works:* Doctors, nursing and allied health sciences staff can be the carrier of infection.
   b. *Environmental sources:* It includes air, water, food, hospital environment, objects and equipments, bed pans, contaminated surfaces, body fluids, etc.

Microorganisms Responsible for HAIs

Nosocomial pathogens include bacteria, viruses and fungi and parasites. Bacteria are the most common pathogens responsible for nosocomial infections. Some belong to natural flora of the patient and cause infection only when the immune system of the patient becomes prone to infections.

The **ESKAPE** pathogens are the commonly responsible for nosocomial infections; the infections are particularly dangerous due to the ability of pathogens to resist the action of currently used antimicrobial agents.

- ***E**nterococcus faecium*
- ***S**taphylococcus aureus*
- ***K**lebsiella pneumoniae*
- ***A**cinetobacter baumannii*
- ***P**seudomonas aeruginosa*
- ***E**nterobacter* species

Other bacteria responsible are E. coli, M. tuberculosis.

- Amongst fungus, *Candida* species (*C. albicans, C. parapsilosis, C. glabrata*) are the most commonly fungal organisms associated with HAI. Other fungal is *Aspergillus fumigatus*.
- Infections due to viral pathogens are the least reported, common viral agents responsible for HAIs are COVID-19, influenza viruses, Ebola virus.

Mode of Transmission of HAIs

The various routes of HAI as are as the following:

Through Direct and Indirect Contact

Direct contact: Skin-to-skin contact through hands of infected persons is the most common mode of transmission of HAIs. Hospital staff and other healthcare workers are the main source of infection of HAIs and transfer the infection through contaminated hands.

Indirect contact: When a person gets infected by contact with infected objects, such as dressing pads, instruments, through needle stick injury, sharp pricks, etc.

Through Air

Infection can also be acquired through air contaminated with infective agents. Droplets from infective patients can be inhaled by other person and gets infection. Dust particles while shedding bed covers, etc., can also transmit HAIs. Aerosols arising from use of nebulizer or any other apparatus can also contribute to HAIs.

Through Vector

In case of poor infection control practices, vectors, such as mosquitoes, flies, etc., carrying infective organisms can cause HAIs, such as malaria, dengue, etc., but this mode is less common.

TYPES OF HOSPITAL ACQUIRED INFECTIONS

The Centers for Disease Control and Prevention (CDC) broadly categorizes the types of HAIs in following categories:
1. Central line-associated bloodstream infections (CLABSI)
2. Catheter-associated urinary tract infections (CAUTI)
3. Surgical site infections (SSI)
4. Ventilator-associated event (VAE)

Other types of HAI include:
- Non-ventilator-associated hospital-acquired pneumonia (NV-HAP)
- Gastrointestinal infections
- HAI can also be caused by various other organs like ear, eye, nose and throat infections, lower respiratory tract infections (including bronchitis, tracheobronchitis, bronchiolitis, tracheitis, lung abscess or empyema without evidence of pneumonia), skin and soft-tissue infections, cardiovascular infection, bone and joint infections, central nervous systems infection, and reproductive tract infections.

1. Central Line-associated Blood Stream Infections (CLABSI)

Definition: Central line-associated BSI (CLABSI)—a laboratory-confirmed bloodstream infection (LCBI) where central line (CL) was in place for >2 calendar days on the date of event, with day of device placement being Day 1, central line was in place on the date of event or the day before. If a CL was in place for >2 calendar days and then removed, the date of event of the LCBI must be the day of discontinuation or the next day.

Femoral Lines are not Considered Central Lines

As per the latest guidelines of Centre for Disease Control National Healthcare Safety Network (CDC-NHSN), criteria for Laboratory-Confirmed Bloodstream Infection (LCBI) are as shown in **Table 5.1**.

TABLE 5.1: Criteria for laboratory—confirmed blood stream infections (LCBI).	
LCB 1	Patient has a recognized pathogen cultured from one or more blood cultures and organism cultured from blood is not related to an infection at another site.

Mode of Infection through Central Lines

The various routes through which an organism reaches in the body through catheter are as following:
1. Normal flora of the patient during the insertion of catheter may get along with catheter tip if proper aseptic techniques are not applied.
2. Contamination of catheter by healthcare worker with hands while insertion
3. Hematogenous route
4. Catheter contamination at production level.

Once the microbe enters into the central line and immune response is generated at the site of catheter in order to prevent the infection. Microbes get attached and form colonies following which biofilm formation is done on the catheter surface which prevents the microbe to be killed by antimicrobial therapies.

Risk Factor

- Long-term duration of catheterization
- Heavy microbial colonization at the insertion site and/or catheter hub
- Femoral vein catheterization in adults
- Reduced nurse-to-patient ratio in the ICU
- Immunocompromised patient. Patients on total parenteral nutrition
- Disturbance in cutaneous microbial flora
- Lack of proper hygiene
- Lack of following bundle approach

Main Causative Agents

- Gram positive bacteria—Staphylococci (*S. aureus*, coagulase negative *Staphylococcus*), *Enterococcus* species
- Gram negative bacteria (e.g., *E. coli, Pseudomonas aeruginosa, Klebsiella pneumoniae*)
- *Candida* species

Maintenance and Care Bundle Approach for CLABSI's

Insertion Bundle Approach

- Proper hygiene should be maintained during and after insertion of central line, such as hand washing, etc.
- Use of personal protective equipment (PPE)—surgical masks, sterile gloves, cap, sterile gown, and large sterile drapes.
- Selection of proper site, i.e., use of subclavian instead of femoral vein.
- Proper disinfection of the skin using appropriate antiseptic solution, such as chlorhexidine. Use of transparent catheter. Follow up of standard guidelines.
- Documentation of all the steps performed in a bundle checklist and recorded properly.

Maintenance Bundle Approach

- Removal of unnecessary central lines and daily assessment of centerline.
- Hand washing before the routine checkup of central lines by staff
- Disinfect catheter hubs, ports, connectors, etc., before using the catheter
- Change dressings and disinfect site with alcohol-based chlorhexidine every 5–7 days or as per need.
- Replace administration sets within 96 hours (immediately if used for blood products or lipids)
- Proper nurse patient ratio in ICUs.

Treatment

- Removal of central line.
- Start of empirical microbial therapy as soon as CRBSI is suspected followed by antimicrobial susceptibility testing.
- The antibiotic duration for central line-associated bloodstream infections is dependent on whether the infection is complicated or uncomplicated and whether the catheter is retained or removed.

2. Catheter-associated Urinary Tract Infection (CAUTI)

Definition

Catheter-associated urinary tract infection (CAUTI): A laboratory-confirmed urinary tract infection (UTI) as per either criterion listed below in **Table 5.2**:

TABLE 5.2: Criteria for catheter-associated urinary tract infections (CAUTI).	

Criterion A	Criterion A includes 1, 2 and 3 below:
	1. Patient has an indwelling urinary catheter in place for the entire day on the date of event and such catheter had been in place for >2 calendar days, on that date (day of device placement = Day 1)
	2. Patient has at least one of the following signs or symptoms:
	  – Fever (>38.0°C)
	  – Suprapubic tenderness
	  – Costovertebral angle pain or tenderness
	3. Patient has a urine culture with not more than two species of organisms, at least one of which is a bacteria of >10^5 CFU/mL.

Criterion B	Criterion B includes 1, 2, and 3 below:
	1. Patient had an indwelling urinary catheter in place for >2 calendar days which was removed on the day of, or day before the date of event
	2. Patient has at least one of the following signs or symptoms:
	  – Fever (>38.0°C)
	  – Suprapubic tenderness
	  – Costovertebral angle pain or tenderness
	  – Urinary urgency
	  – Urinary frequency
	  – Dysuria

Main causative organisms:
- Gram negative bacteria especially *E. coli* is the most common causative agent.
- Gram positive bacteria include *Staph. aureus, Enterococcus.*
- Fungi; *Candida* albicans

Risk Factors of CAUTI
- Long-term catheterization
- Type of material used, such as latex catheters have high CAUTI risk then silicon catheters
- Female gender is at high risk due to anatomical location.
- Immunocompromised state of patient. Underlying illness, such as diabetes mellitus
- Extreme ages
- Lack of personal hygiene
- Lack of proper aseptic techniques while catheterization

Pathogenesis

In CAUTI, duration of catheterization is the most important determinant of bacteriuria, and CAUTI risk increases by 3–7% each day after placement of an indwelling urinary catheter. In catheterized patients the causative agent can reach to the bladder through the following main routes:
- **Extraluminal spread:** If proper hygienic environment or aseptic conditions are not maintained during the catheter placement there is a risk that bacteria from the external sources, such as normal flora, hands of healthcare workers, etc., may get migrated and cause disease.
- **Intraluminal spread:** In case the drainage urine bag is open type, or the catheter has any leakages or hole there is a risk that the contaminated urine from the bag may get back and cause disease.

Maintenance of the Bundle Approach
- Catheter care should be given on regular basis by proper techniques, hand hygiene and use of gloves is must while giving the care.
- It should be regularly checked that catheter is properly secured all the times.

- Drainage bag should always be below the bladder and above the floor
- Documentation and records of daily catheter care should be maintained by the nurse on duty

Nursing Interventions to Reduce the Risk of Catheter-associated Urinary Tract Infection

- Staff education about catheter management, combined with regular monitoring of CAUTI incidence. Facility-wide program to ensure catheterization only when indicated and prompt removal of indwelling catheters, daily cleansing of the urethral meatus using soap and water or perineal cleanser.
- Maintenance of a closed urinary drainage system.
- Routine catheter changes every 4–6 weeks reduce CAUTI incidence in patients managed by long-term catheterization.
- Documentation and records of daily catheter care is mandatory.

Prevention of CAUTI

The most effective way to reduce the incidence of CAUTI is to reduce the use of urinary catheterization by restricting its use to patients who have clear indications and by removing the catheter as soon as it is no longer needed.

The various ways by which the CAUTI can be reduced are as following:

- By following the bundle care approach. Limiting unnecessary catheterization.
- Alternatives to indwelling catheter. In males, where urinary catheter is indicated and who have minimal post-void residual urine, condom catheterization should be considered as an alternative to short-term.
- Intermittent catheterization should be considered as an alternative to short- or long-term indwelling urethral catheterization. A closed catheter drainage system, with ports in the distal catheter for needle aspiration of urine, should be used to reduce.
- Indwelling catheters should be removed as soon as they are no longer required to reduce the risk of CA-bacteriuria and CA-UTI
- In patients with short-term indwelling urethral catheterization, antimicrobial (silver alloy or antibiotic)–coated urinary catheters use, lowers the risk of CAUTI. Daily meatal cleansing with povidone-iodine solution, silver sulfadiazine, polyantibiotic ointment or cream, or green soap and water is not recommended for routine use in men or women with indwelling urethral catheters to reduce CA-bacteriuria.
- Routine addition of antimicrobials or antiseptics to the drainage bag of catheterized patients should not be used to reduce CA-bacteriuria or CA-UTI.
- Prophylactic antimicrobials, given systemically or by bladder irrigation, should not be administered routinely to patients at the time of catheter placement to reduce CA-UTI or at the time of catheter removal or replacement to reduce CA-bacteriuria.

Management/Treatment

- Removal of catheter
- Appropriate antimicrobial therapy following antimicrobial sensitivity testing.

3. Ventilator-associated Event (VAE)

Ventilator: A device to assist or control respiration continuously through a tracheotomy or by endotracheal intubation. Lung expansion devices, such as those that provide intermittent positive pressure breathing, nasal positive end-expiratory pressure, and continuous nasal positive airway pressure are not considered ventilators unless they provide assistance or control through tracheostomy or endotracheal intubation.

VAE: According to the latest guidelines of Centre for Disease Control National Healthcare Safety Network (CDC-NHSN), Ventilator associated Event (VAE) includes:

Ventilator-associated Condition (VAC)

Patient has a baseline period of stability or improvement on the ventilator, defined by >2 calendar days of stable or decreasing daily minimum FiO_2 or PEEP values. The baseline period is defined as the 2 calendar days immediately proceeding the first day of increased daily minimum PEEP or FiO_2 and after a period of stability or improvement on the ventilator, the patient has at least one of the following indicators of worsening oxygenation:

- Increase in daily minimum FiO_2 of >0.20 (20 points) over the daily minimum FiO_2 in the baseline period, sustained for >2 calendar days.
- Increase in daily minimum PEEP values of >3 cm H_2O over the daily minimum PEEP in the baseline period, sustained for >2 calendar days.

Infection-related Ventilator-associated Complication (IVAC)

Patient meets criteria for VAC.

Patient has a baseline period of stability or improvement on the ventilator, on or after calendar day 3 of mechanical ventilation and within 2 calendar days before or after the onset of worsening oxygenation, the patient meets both of the following criteria:
1. Temperature >38°C or <36°C, OR
2. White blood cells count >12,000 cells/mm^3 or <4,000 cells/mm^3
3. A new antimicrobial agent(s) is started, and is continued for >4 calendar days.
Possible VAP—Possible ventilator-associated pneumonia.

Patient meets criteria for VAC and IVAC

Patient has a baseline period of stability or improvement on the ventilator, on or after calendar day 3 of mechanical ventilation and within 2 calendar days before or after the onset of worsening oxygenation, with ONE of the following criteria is met:
- **Criterion 1:** Positive culture of one of the following specimens, meeting quantitative or semi-quantitative thresholds, without requirement for purulent respiratory secretions:
  - Endotracheal aspirate >10^5 CFU/mL or corresponding semi-quantitative result
  - Bronchoalveolar lavage >10^4 CFU/mL or corresponding semi-quantitative result
  - Lung tissue >10^4 CFU/g or corresponding semi-quantitative result
  - Protected specimen brush, >10^3 CFU/mL or corresponding semi-quantitative result.
- **Criterion 2:** Purulent respiratory secretions (defined as secretions from the lungs, bronchi, or trachea that contain >25 neutrophils and <10 squamous epithelial cells per low power field plus a positive culture of one of the following specimens (qualitative culture, or quantitative/semi-quantitative culture without sufficient growth to meet criterion #1):
  - Sputum
  - Endotracheal aspirate
  - Bronchoalveolar lavage
  - Lung tissue
  - Protected specimen brush
- **Criterion 3:** One of the following positive tests:
  - Pleural fluid culture (where specimen was obtained during thoracocentesis or initial placement of chest tube and NOT from an indwelling chest tube)
  - Lung histopathology, defined as:
    - Abscess formation or foci of consolidation within neutrophil accumulation in bronchioles and alveoli
    - Evidence of lung parenchyma invasion by fungi (hyphae, pseudohyphae or yeast forms)
    - Evidence of infection with the viral pathogens listed below based on results of immunohistochemical assays, cytology, or microscopy performed on lung tissue,
  - Diagnostic test for *Legionella* species
  - Diagnostic test on respiratory secretions for influenza virus, respiratory syncytial virus, adenovirus, parainfluenza virus, rhinovirus, human metapneumovirus, coronavirus.

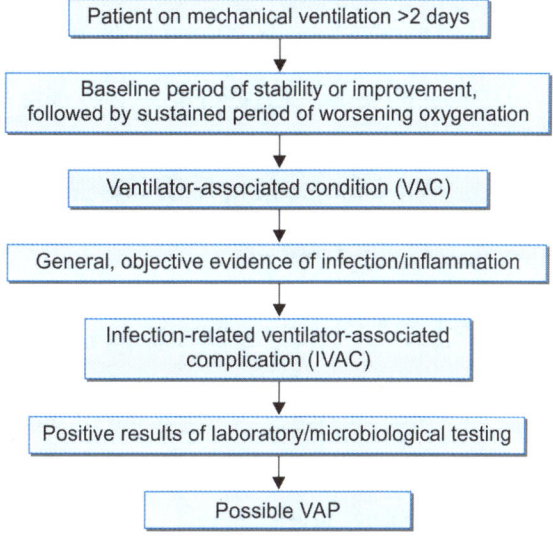

TABLE 5.3: Clinical Pulmonary Infection Score (CPIS).			
Modified CPIS used for ventilator-associated pneumonia			
CPIS points	**0**	**1**	**2**
Temperature	≥36.5°C or ≤38.5°C	≥38.5°C or ≤38.9°C	≥39°C or ≤36°C
Leukocyte count/mm^3	4,000–11,000	<4,000 or >11,000	<4,000 or >11,000 and band forms ≥50%
Tracheal secretions	Rare	Non-purulent	Abundant and purulent
Oxygenation PaO$_2$/FiO$_2$ mm Hg (PaO$_2$ = arterial partial pressure of oxygen) (FiO$_2$ = fraction of inspired oxygen)	>240 with acute respiratory distress syndrome (ARDS)	–	≤240 ADRS
Chest radiography	No infiltrate	Diffuse or patchy infiltrate	Localized infiltrate
Tracheal aspirate culture report	Light growth or no growth	Moderate or heavy growth of pathogenic bacteria	Moderate or heavy growth of bacteria and presence of bacteria with similar morphology on gram stain

VAP can be classified into following types:
1. **Early onset VAP:** It occurs in first 4 days of mechanical ventilation.
2. **Late onset VAP:** It occurs after ≥5 days of ventilation

Diagnosis

This is based on the combined clinical, microbiological, and radiological criteria. Clinical pulmonary infection score (CPIS) is the most scoring system which is based on six parameters with a score scale from 0–2. In this, the maximum score which can be obtained is 12 and a score >6 is diagnosis of VAP. **Table 5.3** depicts the same.

Treatment/Management

Treatment of VAP include the start of combination antimicrobial therapy according to the antimicrobial susceptibility (AST) pattern report and the choice of empirical regime should based on local antimicrobial resistance pattern of the hospital.

Preventive Measures/Care Bundle for VAP

- Effective infection control measures which include education and training of HCWs, high compliance with alcohol-based hand rubbing (70% ethyl alcohol) as the main measure of hand hygiene and isolation to reduce cross infection.
- Surveillance of high-risk patients to determine trends and outbreaks of VAP within the ICU. Infection rates should be reported to ICU physicians and nurses on regular basis.
- Maintaining proper level of nursing staff in ICU.
- Keeping the teeth and mouth clean, preventing the formation of dental plaque on teeth. Effective oral hygiene care (OHC) with chlorhexidine 2% is important for ventilated patients.
- Limiting the use of continuous sedation and paralytic agents/drugs that depress cough coupled with sedation.
- Elevation of head of bed 30–40° to prevent oropharyngeal aspiration to respiratory tract.
- Unnecessary intubation and repeated intubation should be avoided. Non-invasive positive pressure ventilation (NIPPV) should be used whenever possible.
- Endotracheal tube cuff pressure should be maintained at approximately 20–30 cm H$_2$O.
- Contaminated condensers should be carefully removed from ventilator circuits and should be avoided to enter the endotracheal tube or inline medication nebulizer.
- Sterilization and appropriate maintenance of equipments
- Use of proper PPE while handling the patient.
- Change of filters in the breathing circuits every 7 days.
- Use of probiotics
- Deep vein thrombosis (DVT) prophylaxis should be provided, if needed.
- Daily assessment of readiness to remove mechanical ventilator should always documented.

4. Surgical Site Infection (SSI)

Definition

Superficial Incisional SSI

Infection occurs within 30 days after the operative procedure and involves skin and subcutaneous tissue of the incision; and meets the following criterion as shown in **Table 5.4**.

30-day surveillance (Box 5.1): Infection occurs within 30 days after any operative procedure (where day 1 = the procedure date) and involves deep soft tissues of the incision (e.g., fascial and muscle layers) and/or part of the body deeper than the fascial/muscle layers, that is opened or manipulated during the operative procedure; and meets either of the following criteria (A or B).

TABLE 5.4: Criteria for surgical site infection.

Criteria A	Patient has at least one of the following: Infection occurs within 30 days after any operative procedure (where day 1 the procedure date) AND Involves only skin and subcutaneous tissue of the incision AND Patient has at least one of the following: • Purulent drainage from the superficial incision. • A deep incision that spontaneously dehisces, or is deliberately opened or • Aspirated by a surgeon and is culture positive or not cultured AND patient has at least one of the following signs or symptoms: fever (>38°C); localized pain or tenderness. A culture negative finding does not meet this criterion • An abscess or other evidence of infection involving the deep incision that is detected on gross anatomical or histopathology exam, or imaging test
Criteria B	Infection occurs within 30 days after the operative procedure (where day 1 = the procedure date) AND Infection involves any part of the body deeper than the fascial/muscle layers, that is opened or manipulated during the operative procedure AND Patient has at least one of the following: • Purulent drainage from a drain that is placed into the organ/space (e.g., closed suction drainage system, open drain, T-tube drain, CT-guided drainage) organisms isolated from an aseptically-obtained culture from the superficial incision or subcutaneous tissue • Superficial incision that is deliberately opened by a surgeon and is culture positive or not cultured AND patient has at least one of the following signs or symptoms—pain or tenderness; localized swelling; erythema; or heat. A culture negative finding does not meet this criterion • Diagnosis of a superficial incisional SSI by the surgeon

BOX 5.1: List of operative procedures for 30 day surveillance.

- Abdominal aortic aneurysm repair
- Limb amputation
- Appendix surgery
- Shunt for dialysis
- Bile duct, liver or pancreatic surgery
- Carotid endarterectomy
- Gallbladder surgery
- Colon surgery
- Cesarean section
- Gastric surgery
- Heart transplant
- Abdominal hysterectomy
- Kidney transplant
- Laminectomy
- Liver transplant
- Neck surgery
- Kidney surgery
- Ovarian surgery
- Prostate surgery
- Rectal surgery
- Small bowel surgery
- Spleen surgery
- Thoracic surgery
- Thyroid and/or parathyroid surgery
- Vaginal hysterectomy
- Exploratory laparotomy

Deep SSI

90-day surveillance: Infection occurs within 90 days after any operative procedure listed in **Table 5.5** (where day 1 = the procedure date) and involves deep soft tissues of the incision (e.g., fascial and muscle layers) and/or part of the body deeper than the fascial/muscle layers, that is opened or manipulated during the operative procedure and meets either of the following criteria (A or B), shown in **Table 5.5**:

TABLE 5.5: Criteria for deep surgical site infections.	
Criteria A	Infection occurs within 90 days after the operative procedure (where day 1 = the procedure date) AND Involves deep soft tissues of the incision (e.g., fascial and muscle layers) AND Patient has at least one of the following: • Purulent drainage from the deep incision. • A deep incision that spontaneously dehisces or is deliberately opened aspirated by a surgeon and is culture positive or not cultured AND patient has at least one of the following signs or symptoms: fever (>38°C); localized pain or tenderness. A culture negative finding does not meet this criterion. • An abscess or other evidence of infection involving the deep incision that is detected on gross anatomical or histopathologic exam, or imaging test
Criteria B	Infection occurs within 90 days after the operative procedure (where day 1 = the procedure date) AND Infection involves any part of the body deeper than the fascial/muscle layers, that is opened or manipulated during the operative procedure AND Patient has at least one of the following: • Purulent drainage from a drain that is placed into the organ/space (e.g., closed suction drainage system, open drain, T-tube drain, CT-guided drainage) • Organisms isolated from an aseptically obtained culture of fluid or tissue in the organ/space • An abscess or other evidence of infection involving the organ/space that is detected on gross anatomical or histopathologic exam, or imaging test AND meets at least one criterion for a specific organ/space infection site listed in **(Box 5.2)**

BOX 5.2: List of operative procedures for 90-day surveillance.

- Breast surgery
- Cardiac surgery
- Coronary artery bypass graft with both chest and donor site incisions
- Coronary artery bypass graft with chest incision only
- Craniotomy
- Spinal fusion
- Open reduction of fracture
- Hernioplasty
- Hip prosthesis
- Knee prosthesis
- Pacemaker surgery
- Peripheral vascular bypass surgery
- Refusion of spine

Pathogenesis of SSI

Risk Factors

- Immunocompromised or immunosuppressed patient.
- Lack of proper disinfection of surgical site before surgery
- Inadequate or improper surgical scrub
- Extreme age >60 years
- Underlying disease, such as diabetes, leukopenia, etc.
- Long operation times
- Malnutrition, history of obesity, smoking, etc.
- Duration of hospital stay
- Ability of bacteria to form biofilm
- Contaminated surgical instruments
- Lack of proper ventilation system
- High level of wound class
- Emergency surgeries

Wound Class Type

The degree of risk for an SSI depends on the type of surgical wound. Which can be classified in the following categories:
- **Class I/Clean wounds:** These are not inflamed or contaminated and do not involve operating on an internal organ. They are usually closed and if necessary drained with closed drainage, here the rate of SSI is usually less than 2%.
- **Class II/Clean-contaminated wounds:** These are the operative wounds in which the respiratory, genital or urinary tracts are entered under controlled conditions. Operations, such as appendix, etc., are categorized in this category. Here the SI rate is 3–11.
- **Class III/Contaminated wounds:** These involve operating on an internal organ with a spilling of contents from the organ into the wound. It includes open fresh accidental wounds, open cardiac massage, colon surgeries. Here the SSI rate is >10%.
- **Class IV/Dirty wounds:** These are wounds in which a known infection is present at the time of the surgery. Example, intra-abdominal abscess, etc., SSI rate here exceeds 20–40%.

Maintenance and Care Bundle Approach for SSIs

7 "S" Bundle to Prevent SSI

1. **Safety:** Operative room should be safe, i.e., all the factors, such as oxygen, pressure, temperature, persons in the operative room, etc., should be maintained. **Table 5.6** depicts some recommendations.
2. **Screen:** Screening for risk factors and presence of MRSA and MSSA and others screening tests, such as blood glucose level, triple serology, etc., should be done before surgery.
3. **Showers:** Preoperative bathing should be performed using antimicrobial soap to reduce bacterial load.
4. **Skin prep:** The skin prepping with alcohol-based antiseptics, such as **chlorhexidine** gluconate (CHG) or Iodophor should be done.
5. **Solution:** Irrigating the tissues prior to closure to remove exogenous contaminants using CHG.
6. **Sutures:** Closing tissues with antimicrobial sutures.
7. **Skin closure:** Sealing the incision or covering with an antimicrobial dressing to prevent exogenous contamination. Hair removal should be done according to the surgical site, hair should never b shaved but removed only by clipping.

TABLE 5.6: Recommendations to prevent SSI in OTs.

Properties	Recommendations
Air changes per hour	Minimum 20/h out of which 4 should be fresh air
Air velocity	20–25 FPM 9 feet per minute). It is checked by anemometer
Air direction	Unidirectional and downward from OT table
Temperature	21 +/– 3°C (general OT) 18 +/– 2°C (ortho OT)
Relative humidity	20–60%
Occupancy	Maximum 5–8 persons at any time in OT is allowed

Device days for a particular area can be calculated as follows:

Date	No. of patients with Indwelling urinary catheter	No. of patient with Central line(s)	No. of patients on Ventilator

Device-associated Infection Rates

These are calculated monthly and expressed per 1000 device-days.

- VAP = $\dfrac{\text{Number of ventilator-associated pneumonias}}{\text{Number of ventilator-days}} \times 1000$

- ClABSI = $\dfrac{\text{Number of central line-associated BSIs}}{\text{Number of central line-days}} \times 1000$

- CAUTI = $\dfrac{\text{Number of urinary foley catheter-associated UTIs}}{\text{Number of urinary catheter-days}} \times 1000$

Device Utilization Ratios

It is advisable to calculate the utilization ratio of devices.

- Ventilator utilization ratio = $\dfrac{\text{Number of ventilator days}}{\text{Number of patient days}}$

- Central line utilization ratio = $\dfrac{\text{Number of central line day}}{\text{Number of patient days}}$

- Central catheter utilization ratio = $\dfrac{\text{Number of Foley's catheter day}}{\text{Number of patient days}}$

Surgical Site Infection Rate

It is calculated monthly and expressed per 100 procedures performed.

- Superficial incision SST = $\dfrac{\text{Number of superficial surgical site infections}}{\text{Number of surgeries performed}} \times 100$

- Deep SSI (30-day surveillance) = $\dfrac{\text{Number of infections (deep incisional/organ/space)}}{\text{Number of surgeries (as per \textbf{Box 5.1})}} \times 100$

- Deep SSI (90-day surveillance) = $\dfrac{\text{Number of infections (deep incisional/organ/space)}}{\text{No. of surgeries in month of initial surgery (\textbf{Box 5.2})}} \times 100$

Calculation of Device Days

Total number of days of exposure to the device (central line, ventilator, or urinary catheter) by all of the patients in the selected population during the selected time period at the same time each day. (One or more central lines in a patient are to be taken as one)

SURVEILLANCE OF HAI-INFECTION CONTROL TEAM AND INFECTION CONTROL COMMITTEE

Surveillance involves a continuous and systematic process of collecting, analyzing, interpreting, and disseminating descriptive information to monitor health problems.

The actions are related to improvement in prevention or control of the condition. Surveillance for healthcare-associated infections (HAIs) is normally performed by trained infection prevention and control professionals or hospital epidemiologists. **Figure 5.1** depicts the surveillance cycle.

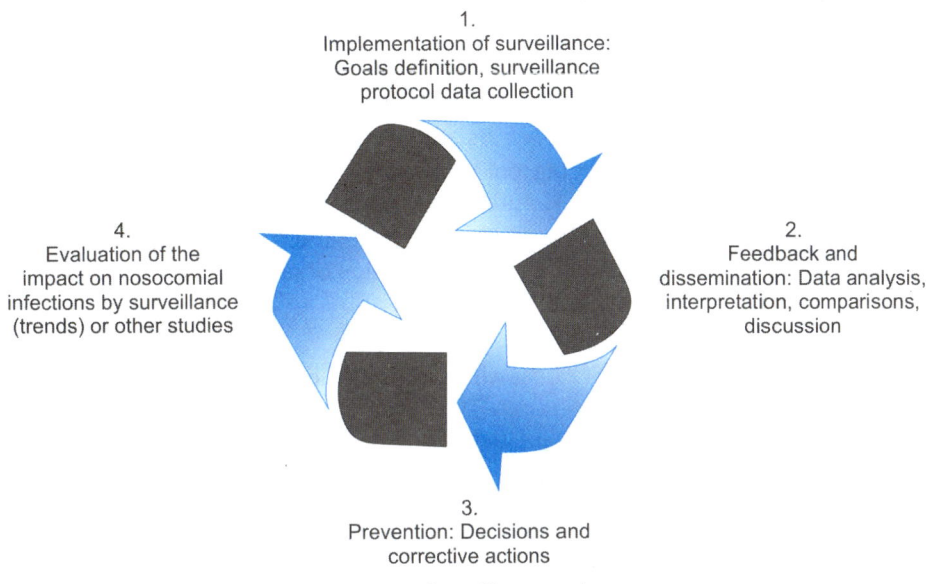

Fig. 5.1: Surveillance cycle.

Objectives

1. It provides the baseline HAI rate and information on type of HAI in hospital,
2. Data can be compared with other hospitals also.
3. It can identify the root cause of HAI and also provide the solution to that particular problem.
4. Help full in implementing infection control programs and identifying the weakness in ongoing program.
5. Provides timely feedback to clinicians through which they can adopt best practices.

The Healthcare-associated Infections Surveillance Network (HAI-Net) is a European network for the surveillance of HAI, coordinated by the European Centre for Disease Prevention and Control (ECDC) provides the following guidelines for surveillance of HAIs.

- **From where to conduct/start:** The surveillance of HAI should be conducted only for the high-risk areas, such as ICUs, etc.
- **The type of HAI to be monitored:** Usually only major type of HAIs (CAUTI, CLABSI, VAP, SSI) can be monitored due to technical difficulty.
- **Conducted by:** The Infection Control Nurses (ICNs) under supervision of Infection Control Officer of hospital infection control committee will conduct HAI surveillance.

Healthcare-associated Infections Surveillance

There are various established components to an active, effective surveillance system are as following:

Planning

It is not feasible to monitor all types of infections at all times, choosing which infections will be surveyed is based upon an initial assessment that will establish the priorities for the surveillance system. An initial assessment will include:
- The types of patients/residents that are served by the healthcare setting.
- The key medical interventions and procedures that are provided in the healthcare setting
- The frequency of particular types of infections within a particular healthcare setting

- The impact of the infection (including percent case fatality and excess costs associated with the infection)
- The preventability of the infection required mandatory reporting elements (e.g., antibiotic-resistant organisms, ventilator-associated pneumonia).
- Required mandatory reporting elements (e.g., antibiotic-resistant organisms, ventilator-associated pneumonia).

Data Collection

- The infection control nurse (ICN) should visit daily to the high-risk areas (ICUs) and collect the clinical data of patient on devices and the patients admitted following surgeries.
- Collection of infection data for surveillance purposes must be done using validated, published definitions for HAIs.
- In order to generate valid HAI rates, information must be collected on those who are at risk of getting an HAI (denominator) and those who actually develop an HAI (numerator).
- Electronic screening of patient records is an emerging tool for identification of potential HAIs. These computerized systems of case finding reduce the time spent by Infection Control Professionals (ICPs) in case finding.
- Post-discharge surveillance for surgical site infection is important component of a surveillance system in acute care, due to shorter hospital stays following surgeries and an increasing proportion of surgeries taking place in the outpatient setting.

Interpretation of Data

- Surveillance data require interpretation to identify areas where improvements to infection prevention and control practices can be implemented to lower the risk of HAI.
- HAI rates may be compared for the same location across different time frames, or between different locations of same or different hospitals during same time frame.
- When comparing HAI rates to those of other healthcare settings, it is essential that the same case finding methods are used, the same case definitions are applied and the same methods for risk stratification are employed.

Communication of Result/Data Dissemination

The monthly HAI surveillance report generated should be shared with:
- All the clinical department and administration,
- A healthcare setting's Infection Prevention and Control Committee, which provides an aggregate picture of all infections of interest in the hospital.
- A particular patient area, focused on the risk of specific types of infections that are of importance to these groups.
- Patient/resident care staff following the identification of an emerging risk of infection, to notify or notify of the required precautions in infection prevention and control
- Local public health unit when there is a reportable communicable disease event.

HOSPITAL INFECTION CONTROL COMMITTEE (HICC) AND INFECTION CONTROL TEAM (ICT)

The HICC is an integral component of the patient safety program of the healthcare facility and is responsible for establishing and maintaining infection prevention and control, its monitoring, surveillance, reporting, research and education.

Infection control program operates at two levels:
1. **Advisory body:** Comprises of Hospital Infection Control Committee (HICC)
2. **Executive body:** Comprises of Infection Control Team (ICT)

The HICC is run an organized by Hospital Chief Administrator for which his/she constitutes the infection control committee. This committee includes wide representation from all relevant disciplines or departments in the facility. The committee has one elected chairperson who is the hospital administrator or a person who has direct access to the head of the hospital.

Structure

- **Chairperson:** Head of the Institute (preferably Medical Suprintendent)
- **Member secretary:** Senior Microbiologist (usually the Head of Department of Microbiology)
- **Hospital infection control officer (ICO):** Usually a representative from department of microbiology
- Hospital infection control nurse (ICN)

- Head of all the clinical, i.e., all medical and surgical departments
- Clinical staff head
- OT supervisor
- In-charge central sterilization department (CSSD)
- In-charge biomedical waste management (BMW)
- In-charge pharmacist
- Epidemiologist
- Relevant medical faculties
- **Support services:** (Housekeeping/Sanitation, engineering, store officer/Materials department)

Functions of Hospital Infection Control Committee (HICC)

Prevention of HAIs in patients is a concern of everyone involved in the patient care and is the responsibility of all individuals and services providing health care. The role of the hospital infection control committee is to implement the annual infection control program and policies. Some of the roles of HICC are as following:
- HAI surveillance: CAUTI, CLABSI, VAP, SSI
- Develops a system for identification, reporting, analyzing and controlling HAI
- Review and update hospital infection control policies and procedures from time to time.
- Making policies for proper antibiotic usage. Implementing Antimicrobial Stewardship Program
- Outbreak management. Develop strategies to control outbreaks **(Fig. 5.2)**.

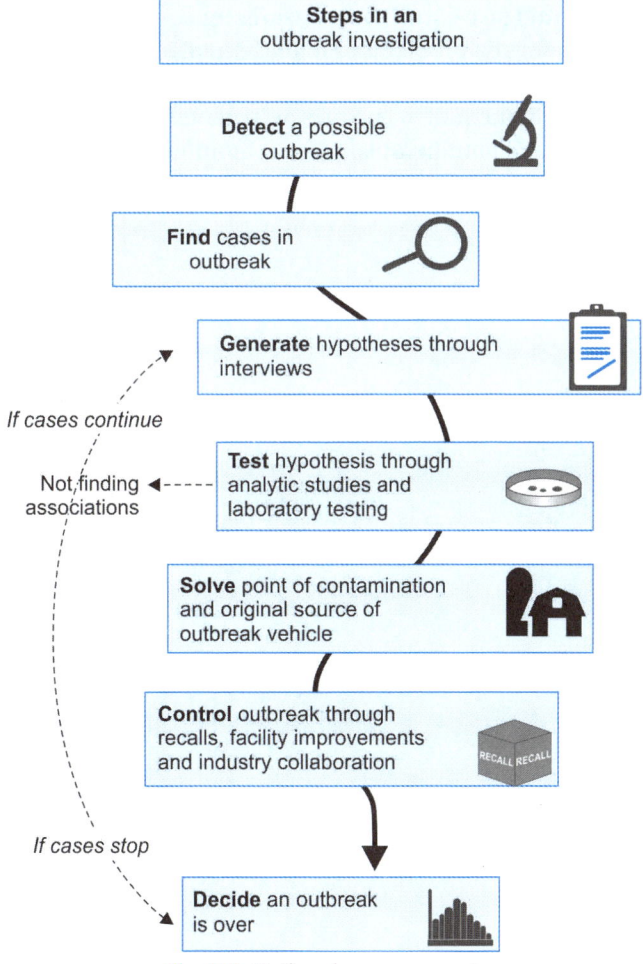

Fig. 5.2: Outbreak management.

- Develop and implement preventive and corrective programs in specific situations where infection hazards exist.
- Advice the Medical Superintendent on matters related to the proper use of antibiotics, develop antibiotic policies and recommend remedial measures when antibiotic resistant strains are detected.
- Conduct teaching sessions for healthcare workers regarding matters related to HAIs
- Monitor staff health activities regarding matters related to HAIs, such as needle stick injury prevention, hepatitis B vaccination, etc.
- Review risk associated with new technologies and monitor infection risk of new devices and products before to their use.

HICC shall meet regularly—once a month and as often as required. The committee is responsible for establishing and maintaining infection prevention and control, its monitoring, surveillance, reporting, research and education.

Infection Control Team (ICT)

The infection control team comprise an Infection Control Officer, a microbiologist and infection control nurse. ICT takes daily measures for the prevention and control of infection in hospital.

Responsibilities of ICT

The various responsibility of ICT is as following:
- To develop a standard operating procedure (SOP) of policies and procedures for aseptic, isolation and antiseptic techniques.
- To advise staff on all aspects of infection control and maintain a safe environment for patients and staff
- To supervise and monitor cleanliness and hygienic practices
- To oversee sterilization and disinfection and monitor the use and quality control of disinfectants
- To advise management of at risk patients and supervision of isolation procedures
- To investigate outbreaks of infection and take corrective measures for control and prevention of outbreak.
- To provide relevant information on infection problems to management
- To assist in training of all new employees as to the importance of infection control and the relevant policies and procedures.
- To organize regular training program for the staff to ensure implementation of infection control practices
- To audit infection control procedures and antimicrobial usage—monitors healthcare workers safety program

CHAPTER 6

Isolation Precautions and Use of Personal Protective Equipments

Chapter Outline

- Isolation Precautions
- Personal Protective Equipment
- Donning and Doffing

ISOLATION PRECAUTIONS

To define various categories for isolation and also indications and requirements for each category for isolation.

Routes of Transmission

Microorganisms are transmitted by various routes. Five main routes of transmission—contact, droplet, airborne, common vehicle, and vector borne.

A. Contact Transmission

This is the most important and frequent means of transmission of nosocomial infections and can be divided into two subgroups—direct contact and indirect contact.

I. Direct Contact

Involves direct physical transfer between a susceptible host and an infected or colonized person, such as occurs when hospital personnel turn patients, give baths, change dressings, or perform other procedures requiring direct personal contact.

Direct contact can also occur between two patients, one serving as the source of infection and the other as a susceptible host.

II. Indirect Contact

Involves personal contact of the susceptible host with contaminated intermediate object, usually inanimate, such as bed linens, clothing, instruments, dressings, contaminated hands not washed and gloves that are not changed.

B. Droplet Transmission

Droplets (more than 5 µm, in size) are generated from the source patient mainly through coughing, sneezing and talking as well as aerosolizing procedures as suctioning. Transmission occurs when droplets containing the infective agent are coughed, etc., through the air and deposited on mucous membranes of susceptible person. Droplets do not remain suspended in the air, thus special ventilation is not necessary.

C. Air-borne Transmission

Occurs by dissemination of either droplet nuclei (less than 5 µm, in size, residue of evaporated droplets that may remain suspended in the air for long periods of time) or dust particles in the air containing the infectious agent. Organisms carried in this manner can be widely dispersed by air currents before being inhaled by or deposited on the susceptible host. Special air handling (6–12 air changes/hour, monitored HEPA filters, discharge of air outdoors) is needed to prevent this transmission.

D. Common Vehicle Route

Diseases transmitted through contaminated items, such as:
- Food (Salmonellosis)
- Water (Legionellosis)
- Drugs (Bacteremia resulting from infusion of a contaminated infusion product)
- Blood (Hepatitis B, Hepatitis C, HIV)

E. Vector-borne Transmission

Occurs when vectors, such as flies, mosquitoes transmit disease. Isolation precautions are designed to prevent the spread of microorganisms among patients, personnel, and visitors. Since agent and host factors are more difficult to control, interruption of the chain of infection in the hospital is directed primarily at transmission.

Recommendations for Isolation Precautions

These recommendations are designed to prevent transmission of infectious agents among patients and healthcare personnel in all settings where healthcare is delivered.

Standard Precautions

- Standard precautions apply to—(1) blood; (2) all body fluids, secretions, and excretions except sweat, regardless of whether or not they contain visible blood; (3) non-intact skin; and (4) mucous membranes.
- Standard precautions are designed to reduce the risk of transmission of microorganisms from both recognized and unrecognized sources of infection in hospitals. Every person is potentially infected or colonized with an organism that could be transmitted in the healthcare setting.

Key Components

- Hand hygiene and hand hygiene moments **(Fig. 6.1 and Table 6.1)**
- Personal protective equipment
- Respiratory hygiene
- Patient placement
- Patient-care equipment and instruments/devices
- Care of environment
- Care of textiles/laundry
- Safe injection practices
- Handling needles and sharps

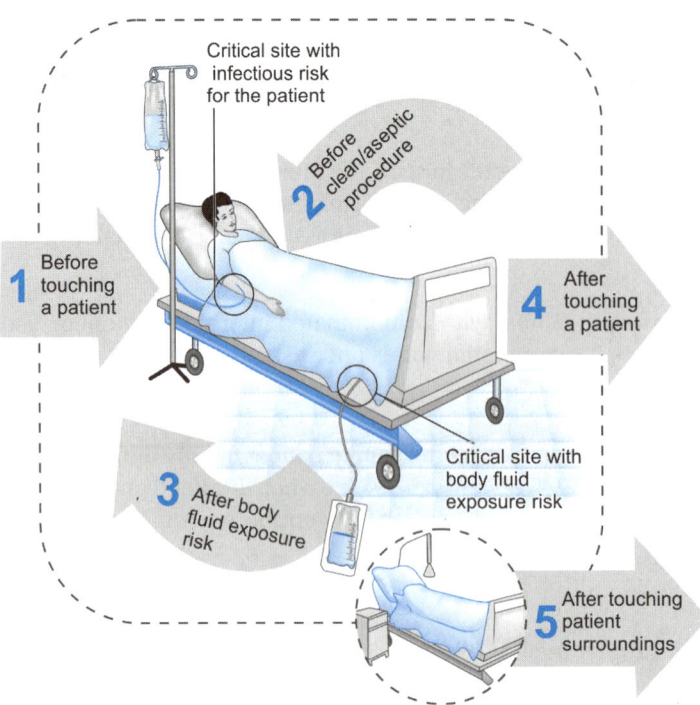

Fig. 6.1: Five moments of hand hygiene.

TABLE 6.1: Hand hygiene: Five moments.	
Key moments	**Situations when moment applies**
1. Before patient contact	• Before shaking hands • Before assisting a patient in personal care activities: To move, to take bath, to eat, to get dressed • Before delivering care and other non-invasive treatment: Applying oxygen mask • Before performing a physical non-invasive examination: Taking pulse, BP, chest auscultation, recording ECG
2. Before clean/aseptic procedure	• Before brushing the patient teeth, instilling eye drops, examining mouth, nose, ear with/without know instrument, inserting a suppository/pessary, suctioning mucous • Before dressing a wound with/without instrument, applying ointment on vesicle, making a percutaneous injection/puncture. • Before inserting an invasive medical device (nasal cannula, NG tube, endotracheal tube, urinary probe, percutaneous catheter, drainage), opening any circuit of an invasive medical device (for load medication, draining, suctioning, monitoring purposes) • Before preparing food, medications, pharmaceutical products, sterile material
3. After body fluid exposure risk	• When the contact with a mucous membrane and with non-intact skin ends • After a percutaneous injection or puncture, after inserting an invasive medical device (vascular access, catheter, tube, drain, etc.), after disrupting and opening an invasive circuit. • After removing an invasive medical device • After removing any form of material offering protection • (Napkin, dressing, gauze, sanitary towel, etc.) • After handling a sample containing organic matter, after cleaning excreta and any other body fluid, after cleaning any contaminated surface and soiled material (soiled bed linen, dentures, instruments, urinal, bedpan, lavatories, etc.)
4. After touching a patient	• After shaking hands, stroking a child's forehead • After you have assisted the patient in personal care activities, to move, to bath, to eat, to dress, etc. • After delivering care and other non-invasive treatment, changing bed linen as patient is in, applying oxygen mask, giving a massage • After performing a physical non-invasive examination—taking pulse, BP, chest auscultation, recording ECG.
5. After touching patients surroundings	• After an activity involving physical contact with patients immediate environment, changing bed linen with the patient out of bed, holding a bed rail, clearing a bedside table • After a care activity, adjusting perfusion speed, clearing a monitoring alarm • After other contacts with surfaces or inanimate objects—leaning against a bed/night table/bedside table

PERSONAL PROTECTIVE EQUIPMENT

Personal protective equipment (PPE) is specialized clothing or equipment, worn by an employee for protection against infectious materials **(Fig. 6.2)**.

Principles of Use

- Wear PPE when the nature of the anticipated patient interaction indicates that contact with blood or body fluids may occur.
- Prevent contamination of clothing and skin during the process of removing PPE
- Before leaving the patient's room or cubicle, remove and discard PPE. Do not share PPE

Selection of PPE

- **Types of isolation precautions applied**
- **Durability** of the PPE, it must be fit the individual accurately
- **Appropriate use of PPE**
- **Training:** The user should have an appropriate knowledge how to use the PPE
- **Disposal or should be done accordingly.**
- Selection of PPE is determined by the type of anticipated exposure, such as touch, splashes or sprays, or large volumes of blood or body fluids that might penetrate the clothing.

Section II: Infection Control and Safety

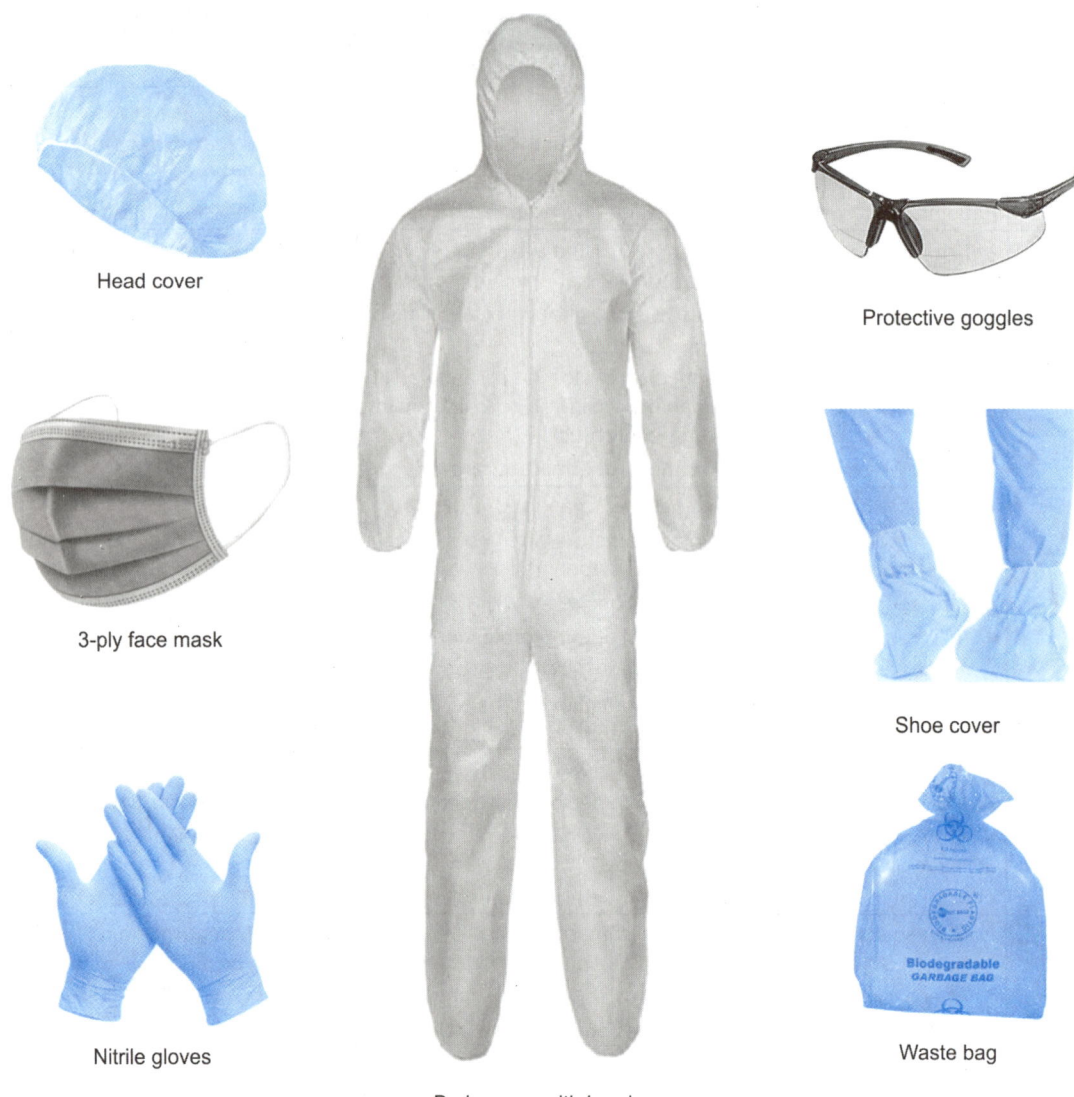

Fig. 6.2: Personal protective equipment.

Components

Personal protective equipment includes:
- Gloves
- Protective eye wear (goggles)
- Masks and respirators
- Apron
- Gown
- boots/shoe covers; and
- Cap/hair covers

DONNING AND DOFFING (FIGS. 6.3 AND 6.4)

This is an important step in order to minimize the risk of transmission of infection.

Donning **(wearing)** and doffing **(removing)** must should be performed in a particular sequence.

- **Donning (wearing):** Gown first → mask or respirator → goggle or face shield → gloves.
- **Doffing (removing):** Gloves first → goggle or face shield → gown → mask or respirator.

Sequence for PUTTING ON personal protective equipment (PPE)

The type of PPE used will vary based on the level of precautions required, such as standard and contact droplet or airborne infection isolation precautions. The procedure for putting on and removing PPE should be tailored to the specific type of PPE

1. Gown
- Fully cover torso from neck to knees, arms to end of wrists, and wrap around the back
- Fasten in back of neck and waist

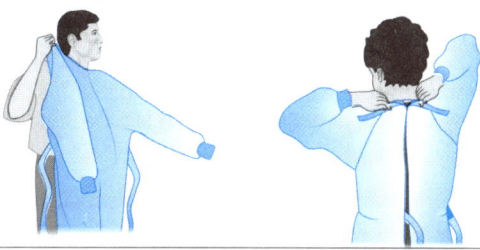

2. Mask or respirator
- Secure ties or elastic bands at middle of head and neck
- Fit flexible band to nose bridge
- Fit snug to face and below chin
- Fit-check respirator

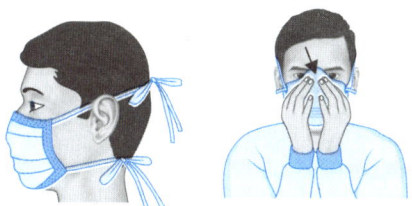

3. Goggles or face shield place over face and eyes and adjust to fit

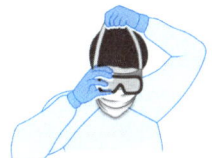 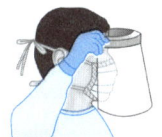 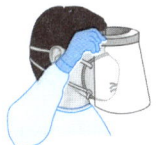

4. Gloves extend to cover wrist of isolation gown

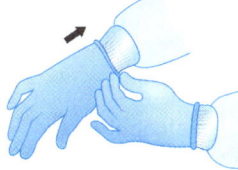

Use safe work practices to protect yourself and limit the spread of contamination

- Keep hands away from face
- Limit surfaces touched
- Change gloves when torn or heavily contaminated
- Perform hand hygiene

Fig. 6.3: Donning of PPE.

How to safely remove personal protective equipment (PPE)

There are a variety of ways to safely remove PPE without contaminating your clothing, skin, or mucous membranes with potentially infectious materials. Here is one example. Remove all PPE before exiting the patient room except a respirator, if worn. Remove the respirator after leaving the patient room and closing the door. Remove PPE in the following sequence:

1. Gloves
- Outside of gloves are contaminated!
- If your hands get contaminated during glove removal, immediately wash your hands or use an alcohol-based hand sanitizer
- Using a gloved hand, grasp the palm area of the other gloved hand and peel off first glove
- Hold removed glove in gloved hand
- Slide fingers of ungloved hand under remaining glove at wrist and peel off second glove over first glove
- Discard gloves in a waste container

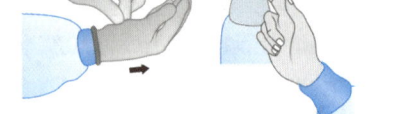

2. Goggles or face shield
- Outside of goggles or face shield are contaminated!
- If your hands get contaminated during goggle or face shield removal, immediately wash your hands or use an alcohol-based hand sanitizer
- Remove goggles or face shield from the back by lifting head band or ear pieces
- If the item is reusable, place in designated receptacle for reprocessing. Otherwise, discard in a waste container

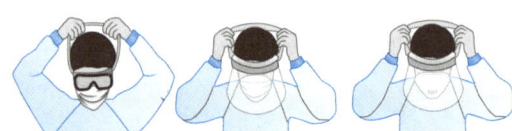

3. Gown
- Gown front and sleeves are contaminated!
- If your hands get contaminated during gown removal, immediately wash your hands or use an alcohol-based hand sanitizer
- Unfasten gown ties, taking care that sleeves do not contact your body when reaching for ties
- Pull gown away from neck and shoulders, touching inside of gown only
- Turn gown inside out
- Fold or roll into a bundle and discard in a waste container

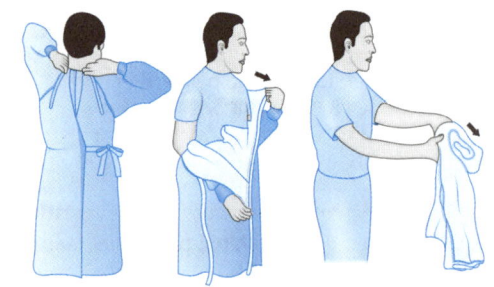

4. Mask or respirator
- Front of mask/respirator is contaminated — DO NOT TOUCH!
- If your hands get contaminated during mask/respirator removal, immediately wash your hands or use an alcohol-based hand sanitizer
- Grasp bottom ties or elastics of the mask/respirator, then the ones at the top, and remove without touching the front
- Discard in a waste container

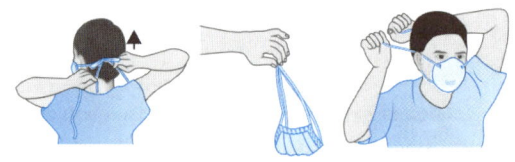

5. Wash hands or use an alcohol-based Hand sanitizer immediately after Removing all PPE

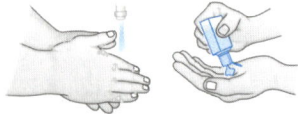

Perform hand hygiene between steps if hands become contaminated and immediately after removing all PPE

Fig. 6.4: Doffing of PPE.

Gloves (Tables 6.2 and 6.3)

- Wear gloves when it can be reasonably anticipated that contact with blood or other potentially infectious materials, mucous membranes, non-intact skin, or potentially contaminated intact skin could occur.
- Wear gloves with fit and durability appropriate to the task
- Wear disposable medical examination gloves for providing direct patient care.
- Wear disposable medical examination gloves or reusable utility gloves for cleaning the environment or medical equipment.
- Remove gloves after contact with a patient and/or the surrounding environment (including medical equipment) using proper technique to prevent hand contamination
- Do not wear the same pair of gloves for the care of more than one patient.
- Change gloves during patient care if the hands will move from a contaminated body-site (e.g., perineal area) to a clean body-site (e.g., face), or if the gloves are damaged.

TABLE 6.2: Types of gloves.

Type of glove	Indication
Latex	• Used in activity with high biological risk, that is, when it is necessary to handle blood or body fluids in a repeated or prolonged way. • Provides good protection against pathogen. • High tensile strength, extremely flexible • Contraindicated in latex allergy; should not be used with organic soils, oils, gas, or grease
Nitrile	• Alternative to latex, especially if allergic to latex, for high-biological-risk procedures • Moderate protection against pathogens • High puncture and chemical resistance; good comfort, soft and flexible, but stiffer than latex • More-expensive option
Vinyl–polyvinyl	• Use in case of low biological risk (low protection against pathogens), for patient cleaning activities. • Food prep (low heat) • Average resistance to chemicals (alcohols), low tensile strength • Less-expensive option
Polyethylene	• Only maneuvers where one-handed and short-lasting sterility is required (intravesical catheterization, endotracheal aspiration) • Loose fit, ideal for frequent glove change, but low protection against hazardous materials • Very economical
Rubber or neoprene	• Used to prepare surgical instruments and endoscopes for disinfection, cleaning of environments. • High mechanical resistance

TABLE 6.3: Classification of gloves according to their use with clinical situations.

Types of gloves	Indication of use	Example
Nonsterile gloves	Used if there is risk of transmission of infection from patient to HCWs • Potential for exposure to body, body fluids, secretions, or excretions • Contact with non-intact skin or mucous membranes	• Venipuncture • Vaginal examination • Dental examination • Emptying urinary catheter bag • Nasogastric aspiration • Management of minor cuts and abrasions
Sterile gloves	Used for procedure where sterile environment is required and prevents the transmission of organism from patients to HCWs and HCWs to patients	Surgical aseptic technique procedures: • Urinary catheter site dressing • Central venous line insertion site dressing • Lumbar puncture • Clinical care of surgical wounds or drainage sites • Dental procedures
Reusable utility gloves	Used for non-patient care activities	• Cleaning or handling of contaminated equipments • Housekeeping duties • Instrument cleaning in CSSD unit

Gowns

- Wear a gown, to protect skin and prevent soiling or contamination of clothing during procedures and patient-care activities when contact with blood, body fluids secretions, or excretions is anticipated.
- Wear a gown for direct patient contact if the patient has uncontained secretions or excretions.
- Remove gown and perform hand hygiene before leaving the patient's environment.
- Do not wear the same gown for the care of more than one patient.

Mouth, Nose, Eye Protection

- Use PPE to protect the mucous membranes of the eyes, nose and mouth during procedures and patient-care activities that are likely to generate splashes or sprays of blood, body fluids, secretions and excretions. Select masks, goggles, face shields, and combinations of each according to the need anticipated by the task performed.
- During aerosol-generating procedures (e.g., bronchoscopy, suctioning of the respiratory tract, endotracheal intubation) in patients who are not suspected of being infected with an agent for which respiratory protection is otherwise recommended (e.g., *M. tuberculosis*), wear one of the following—a face shield that fully covers the front and sides of the face, a mask with attached shield, or a mask and goggles (in addition to gloves and gown).
- If available, wear N95 or higher respirators for potential exposure to infectious agents transmitted via the airborne route (e.g., tuberculosis).

Caps

In aseptic units, operating rooms, or performing selected invasive procedures, staff must wear caps which completely cover the hair.

Respiratory Hygiene/Face Mask/Respirators (Fig. 6.5)

- Respiratory hygiene is important in source containment of infectious respiratory secretions in symptomatic patients, beginning at initial point of encounter, e.g., triage and reception areas in emergency departments and physician offices.
- Instruct symptomatic persons to cover mouth/nose when sneezing/coughing or sneeze into the crook of elbow.
- Use tissues and dispose.
- Observe hand hygiene after soiling of hands with respiratory secretions.

Composition of Surgical Mask It has three layers		
1. Outer fluid repellent layer	**2. Middle filter layer**	**3. Inner hydrophilic layer**
• It is hydrophobic in nature • It repels water, blood and other body fluids	• It is made of melt-blown material • It filters bacteria/viruses and outer water droplets • Pore size is not standardized	• Hydrophilic (water loving) in nature • It is made up of non-woven fabrics • It absorbs water, sweat and spit

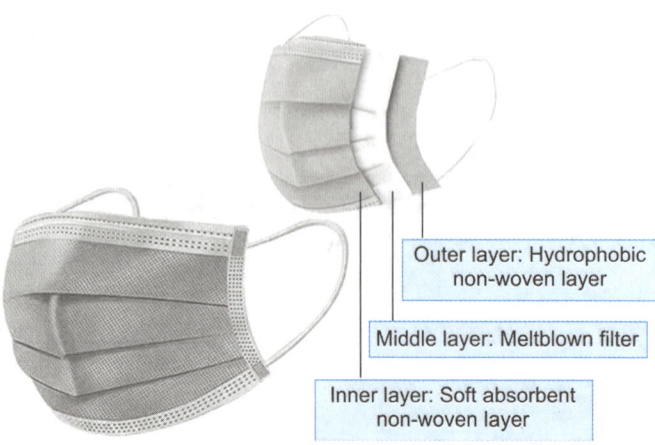

Fig. 6.5: Surgical mask.

N95 Respirator

- N95 means not resistant to oil and ability to filter off 95% of air-borne particles.
- It is comprised of four layers of material (**Fig. 6.6**)
  - *Outer and inner layer:* Made of spun bound polypropylene
  - *Middle two layers:* Made of cellulose/polyester, melt blow polypropylene filter.
- They are described as negative pressure as the pressure inside the face piece is negative during inhalation as compared to pressure outside the respirator.
- They should be removed or changed once in 8 hours or earlier if it gets wet or dirty, deformed or torn.
- It is also for single use, it should not be reused as it cannot be cleaned or disinfected.
- After wearing one must should perform a fit check to ensure if it is properly fitted it include following steps:
  1. *Sealing:* The respirator is compressed to ensure a seal across the face, cheeks and nasal bridge
  2. *Positive pressure seal:* It is checked by gently exhaling, if air escapes the respirator needs to be adjusted.
  3. *Negative pressure seal:* It is cheeked by gently inhaling, if respirator is not drawn toward the face, or air leaks around the face seal then it is readjusted.

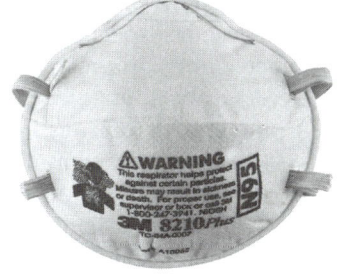

Fig. 6.6: N95 respirator.

Understanding the difference

	Surgical Mask	N95 Respirator
Testing and approval	Cleared by the US Food and Drug Administration (**FDA**)	Evaluated, tested, and approved by NIOSH as per the requirements in 42 CFR part 84
Intended use and purpose	Fluid resistant and provides the wearer protection against large droplets, splashes, or sprays of bodily or other hazardous fluids. Protects the patient from the wearer's respiratory emissions	Reduces wearer's exposure to particles including small particle aerosols and large droplets (only non-oil aerosols)
Face seal fit	Loose-fitting	Tight-fitting
Fit testing requirement	No	Yes
User seal check requirement	No	Yes. Required each time the respirator is donned (put on)
Filtration	Does not provide the wearer with a reliable level of protection from inhaling smaller air-borne particles and is not considered respiratory protection	Filters out at least 95% of air-borne particles including large and small particles
Leakage	Leakage occurs around the edge of the mask when user inhales	When property fitted and donned, minimal leakage occurs around edges of the respirator when user inhales
Use limitations	Disposable, discard after each patient encounter	Ideally should be discarded after each patient encounter and after aerosol-generating procedures. It should also be discarded when it becomes damaged or deformed; no longer forms an effective seal to the face; becomes wet or visibly dirty; breathing becomes difficult; or if it becomes contaminated with blood, respiratory or nasal secretions, or other bodily fluids from patients

Patient Placement

- Place patients who pose a risk for transmission to others (e.g., uncontained secretions, excretions or wound drainage; infants with suspected viral respiratory or gastrointestinal infections) in a single-patient room when available or patients infected or colonized by the same organism can be cohered (sharing of room/s).
- **Determine patient placement based on the following principles:**
  - Route(s) of transmission of the known or suspected infectious agent
  - Risk factors for transmission in the infected patient
  - Risk factors for adverse outcomes resulting from an HAI in other patients
  - Availability of single-patient rooms
  - Patient options for room-sharing (e.g., chortling patients with the same infection)

Patient-care Equipment and Instruments/Devices

- Handle in a manner that prevents transfer of microorganisms to others and to the environment; wear gloves if visibly contaminated; perform hand hygiene.
- Remove organic material from critical and semi-critical instrument/devices, using recommended cleaning agents before high level disinfection and sterilization to enable effective disinfection and sterilization processes.

Care of Environment

- Clean and disinfect surfaces that are likely to be contaminated with pathogens, including those that are in close proximity to the patient (e.g., bed rails, over bed tables) and frequently touched surfaces in the patient care environment (e.g., door knobs, surfaces in and surrounding toilets in patients' rooms) on a more frequent schedule compared to that for other surfaces.
- Use hospital approved disinfectants. Use in accordance with manufacturer's instructions.

Care of Textiles/Laundry

Handle used textiles and fabrics with minimum agitation to avoid contamination of air, surfaces and persons.

Safe Injection Practices

The following recommendations apply to the use of needles, cannulas that replace needles, and, where applicable intravenous delivery systems **(Fig. 6.7)**:

- Use aseptic technique to avoid contamination of sterile injection equipment.
- Do not administer medications from a syringe to multiple patients, even if the needle or cannula on the syringe is changed. Needles, cannula and syringes are sterile, single-use items; they should neither be reused for another patient nor to access a medication or solution that might be used for a subsequent patient. Use fluid infusion and administration sets (i.e., intravenous bags, tubing and connectors) for one patient only and dispose appropriately after use. Consider a syringe or needle/cannula contaminated once it has been used to enter or connect to a patient's intravenous infusion bag or administration set.

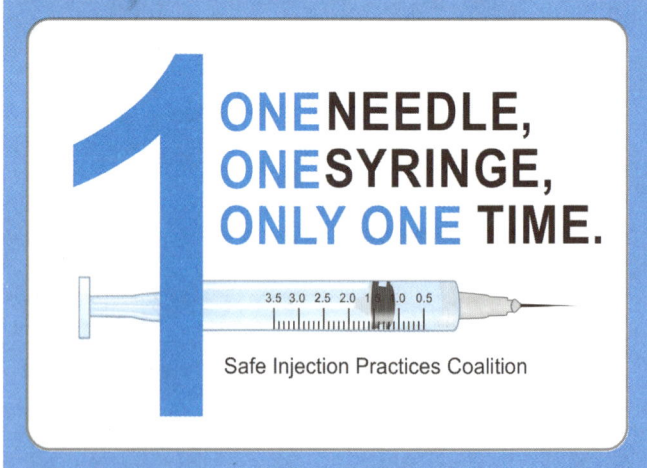

Fig. 6.7: Safe injection practices.

- Do not administer medications from single-dose vials or ampules to multiple patients or combine leftover contents for later use.
- If multidose vials must be used, both the needle or cannula and syringe used to access the multidose vial need be sterile.
- Do not keep multidose vials in the immediate patient treatment area and store in accordance with the manufacturer's recommendations; discard if sterility is compromised or questionable.

CHAPTER 7

Hand Hygiene

Chapter Outline

- Methods of Hand Hygiene
- Hand Hygiene Products
- WHO Hand Hygiene Promotion
- Strategies to Improve Hand Hygiene

INTRODUCTION

Hand hygiene is the primary measure proven to be effective in preventing healthcare associated infections (HAIs) and the spread of antimicrobial resistance. Failure to perform appropriate hand hygiene is considered to be the leading cause of HAIs and the spread of multi-resistant organisms and has been recognized as a significant contributor to outbreaks.

As defined by CDC, hand hygiene encompasses the cleansing of hands with soap and water, antiseptic hand washes, antiseptic hand rubs, such as alcohol-based hand sanitizers, foams or gels, or surgical hand antisepsis.

Hand washing is the act of washing hands with soap, either antimicrobial or non-antimicrobial, and water for at least 15 to 20 seconds with a vigorous motion to cause friction making sure to include all surfaces of the hands and fingers.

Indication of Hand Hygiene

My 5 Moments of Hand Hygiene

My 5 moments of hand hygiene, is an approach by WHO which defines the important moments when the HCWs should perform hand hygiene. This is an evidence and research based, field tested approach designed make the learning easy in a wide range of healthcare settings.

My 5 moments of hand hygiene as per WHO **(Fig. 7.1)**:

- **Moment 1**: Before touching a patient
- **Moment 2:** Before clean/aseptic procedures
- **Moment 3**: After body fluid exposure/risk
- **Moment 4:** After touching patient
- **Moment 5**: After touching patient surroundings

METHODS OF HAND HYGIENE

The hand washing methods are of three types **(Table 7.1)**:
1. Hand rub
2. Hand wash
3. Surgical hand scrub

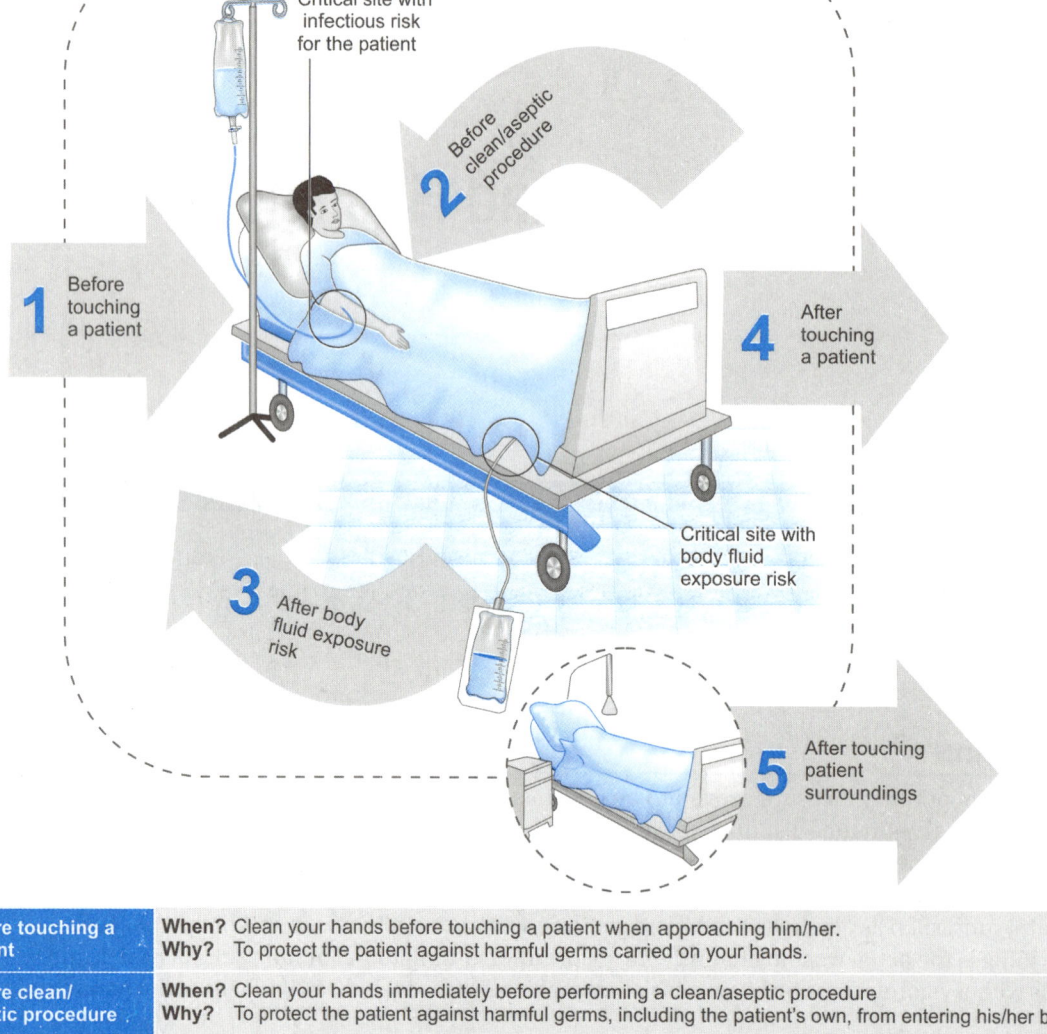

1 Before touching a patient	When?	Clean your hands before touching a patient when approaching him/her.
	Why?	To protect the patient against harmful germs carried on your hands.
2 Before clean/aseptic procedure	When?	Clean your hands immediately before performing a clean/aseptic procedure
	Why?	To protect the patient against harmful germs, including the patient's own, from entering his/her body.
3 After body fluid exposure risk	When?	Clean your hands immediately after an exposure risk to body fluids (and after glove removal)
	Why?	To protect yourself and the healthcare environment from harmful patient germs.
4 After touching a patient	When?	Clean your hands after touching a patient and her/his immediate surroundings, when leaving the patient's side.
	Why?	To protect yourself and the healthcare environment from harmful patient germs.
5 After touching patient surroundings	When?	Clean your hands after touching any object or furniture in the patient's immediate surrounding. when leaving—even if the patient has not been touched.
	Why?	To protect yourself and the healthcare environment from harmful patient germs.

Fig. 7.1: Five moments of hand hygiene.
Source: WHO Guidelines on hand hygiene in health care: A Summary (2009).

TABLE 7.1: Indications for using hand hygiene methods.

Hand rub	Hand wash	Surgical hand scrub
• This should be used during routine clinical rounds and while handling the patients. • If the hands are not visibly dry, not contaminated with blood or body fluids, etc.	• If the hands are visibly dry, contaminated with blood or body fluids, etc. • Potential exposure to organisms especially spore forming (e.g., *Clostridioides difficile*), non-enveloped virus, such as norovirus, rotavirus, etc. • Handling diarrhea patient • After using restroom • Before handling medication or food	Before any surgical procedure and also in between the cases

HAND HYGIENE PRODUCTS

These are mainly designed for hand washing or handrub. Hand wash refers to the application of soap (plain or antimicrobial) and water on the hands for duration of 40–60 seconds.

Hand Wash Products

Water and Soap

It removes dirt and organic matter as well as microbial contamination of hand by mechanical action. **Plain soap with** neutral pH has minimal antimicrobial activity but it can be still used for hand washing. It acts through its detergent property. Liquid soap is preferred over soap bar.

Antiseptic Handwash

These are more effective than soap and water in removing residential normal flora.
- Chlorhexidine gluconate **(CHG 4%)** is recommended for hand washing.
- Povidone-iodine solution
- Triclosan

Handrub Products

Alcohol and chlorhexidine are widely used handrub products among the various handrub products available.

Alcohol-based Handrub (AHBR)

- This removes organism more effectively, requires less time and irritates skin less as compared to soap and other antiseptic agents and water.
- They act by denaturing the proteins (mechanism of action)
- Minimum 20–30 seconds of duration is recommended by WHO
- No fixed volume recommended; it depends as per need.
- It is available in the form of gel, rinses or liquid and foam (liquid is preferred)

Surgical Hand Disinfection

AHBR can also be used for surgical hand preparations. It requires a specific skill set to ensure proper technique.

Chlorhexidine Hand Rub

- Chlorhexidine-based alcohol handrubs are the second most common handrubs used in hospitals.
- They act by disruption of cytoplasmic membrane (mechanism of action)
- The immediate effect of alcohol and slow but persistent activity of chlorhexidine complement each other and therefore CHG handrub is preferred in high-risk locations, such as ICUs (synergistic effect).

THE WORLD HEALTH ORGANIZATION (WHO) RECOMMENDS 6 STEPS IN HAND HYGIENE

This includes **(Fig. 7.2)**.
1. Palm to palm,
2. Right palm over the left dorsum and vice versa
3. Palm to palm with fingers interlaced,
4. Backs of fingers to opposing palms,
5. Rubbing of thumbs and
6. Rubbing of fingertips.

    When rinsing off water remember to keep hands down and elbows up, then dry hands and wrists entirely with clean or disposable towels **(Fig. 7.3)**.

Hand Hygiene for Surgery

This follows specific vital steps using either an antimicrobial soap or an alcohol-based hand sanitizer before donning sterile gloves for surgical procedures. In contrast to hygienic hand washing, surgical hand preparation must remove the transient flora and reduce the presence of resident flora.

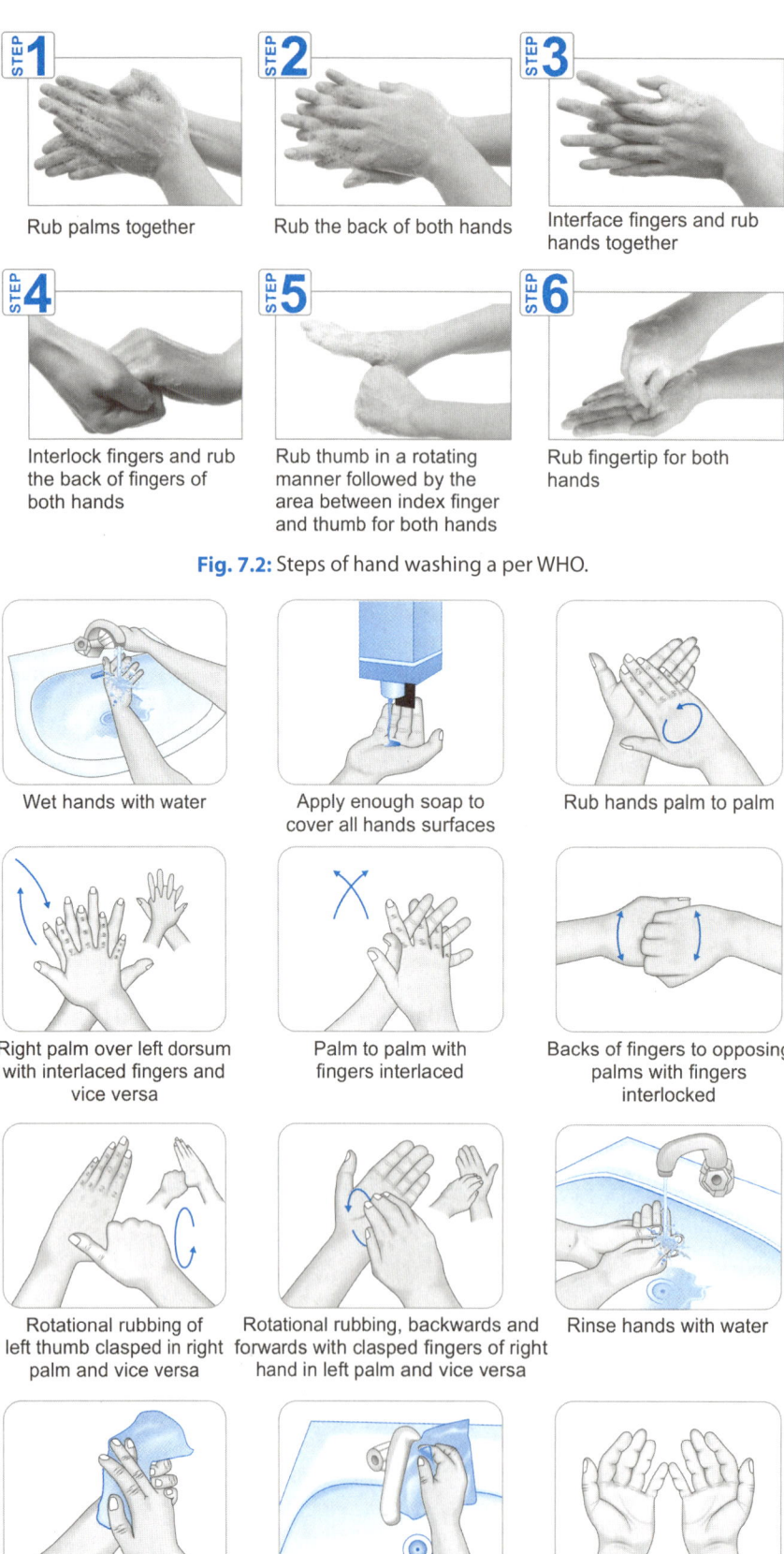

Fig. 7.2: Steps of hand washing a per WHO.

Fig. 7.3: Steps of hand wash.

Chapter 7: Hand Hygiene 141

STRATEGIES TO IMPROVE HAND HYGIENE

1. **Educating and training:** Continuous training and education is an important step for improving the hand hygiene. It should be done in appropriate language and pre-test and post-test should be conducted.
2. **Audit and feedback**
3. **Reminders:** Visual or auditory reminders should be installed like use of easy understanding poster and bright colored signs, eye catching screen savers, taking walls, voice mail messages, labels on equipment and supplies, etc.
4. **Reward-punish policy:** This should be followed by the organization to develop interest among HCWs for hand hygiene.
5. **Education sessions**
6. **Observation through CCTV cameras.**
7. **Electronic monitoring**

WHO HAND HYGIENE PROMOTION WORLD HAND HYGIENE DAY (5 MAY) (FIGS. 7.4A AND B)

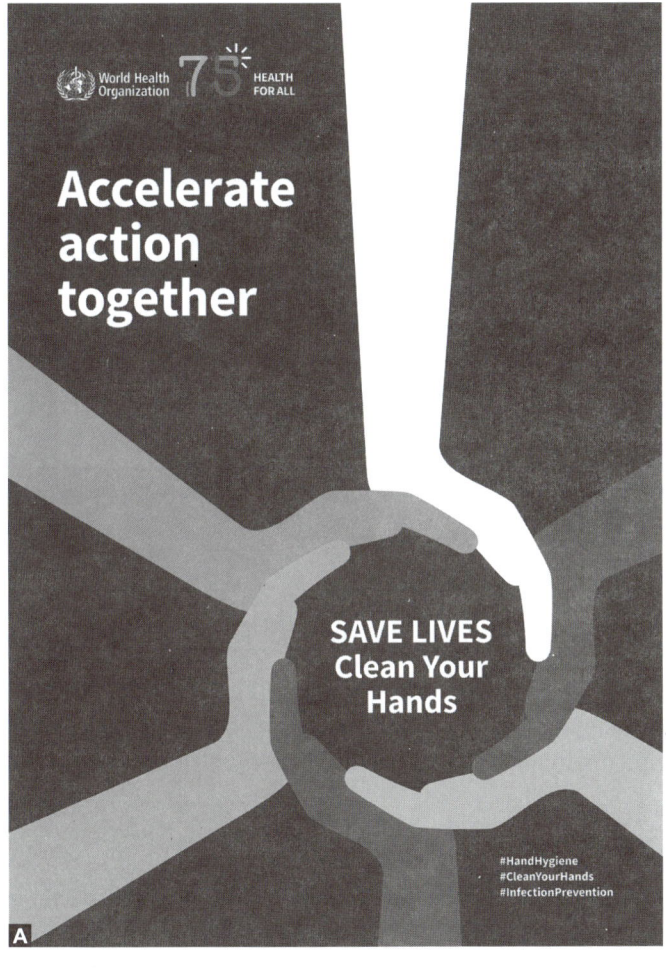
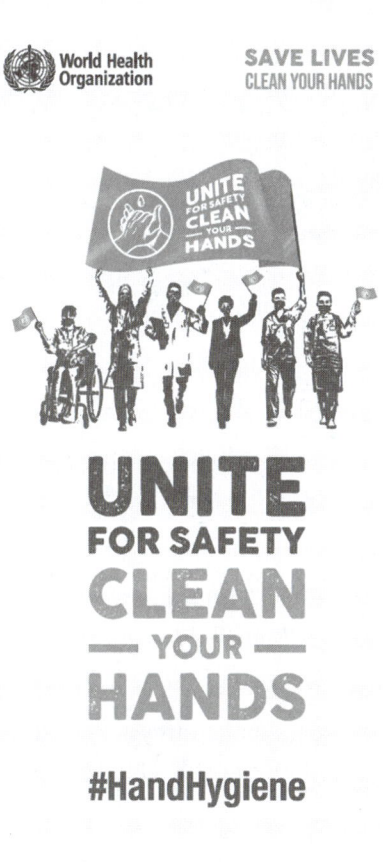

Figs. 7.4A and B: (A) WHO Hand Hygiene Promotion 2023; (B) WHO Hand Hygiene Promotion 2022.

CHAPTER 8

Disinfection and Sterilization

Chapter Outline

- Definitions
- Classification of Different Methods of Sterilization
- Rationale Approach of Sterilization for Equipment
- Spaulding's Principle
- Spaulding's Classification of Equipment Decontamination

DEFINITIONS

Microorganisms are responsible for contamination and infection. Sterilization aims to destroy them from materials or from surfaces.

Sterilization

It is a process by which all living and dead microorganisms, including viable spores are either destroyed or removed from an article, body surface or medium.

Disinfection

It refers to the process that destroys or removes all the pathogenic organisms but not bacterial spores. Primary action of a disinfectant is to destroy potential pathogens.

Antiseptic

It is an agent that can be safely applied on the skin or mucus membrane to prevent infection by inhibiting the growth of bacteria.

Decontamination (Sanitization)

It refers to the reduction of pathogenic microbial population to a level at which items are considered as safe to handle without protective attire.
- *Suffix 'cide' is used for agents who can kill microorganisms.*
- *Suffix 'static' is used for agents that do not kill but inhibit the microbial growth*

CLASSIFICATION OF DIFFERENT METHODS OF STERILIZATION

A. Physical Methods

1. Sunlight

2. Heat

Dry heat and moist heat

Dry Heat

- **Flaming:** Items are held in flame of Bunsen burner—long time exposure till they become red hot-inoculating wires and loops. Short time exposure for fragile items, such as mouth of test tubes.
- **Incineration:** Used for disposal of biomedical waste materials. It burns the anatomical and microbiology waste by providing very high temp 870–1200°C, thereby converting the waste into ash, flu gas and heat.
- **Hot air oven:** Widely used method of sterilization by dry heat (Fig. 8.1).
- **Temperature:** Holding temperature of 160°C for 2 hours is required for sterilization.
- **Materials sterilized:** Glassware, such as glass syringes, petri dishes, flasks, pipettes and test tubes. Surgical instruments, such as scalpels, forceps. Chemicals life paraffin, fats, glycerol, glove powder.

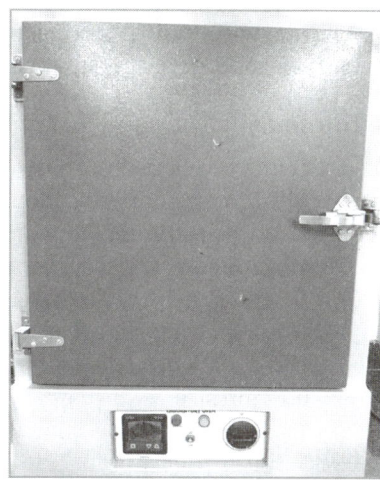

Fig. 8.1: Hot air oven.

Moist Heat

I. At temperature below 100°C

- **Pasteurization:** It is a method used for control of microorganisms in milk, juices and beer. Two methods are available
  - *Holder's method:* Milk is heated at 63°C for 30 mins
  - *Flash method:* Milk is heated at 72°C for 15–20 seconds followed by rapid cooling to 13°C or lower
- **Inspissation:** It is a process of heating an article on 3 successive days at 80–85°C for 30 minutes by an inspissator, e.g., Lowenstein-Jenson medium for *Mycobacterium tuberculosis* and Loeffler's serum slope for *Corynebacterium diphtheriae*.
- **Vaccine bath**

II. At temperature 100°C

- **Boiling:** Boiling of the items in water for 15 minutes can kill most of the vegetative forms but not spores. It is simple method of sterilization.
- **Tyndallization:** Method uses exposure at 100°C for 20 minutes for 3 consecutive days. Used for sterilization of media containing sugars or gelatine.
- **Steam sterilizer:** Used for media which are decomposed at high temperature of autoclave. Articles are kept on a perforated tray and exposed to steam at 100°C at atmospheric pressure for 90 minutes.

III. At temperature above 100°C

Autoclave (Fig. 8.2)

Principle: Water boils when its vapor pressure equals that of surrounding atmosphere. When atmospheric pressure is raised, boiling temperature is also raised. Bacteria are more susceptible to moist heat as bacterial proteins coagulates rapidly. Saturated steam can penetrate porous material easily.

Sterilization conditions:
- **Temperature:** 121°C
- **Chamber pressure:** 15 pounds (lbs) per square inch (psi).
- **Holding time:** 15 mins

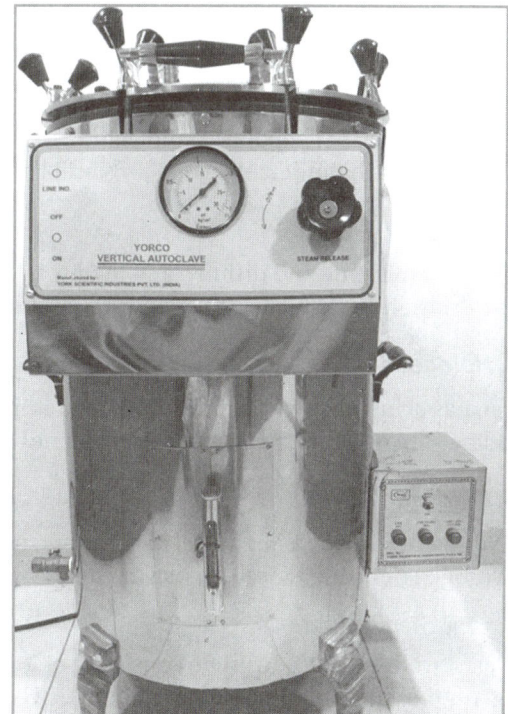

Fig. 8.2: Autoclave.

Uses: For surgical instruments, culture media, autoclavable plastic containers, rubber material, plastic tubes and pipette tips, solutions, biohazardous waste.

3. Ozone

Ozone sterilizer uses oxygen, water and electricity to produce ozone within the sterilizer and provide sterilization without producing toxic chemicals. It runs at lower temperature at 25–35°C. In this device, oxygen molecules are separated into atomic oxygen in presence of intense electrical field. This atomic oxygen combines with other oxygen molecules to form ozone. Ozone provides a good sterility assurance.

4. Filtration

It helps remove bacteria from heat labile liquids, such as sera and solutions of sugars and antibiotics. Different types of filters are:
a. **Candle filters:** For purification of water for drinking and industrial purpose
b. **Sintered glass filters:** Prepared by heat-fusing finely powdered glass particles of graded sizes
c. **Membrane filters:** Used for water purification, analysis, sterilization and sterility testing
d. **Air filters:** Used to deliver bacteria free air. Types of air filters are:
   - *High efficient particulate air filters (HEPA):* Removes 99.9% of particles size of 0.3 µm or more
   - *Ultra-low particulate air filters (ULPA):* Removes 99.99% of dust, pollen, mold, bacteria or any airborne particle of 0.12 µm size.

5. Radiation

- **Ionizing radiation:** Includes X-rays and gamma rays. Causes breakage of DNA without temperature rise. Destroys bacterial spores and vegetative cells but not much effective against viruses.
- **Non-ionizing radiation:** Includes infrared and ultraviolet radiations. Used for disinfection of clean surfaces in OTs, laminar flow hoods and for water treatment.

B. Chemical Methods

1. Alcohols

These are bactericidal, fungicidal and virucidal, e.g.; isopropyl alcohol, ethanol

2. Aldehydes

These are bactericidal, sporicidal and virucidal
- **Formaldehyde** or formalin used for preservation of anatomical specimens, formaldehyde gas used for disinfection of OTs, preparation of toxin.
- **Glutaraldehyde (2% Cidex):** Disinfects objects in 20 minutes. Effective for *Mycobacterium tuberculosis*, fungus and viruses (including HIV, hepatitis B and enteroviruses). It also kills spores. Rapid, broad spectrum, high level disinfectant.
- **Ortho-phthalaldehyde:** Used for sterilization of endoscopes, cystoscopes, mycobactericidal activity also.

3. Phenols

Used as antiseptic and disinfectant, mainly tuberculocidal also. Chlorhexidine gluconate is bactericidal, sporostatic, mycobacteriostatic, virucidal and effective on yeasts and protozoa also.

4. Halogens

Used as skin antiseptic, such as Tincture iodine and Betadine. Betadine is an Iodophor which is prepared by complexing iodine with organic carrier, such as povidone.

5. Oxidizing Agents

Hydrogen peroxide, a high level disinfectant, used to disinfect ventilator, soft contact lenses, tonometer biprisms. Vaporized hydrogen peroxide is used for plasma sterilization.

Plasma Sterilization

Plasma refers to gaseous state consisting of ions, photons and free electrons and neutral uncharged particles. These active agents present in plasma, such as photons of UV rays and radicals are capable of killing microorganisms and spores efficiently.

Peracetic Acid

Used in conjunction with hydrogen peroxide, to disinfect hemodialyzers, sterilizing endoscopes.

6. Salts
Salts of heavy metals, such as mercury, silver, arsenic, zinc and copper are used.

7. Surface Active Agents
Quaternary ammonium compounds are bactericidal, highly effective against gram positive and gram negative compounds

8. Dyes
Aniline and acridine dyes are more active against gram positive bacteria.

9. Gases—Ethylene Oxide (ETO)
It is both microbicidal and sporicidal activity. It has large sterilizing chamber capacity. ETO is highly diffusible, penetrates areas where steam cannot reach.

METHODS OF STERILIZATION FOR EACH OF THE FOLLOWING

1. **Test tube:** Hot air oven
2. **Cystoscopes and endoscopes:** 2% Glutaraldehyde
3. **Surgical dressings and linen:** Autoclave
4. **Disposable catheters and disposable gloves:** Gamma radiation
5. **Rubber gloves:** Autoclave
6. **Disposable syringes:** Gamma radiation, 10% ETO
7. **Glass syringes:** Hot air oven
8. **Pipettes:** Hot air oven
9. **Clinical thermometers:** Isopropyl alcohol
10. **Basal media and Sabouraud's dextrose agar:** Autoclave
11. **Loeffler's serum slope:** Inspissation
12. **Lowenstein Jensen's medium:** Inspissation
13. **Sugar media:** Filtration
14. **Inoculation loop:** Red Heat flaming
15. **Forceps and scalpel:** Hot air oven and flaming.
16. **Scissors and needles:** Hot air oven, flaming
17. **Serum and other body fluids:** Vaccine bath
18. **Antibiotic solutions:** Filtration and ionizing radiation
19. **Vaccines:** Filtration
20. **Dental equipment:** Autoclave and ethylene oxide (ETO)
21. **Suture material:** Autoclave and ethylene oxide (ETO)
22. **Plastic endotracheal tubes:** 2% glutaraldehyde, gamma radiation
23. **Heart lung machine:** Ethylene oxide, 5% cresol
24. **Soiled dressing:** Incineration

Protocol for cleaning/disinfection/sterilization of various instruments (Table 8.1)

TABLE 8.1: General recommendations for sterilization of equipment's.		
Sl. No.	Activity	Recommendations
1.	Hand hygiene	2.5% chlorhexidine v/v + 70% ethyl alcohol v/v (or isopropyl alcohol 70%) + emollients-based hand rub
2.	Skin antisepsis	Povidone Iodine 10% w/v OR Tincture chlorhexidine 2.5% v/v
3.	Surface disinfection (Low level disinfection)	Fourth generation Quaternary ammonium compound OR hydrogen peroxide-based product.
4.	CVP line	2.5% v/v (= 0.5% w/v) Tincture chlorhexidine (Chlorhexidine not to be used <2 months)
5.	Peripheral vein	70% Ethyl/Isopropyl alcohol swabs of appropriate size
6.	High level disinfection	Glutaraldehyde (= or >2.4%) or hydrogen peroxide (7.5% stabilized) or ortho-phthalaldehyde or peracetic acid with hydrogen peroxide

RATIONALE APPROACH TO DISINFECTION AND STERILIZATION

Earle H Spaulding devised a rational approach to disinfection and sterilization of patient-care items and equipment. This classification scheme is so clear and logical that it has been retained, refined, and successfully used by infection control professionals and others when planning methods for disinfection or sterilization. The Spaulding classification scheme places reusable medical instruments or devices into three categories of ascending risk for infection.

1. High-level [semicritical items; (except dental) will come in contact with mucous membrane or nonintact skin]
2. Intermediate level (some semi-critical items and noncritical items)
3. Low-level (noncritical items; will come in contact with intact skin)

SPAULDING'S PRINCIPLE

Figure 8.3 depicts the Spaulding's classification for disinfecting instruments and **Table 8.2** depicts the Spaulding's classification of equipment decontamination.

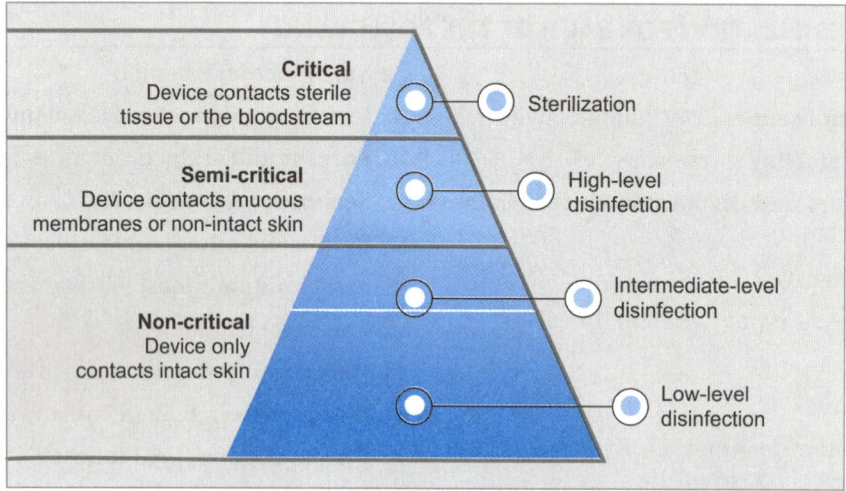

Fig. 8.3: Spaulding's classification for disinfecting instruments.

TABLE 8.2: Spaulding's classification of equipment decontamination.

Category	Definition	Level of microbicidal action	Method of decontamination	Example of common items/equipment
High (critical)	Medical devices involved with a break in the skin or mucous membrane or entering a sterile body cavity	Kills all microorganisms	Sterilization (usually heat if heat-stable or chemical if heat-sensitive)	Surgical instruments, implants, prostheses and devices, urinary catheters, cardiac catheters, needles and syringes, dressing, sutures, delivery sets, dental instruments, rigid bronchoscopes, cystoscopies, etc.
Intermediate (semi-critical)	Medical devices in contact with mucous membranes or non-intact skin	Kills all microorganisms, except high numbers of bacterial spores	High-level disinfection by heat or chemicals (under controlled conditions with minimum toxicity for humans)	Respiratory therapy and anesthetic equipment, flexible endoscopes, vaginal specula, reusable bedpans and urinals/urine bottles, patient bowls, etc.
Low (non-critical)	Items in contact with intact skin	Kills vegetative bacteria, fungi and lipid viruses	Low level disinfection (cleaning)	Blood pressure cuffs, stethoscopes, electrocardiogram leads, etc. Environmental surfaces, including tables or any other environmental surfaces.

CHAPTER 9

Specimen Collection

Chapter Outline

- Specimen—Principle of Collection, Types
- Collection of Various Specimens
- Vacutainer
  — Advantages of Vacutainer System
- — Color Coding of Vacutainers
- — Draw Order of Blood Specimen
- Staff Precautions

INTRODUCTION

The first step in acquiring a quality laboratory test result for any patient is the specimen collection procedure and quality of result depends on the quality of sample. An accurate collection of specimen is essential to reduce the risk of contamination, which can lead to inaccurate results and inappropriate treatment. Specimens must be collected at the right time, using the correct technique and equipment, and be delivered to the laboratory as quickly as possible.

SPECIMEN

It can be defined as a small quantity of a substance which shows the kind and quality of the whole sample.

The various types of specimens collected are as following:

1. Blood
2. Urine
3. Sputum
4. Stool
5. Cerebrospinal fluid (CSF)
6. Sore throat
7. Vaginal swab/urethral swab
8. Pus sample

Beyond these samples the others samples are bronchoalveolar lavage (BAL) fluid, ascetic fluid, pleural fluid, etc. The sample collected is sent for different analysis/diagnosis according to requirements/test ordered. Sample collected can be sent for biochemistry, hematology, clinical pathology, immunology, microbiology.

Collection of Blood Specimen

The act of drawing or removing blood from the circulatory system through a puncture in order to obtain a sample for analysis and diagnosis is called Phlebotomy. Phlebotomy is performed by a nurse or a technician known as a phlebotomist.

Three popular methods of blood collection are:
1. Venipuncture sampling
2. Capillary blood collection
3. Arterial sampling

Choosing the Site

A key element for successful venipuncture is choosing the best vein. To determine the best vein, use both sight and touch. Choosing an appropriate site for venipuncture is crucial for a successful venipuncture. The widest, deepest part of the vein is usually the easiest from which to draw. The veins most often used for venipuncture are located in the antecubital area. Typically the order of choice in vein selection is as follows **(Fig. 9.1)**:
- **Cubital vein:** This vein is usually the largest and fullest vein and is best anchored by the surrounding musculature of the arm.
- **Cephalic vein:** This vein is next largest and next better anchored by the surrounding musculature of the arm.
- **Basilic vein:** This vein is typically smaller than the two above and is not anchored as well by the surrounding musculature.

Phlebotomy Procedure Illustrated
- Patient identification
- Filling out the requisition
- Apply tourniquet and palpate for vein
- Sterilize the site. Insert needle
- Drawing the specimen
- Releasing the tourniquet
- Applying pressure over the vein
- Applying bandage
- Disposing needle into sharps
- Labeling the specimens

Fig. 9.1: Veins of hand.

Anticoagulants are agent that prevents clotting of blood when mixed with blood in appropriate quantity. Anticoagulants are used to prevent clot formation both in vitro and in vivo.

VACUTAINER

Vacutainer is a sterile glass or plastic test tube with a colored rubber stopper creating a vacuum seal inside of the tube, facilitating the drawing of a predetermined volume of liquid **(Fig. 9.2)**.

Advantages of Vacutainer System
- It eliminates the preparation of anticoagulant containing bulbs and tubes.
- It minimizes hemolysis of specimen. The whole system is closed and hence no possibility of leakage of blood.
- Correct blood to anticoagulant ratio is maintained as each tube is designed to draw exactly the right amount of blood.
- Interior of vacutainer is sterile, which prevents microbial growth.
- The vacutainer blood collection system offers early detection of microbial growth by ensuring minimum risk of contamination.
- Reduces time of collection. It is a type of closed blood collection system.

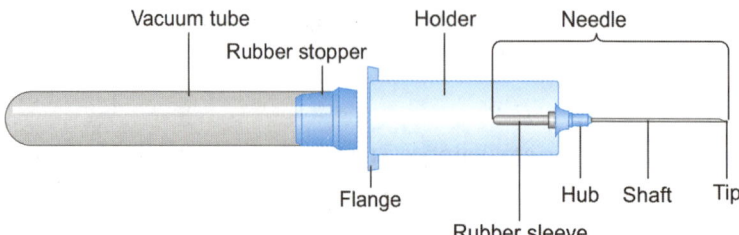

Fig. 9.2: Showing parts of vacutainer.

Color Coding of Vacutainers
See **Table 9.1.**

TABLE 9.1: Tubes commonly used in blood collection and their specifications.

Tube	Color	Name	Additive	Test used for
	Blood culture bottle	Culture bottle	Sodium polyanethol sulfonate (anticoagulant) and growth media for microorganisms	Two bottles are typically collected, in one blood draw; one for aerobic organisms and one for anaerobic organisms
	Light blue	Sodium citrate	3.2% sodium citrate (anticoagulant)	Coagulation tests
	Red	Red or plain	No additive No anticoagulant	Immunology, serological examination
	Gold	Serum separating tube	Serum separating gel and clot activator	All biochemistry test
	Light green	Heparin tube	Sodium heparin or lithium heparin (anticoagulant)	Prevent clotting chromosome testing HLA typing ammonia, lactate
	Purple/lavender	EDTA	Ethylene diamine tetra acetic acid (EDTA) (Anticoagulant)	Hematological examination like complete hemogram
	Pink		Ethylene diamine tetra acetic acid (EDTA) (Anticoagulant) Used only for whole blood sample being send to transfusion lab	Blood typing and cross-matching direct coombs test for autoimmune haemolytic anemia, HIV viral load (G & S) These tubes are preferred for blood bank tests
	Grey	Sodium fluoride	Sodium fluoride (glycolysis inhibitor) Potassium oxalate (anticoagulant)	Glucose, lactate testing
	Yellow	Acid-citrate-dextrose (anticoagulant)		Tissue typing, DNA studies, HIV cultures

(For color version, see Plate 6)

Draw Order of Blood Specimen
The draw order for specimen tubes is as follows:
- Blood culture
- Blue tube for coagulation (sodium citrate)
- Red No gel
- Gold SST (plain tube w/gel and clot activator additive)
- Green and dark green (heparin, with and without gel)
- Lavender (EDTA)
- Pink—blood bank (EDTA)
- Gray (oxalate/fluoride)

BLOOD

A. Technique of Collection (Fig. 9.3)

- Select vein puncture site, then release tourniquet. Cleanse the selected vein puncture site. Rub vigorously with an alcohol prep pad. Let dry 1 minute.
- Apply a 10% povidone-iodine solution over the same area, beginning at the proposed entry site and circling outward to a diameter of approximately 5-cm. Let dry 1 minute.

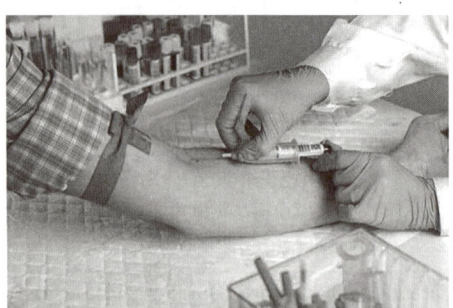

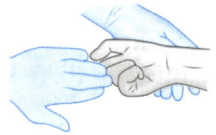
1. Ask the patient to form a first so that the veins are more prominent

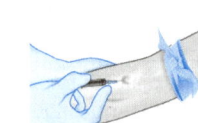
2. Put on well-fitting, non-sterile gloves

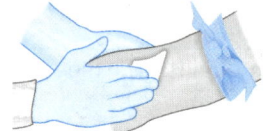
3. Disinfect the site using 70% isopropyl alcohol for 30 seconds and allow to dry completely (30 seconds)

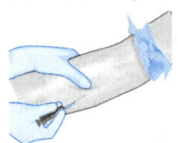
4. Anchor the vein by holding the patient's arm and placing an thumb below the venepuncture site

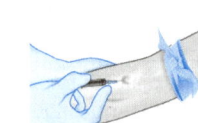
5. Enter the vein swiftly at a 30° angle

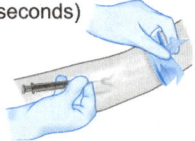
6. Once sufficient blood been collected, released the tourniquet before with drawing the needle

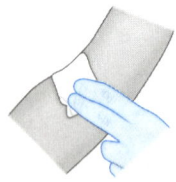
7. Withdraw the needle gently and then give the patient a clean gauze or dry cotton-wool ball to apply to the site with gentle pressure

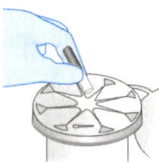
8. Discard the used needle and syringe or blood sampling device into a puncture resistant container

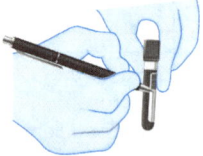
9. Check the label and forms for accuracy

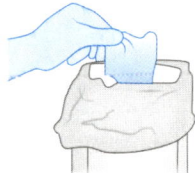
10. Discard the used needle and syringe or blood sampling device into a puncture resistant container

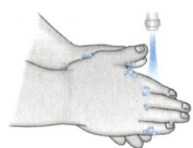
11. Remove gloves and place them in the general waste. perform hand hygiene. If using soap and water, dry hands with single-use towels

Fig. 9.3: Technique of blood sample collection.

- Cleanse the site a second time with an alcohol prep pad to remove the iodine by wiping down the center of the prep area, then down each side. This step is helpful in the event the site must be palpated during the phlebotomy procedure.
- Clean rubber caps of vacutainers and blood culture containers with alcohol. Do not prep rubber stoppers with any other agent, per manufacturer's instructions.
- Retie tourniquet without touching the prepped area, insert needle into vein, and withdraw blood. Repeat the procedure for each blood culture set ordered, selecting a different site for each vein puncture, if possible **(Fig. 9.4)**.

B. Labeling and Transport

All bottles must be labeled in the presence of the patient. Label the vacutainers, aerobic/anaerobic bottles for blood culture of each set with the same accession.

Blood cultures are transported at room temperature. Do not refrigerate blood cultures if there is a delay in transporting to laboratory.

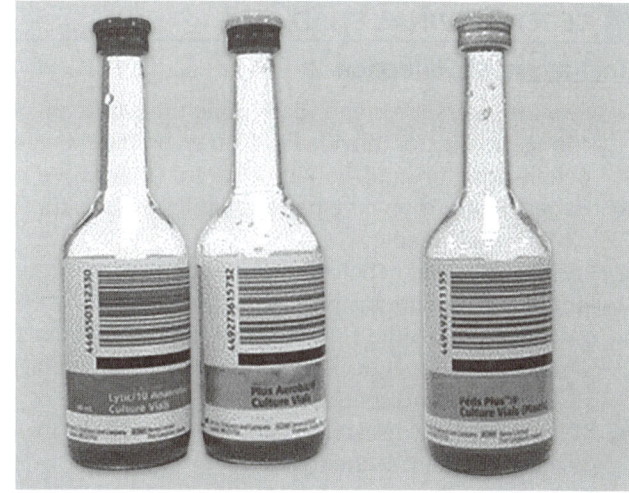

Fig. 9.4: Automated blood culture bottles and its cap color types.

Pyrexia of Unknown Origin

Definition

Any febrile illness with a body temperature more than 38°C or more than 100°F, lasting for more than 3 weeks or longer, without any obvious cause or remain uncertain in spite of investigations.

Causes

A. Bacterial

Localized pyogenic infections:	**Systemic bacterial infections:**
• Appendicitis	Mycobacterial infections
• Cholangitis	Typhoid fever
• Cholecystitis	*Mycoplasma*
• Localized abscess	Chlamydial infections
• Mesenteric lymphadenitis	Brucellosis
• Osteomyelitis	Melioidosis
• Pelvic inflammatory disease	Listeriosis
• Sinusitis	Bartonellosis
• Suppurative thrombophlebitis	Spirochete infections
• Intravascular infections	

B. Virus
Chikungunya fever, dengue fever, cytomegalovirus and EBV infection, coxsackie group B, viral hepatitis, HIV infection.

C. Fungus
Aspergillosis, mucormycosis, blastomycosis, histoplasmosis, coccidioidomycosis, paracoccidioidomycosis, candidiasis, cryptococcosis, pneumocystis infection, sporotrichosis.

D. Parasite
Malaria, amoebiasis, leishmaniasis, Chagas' disease, toxoplasmosis, strongyloidiasis.

CEREBROSPINAL FLUID

Technique of Collection

- Identify interspaces and mark puncture site at the L4-5 interspaces in a perpendicular line from the iliac crest. Using sponge applicator provided in LP tray, prepare the back with chlorhexidine solution, beginning at the site marked for the needle puncture and working outward **(Fig. 9.5)**.
- Repeat twice, drape the patient. Infiltrate the skin and subcutaneous tissue with preservative free 1% lidocaine with a 22–25-gauge needle.
- Insert the spinal needle into the midline of the interspaced with bevel up. Direct the needle on a 10° angle toward the umbilicus (horizontal axis).
- Advance the needle slowly, removing the stylet every 2–3 millimeters to check for CSF flow. Withdraw 2 millimeters, remove stylet and check for CSF. If none, then replace the stylet and remove. Remove the needle to subcutaneous tissue, change angle and continue.
- If repeated bony resistance is noted, discard the needle and replace it. If blood is returned, watch for clearing of fluid; if no clearing, replace the stylet.
- Once CSF flow is established, rotate the needle 90° counterclockwise (bevel in transverse plane) for patients in the lateral decubitus position. 1–2 mL of CSF in a universal container **(Fig. 9.6)**.
- Send samples to the lab for glucose, protein, cell count (culture and Gram staining or other test), cytology tests as indicated with proper labeling.

Meningitis

Meningitis is an inflammation of the meninges surrounding the brain and spinal cord, which implies to infection of subarachnoid space or leptomeninges.

Types of Meningitis

Based on leukocytes in CSF, it is grouped into:
- **Pyogenic meningitis:** Characterized by elevated polymorphonuclear cells in CSF.
  Causes of pyogenic meningitis are:
  - *Neonates or infants of 0–2 months: Escherichia coli*, Group B *Streptococcus, Klebsiella pneumoniae, Listeria monocytogenes*
  - *2–20 years: Neisseria meningitidis, Haemophilus influenzae, Streptococcus pneumoniae*
  - *>20 years: Streptococcus pneumoniae, Haemophilus influenzae* and *Neisseria meningitidis*
- **Aseptic meningitis:** Characterized by elevated lymphocytes in CSF. Causes of aseptic meningitis are:
  - *Bacteria:* M. tuberculosis, Treponema pallidum, Leptospira.
  - *Fungi:* Cryptococcus neoformans
  - *Virus:* Enterovirus, herpes simplex virus 1&2, varicella zoster virus, cytomegalovirus, Epstein-Barr virus, mumps virus, arbovirus, adenovirus, rubella virus and HIV
  - *Parasites: Naegleria fowleri, Acanthamoeba* species, *Toxoplasma gondii*

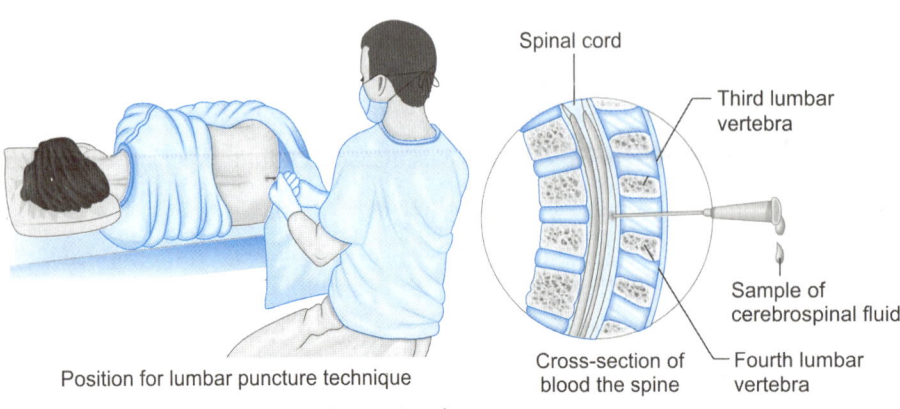

Fig. 9.5: Lumbar puncture.

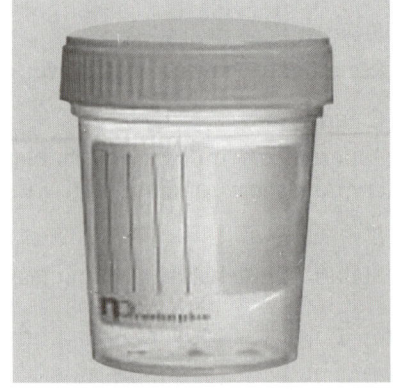

Fig. 9.6: CSF sample collection in universal container.

SPUTUM (FIG. 9.7)

Pneumonia

Pneumonia refers to inflammation of lungs which can be classified as:
- **Community acquired:** Patients acquire organisms from community.
  - *Bacterial causes:* Streptococcus pneumoniae, Mycoplasma pneumoniae, Haemophilus influenzae, Chlamydophila pneumoniae, Legionella, Coxiella brunette (Q fever)
  - *Viral causes:* Influenza virus, adenovirus, respiratory syncytial virus, parainfluenza virus
- **Hospital acquired:** Patients acquire organisms in hospital setting:
  - *Bacterial causes:* MDR non-fermenters (*Pseudomonas* and *Acinetobacter* species), MDR *Enterobacteriaceae* (*E. coli*, *Klebsiella*, *Enterobacter*), Streptococcus pneumoniae, Mycoplasma pneumoniae, Haemophilus influenzae, Chlamydophila pneumoniae, Legionella pneumoniae, Staphylococcus aureus
  - *Viral causes:* Influenza virus, adenovirus, respiratory syncytial virus, parainfluenza virus

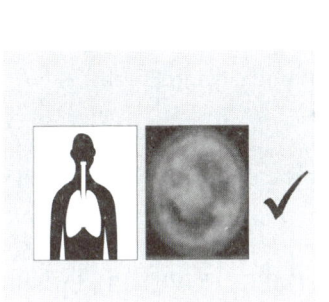
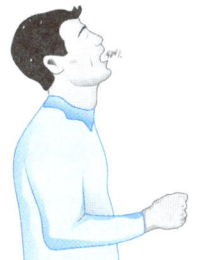

1. Gargle of rinse and then spit out the water you are given

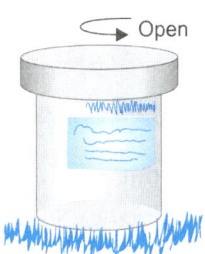

2. Open the sample container

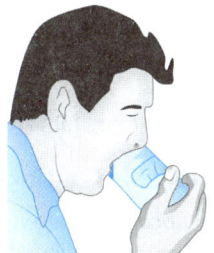

3. Hold the container to your mouth with your lips inside it

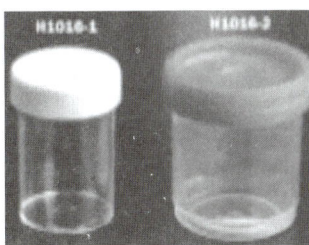
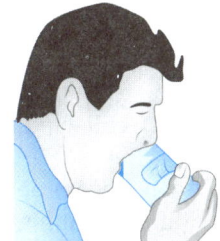

4. Take as deep a breath as you can and cough then spit into the container (do not just spit saliva)

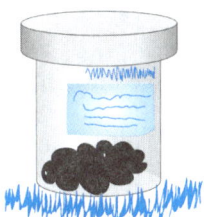

5. The sample you cough should look thick and yellow or green, more than a tablespoon of sample is needed

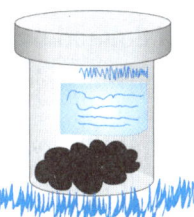

6. Close the container lid tightly and seal with parafilm

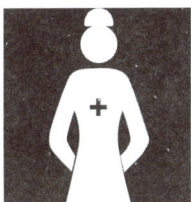

7. Give the sample to your caregiver right away

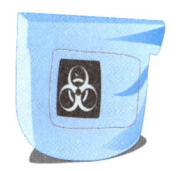

8. If you are at home
   - Put your sample in the plastic bag you were given
   - Close the bag and put it in the fridge right away
   - Return your sample to your caregiver within 24 hours

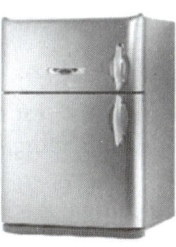

Fig. 9.7: Technique of sputum sample collection.

SORE THROAT

Techniques of sample collection **(Figs. 9.8A and B)**:

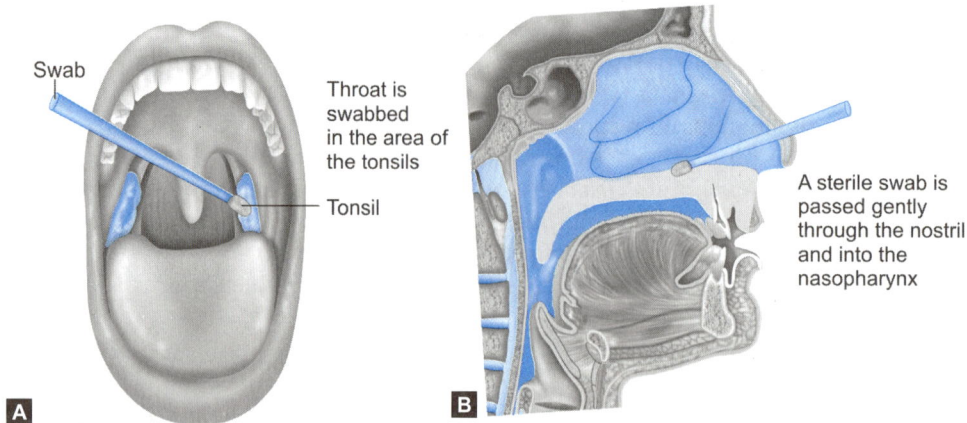

Figs. 9.8A and B: Technique of sample collection; (A) Oropharyngeal; (B) Nasopharyngeal swabs.

Various Organisms Causing Sore Throat

Bacteria: *Streptococcus pyogenes* (most common), *Streptococcus pneumoniae, Corynebacterium diphtheria, Corynebacterium ulcerans, Treponema vincentii, Leptotrichia buccalis, Actinobacterium* species.
Fungal: *Candida albicans*
Viral: Influenza virus, parainfluenza virus, coxsackie virus, rhinovirus, coronavirus (MERS COVID-19), Epstein-Barr virus, adenovirus

URINE

Technique of Collection

- **Clean voided midstream urine:** Most common specimen for UTI, collected after properly cleaning the ureteral meatus or glans **(Fig. 9.9)**.
- **Suprapubic aspiration:** Urine from bladder, most ideal specimen. Recommended for infants or patients in coma.
- In catheterized patients, urine is collected from catheter tube (after clamping and disinfecting); but not from urobag.
- Transportation of urine sample should be done immediately. If delay, it can be refrigerated and stored by adding boric acid

Various Causative Agents of Urinary Tract Infection—KASS Criteria

Definition: Urinary tract infection is defined as disease caused by microbial invasion of the urinary tract that extends from renal cortex of kidney to urethral meatus. UTI is classified into two types:
1. **Upper UTI:** Involves kidney and ureter.
2. **Lower UTI:** Involves urethra and bladder

Causes
- **Bacteria:**
  - *Gram-negative: Escherichia coli, Klebsiella pneumoniae, Proteus mirabilis, Pseudomonas aeruginosa, Acinetobacter* species, *Enterobacter* species, *Serratia* species
  - *Gram-positive cocci: Staphylococcus saprophyticus, Staphylococcus aureus, Staphylococcus epidermidis, Enterococcus* species
- **Viral:** Herpes simplex virus, adenovirus, JC and BK virus, cytomegalovirus
- **Fungal:** *Candida albicans*
- **Parasitic:** *Schistosoma haematobium, Trichomonas vaginalis*
- **KASS criteria (significant bacteriuria):** Presence of bacteria more than 10^5 CFU/mL in a midstream urine sample by standard loop technique on blood agar/CLED agar. It indicates active infection.

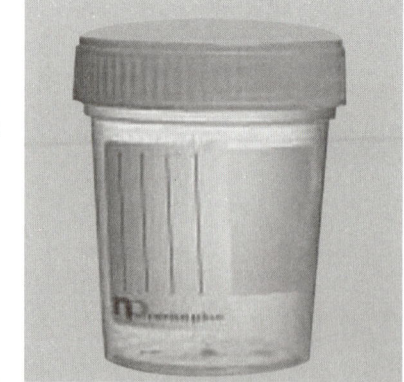

Fig. 9.9: Universal container for collection of fresh midstream urine sample.

VAGINAL SWAB/URETHERAL SWAB

Technique of Collection (**Fig. 9.10**)

High vaginal swab: For cervicitis, vaginitis

Urethral smear/exudates: Syphilis, chancroid, gonorrhea, non-gonococcal urethritis

- The specimen commonly collected for the diagnosis of vaginitis, vaginosis or uterine sepsis is high vaginal swab
- The swab is inserted into upper part of the vagina and rotated there before withdrawing it

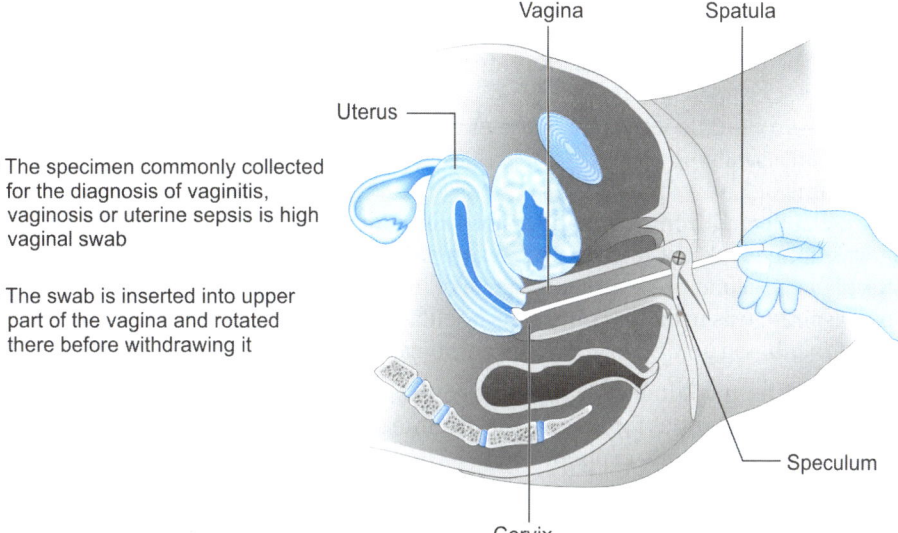

Fig. 9.10: Collection of specimen through vagina.

Various Organisms Causing Sexually Transmitted Diseases and its Laboratory Diagnosis

Sexually transmitted diseases (STD): STDs are group of communicable diseases which are transmitted predominantly or entirely by sexual contact and caused by bacteria, virus, protozoa and fungus.

Classification based on clinical manifestations:

Painless genital ulcer:
- Syphilis: *Treponema pallidum*
- Lymphogranuloma venereum: *Chlamydia trachomatis*
- Donovanosis: *Klebsiella granulomatis*

Painful genital ulcer:
Chancroid: *Hemophilus ducreyi*
Herpes genitals: HSV1&2

Urethral discharge:
- Gonorrhea: *Neisseria gonorrhoeae*
- **Non-gonococcal urethritis:** *Chlamydia trachomatis, Ureaplasma urealyticum, Mycoplasma genitals, Mycoplasma hominis,* herpes simplex virus, *Candida albicans, Trichomonas vaginalis*

Vaginal discharge:
- **Vulvovaginal candidiasis:** *Candida albicans,* non-albicans candida
- **Bacterial vaginosis:** *Gardnerella vaginalis, Mobiluncus* species
- **Trichomonas vaginitis:** *Trichomonas vaginalis*

Genital wart: Human papilloma virus

Systemic manifestations: Pelvic inflammatory disease: *N. gonorrhoeae* and *Chlamydia trachomatis*

No genital lesions: HIV, HBV, HCV

PUS SAMPLE

Technique of Collection

For aerobes:
- Samples of pus are preferred in swabs. However, pus swabs are often received (when using swabs, the deepest part of the wound should be sampled, avoiding the superficial microflora). Swabs should be well soaked in pus. Swabs for bacterial and fungal culture should be placed in the transport medium provided in the tube (Fig. 9.11).
- If possible a few mL of pus in a sterile universal bottle or even a few drops still in a syringe is much better than a swab.
- Ideally, a minimum volume of 1 mL of pus.
- Two wound swabs were collected from the wound and from a drop of aspirate, smear was made on clean glass slide and Gram staining was done for direct microscopic examination under oil immersion 100X objective to know various morphological types of bacteria and presence or absence of inflammatory cells.
- Second swab/drop of aspirate was used for culture by inoculating it on routine media, such as blood agar, nutrient agar and MacConkey's agar, incubated at 37°C for 24 hours aerobically.

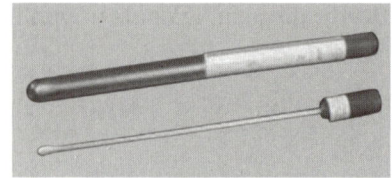

Fig. 9.11: Swab specimen.

For anaerobes: Ideally, a minimum volume of 1 mL (up to 5 mL) of pus should be collected. Large volumes of purulent material maintain the viability of anaerobes for longer. The aspirate should be collected in a sterile syringe—any air bubbles should be expelled. Needle safely and tightly capped.

Etiology of infections of subcutaneous tissue:
Bacteria: *Clostridium perfringens, Clostridium novyi, Clostridium septicum, Bacillus* species, *Bacteroides* species, *Peptostreptococcus* species, *Staphylococcus aureus,* Group A *Streptococcus*
Fungi: *Madurella mycetomatis, Madurella grisea, Candida* species
Parasites: *Taenia solium, Wuchereria bancrofti, Dracunculus medinensis*

Agents causing surgical site wound infections.
- **Bacterial:** *Staphylococcus aureus*, coagulase negative staphylococci, *Enterococcus*
- **Fungal:** *Candida albicans*
- **If bowel integrity compromised:** Gram-negative flora, such as *E. coli*
- **Anaerobic** organisms, such as *Bacteroides, Prevotella*.

Agents causing burn wound infections: *Staphylococcus aureus, Pseudomonas aeruginosa, Staphylococcus epidermidis*.

STOOL

Technique of Collection

In a universal container. Stool should be passed into a clean dry container. Pass stool directly into a sterile wide-mouth, leak-proof container with a tight-fitting lid. Pass stool into a clean, dry bedpan and transfer the stool into a sterile leak-proof container with a tight fitting lid.

Enteric pathogens differ from each other in infective dose:
- **Shigella, Enterohemorrhagic *E. coli*, Giardia or Entamoeba:** 10–100 bacteria or cysts
- ***Vibrio cholerae*:** 10^5–10^8 bacilli
- ***Salmonella*:** 10^3–10^5 bacilli

Various Causes of Diarrhea and Dysentery and its Laboratory Diagnosis

Diarrhea: As per WHO, diarrhea is defined as passage of three or more loose or liquid stools per day, in excess than the usual habitat for that person. Causes are:
- **Bacteria (enterotoxin mediated):** *Vibrio cholerae, Vibrio parahaemolyticus, Escherichia coli* (enterotoxigenic), *Clostridium perfringens, Aeromonas* species
- **Cytotoxin mediated:** *Shigella* species, Enterohemorrhagic *E. coli, Yersinia enterocolitica, Listeria monocytogenes, Clostridium difficile*
- **Neurotoxin mediated:** *Staphylococcus aureus, Bacillus cereus, Clostridium botulinum*
- **Viral:** Rotavirus, Norovirus, Astrovirus, Calicivirus, Norwalk virus
- **Parasite:** *Giardia lamblia, Cryptosporidium parvum, Cyclospora, Microsporidia*.

CHAPTER 10

Biomedical Waste Management

Chapter Outline

- Laundry Management Process and Infection Control and Prevention
  - Change of Linen
  - Segregation at Source
  - Handling and Storage of Used Linen in Ward/Department
  - Transporting Used Linen from Ward/Department to Pick-up Point to Laundry
  - Return of Clean Linen to the User
  - Infection Control Issues in the Laundry
  - Spillage of Contaminated Linen
- Biomedical Waste Management
  - Salient Features of Biomedical Waste Rules 2018
  - Biomedical Waste Segregation
  - Central Storage for HCFs Having Captive Treatment and Disposal System

LAUNDRY MANAGEMENT PROCESS AND INFECTION CONTROL AND PREVENTION

In healthcare settings, it is process by which different textiles and fabrics are cleaned and disinfected. Its purpose is to protect HCWs from exposure of harmful infectious materials during collection, handling and sorting of contaminated textiles.

- **Used linen:** Linen that has been used once but is clean (not contaminated with blood and body fluids)
- **Soiled linen:** Linen that is contaminated with blood and body fluids **(Table 10.1)**.

Change of Linen

- Linen is changed every day for every patient.
- For every new patient
- Visibly dirty
- As per the requirement.

TABLE 10.1: Various Infections transmitted through contaminated linen.

• **Bacterial**
  – *Salmonella* species
  – *Bacillus cereus*
  – *Staphylococcus aureus*
  – *Diphtheroid*
  – *Acinetobacter* species
• **Viral:** HBV
• **Fungal:** *Microsporum canis*
	• **Parasites:** Scabies
	• **Routes of transmission:**
	  – Direct contact with contaminated linen
	  – Aerosol generated while sorting and handling of contaminated linen

Facility Design

The laundry design (constriction) should meet the criteria of American Institute of Architects (AIA) as recommended by CDC.
- The laundry area should be separate, which is divided into two separate divisions:
  1. *Direct area:* It is the area were receiving and handling the soiled laundry is done, the air pressure here should be negative air pressure.
  2. *Clean area:* It is the area where main cleaning process is done. It is further divided into several rooms, such as:
- Laundry processing room—area where cleaning and disinfection of linen is done
- Drying area—area for ironing and disinfection of linen
- Inspection and mending room for clean linen
- Storage area for sorting and issuing of clan lining.
- Hand washing facility should be there.
- PPE should be provided to laundry workers.
- There should be industrial machines and tumble dryers instead of household ones.

Segregation at Source

- All used linen is segregated at the source (wards/ICU/OT—where being used)
- Is segregated into "used" and "soiled" categories as stated in **Table 10.2**.
- The clean and the soiled linen is packed separately and securely and sent to the laundry department.
- In the utility room—soiled linen is disinfected by dipping into 1% sod. Hypochlorite solution for a period of minimum 30 minutes (approximately).

TABLE 10.2: Color coding of the bags.

Sl. No.	Category	Contents of the bags	Bag
1.	Used	• General Items—uniforms, scrubs, etc. • Cleaning mops • Theatre scrubs	Blue bag
2.	Soiled	Items which are soiled with blood and body fluids like uniforms, scrub suits	Yellow plastic bag

Handling and Storage of Used Linen in Ward/Department

- No extraneous items must be placed in the laundry bags, especially sharp objects. This may contribute to a health and safety risk for the laundry workers.
- All linen bags must be placed in the correct color bag as per **Table 10.2**, securely tied, labeled as appropriate and stored in a room or area designated for the purpose, which is safe and separate from patient areas.
- **Label to contain:**
  - Area
  - Time and date
  - Items
  - Quantity
- Labeling is done by GDA under the supervision of housekeeping supervisor.
- Bags must be less than 3/4th full.
- Gloves may also be required if linen is wet. Hands must be washed after handling soiled or infected linen.

Transporting Used Linen from Ward/Department to Pick-up Point to Laundry

- The pick-up point must be dry and secure and separate from the clean linen area.
- Dirty utility rooms are used as "Pick up points".

- The frequency of collection will depend on the volume of laundry but not less than twice daily from all IPD areas. Shift timings have to be allotted.
- Linen handlers must have heavy-duty rubber gloves available. Training on hand washing technique should be mandatory.
- Frequency of collection is twice daily from all departments to laundry department in the designated floor-wise closed trolley.
- The provider is responsible for cleaning and disinfection of the container/vehicle in order to prevent contamination of clean linen:
  – After any spillage
  – After transportation of dirty laundry, if it is to be used for clean laundry next.
  – At least weekly

Return of Clean Linen to the User

Contamination of clean linen must be prevented by:
- Storage in a clean, dry area or cage
- Transport in a clean, dry container/vehicle which is cleaned and disinfected prior to loading with clean linen.

Infection Control Issues in the Laundry

- Restricted the entry of personnel who is suffering from an infection or skin disease, in processing and handling of any article to be supplied to the hospital
- Personal protective equipment should be made available and worn when handling linen. All such clothing must be removed and changed each time the person leaves the department.
- Disposable items must not be re-used. Reusable gloves must be cleaned and dried at least daily.
- A hand washbasin, complete with soap and paper towels, must be available close to the working areas.
- Staff must be aware of the possibility of extraneous items and sharps containers must be available.
- Staff must be aware of actions to take in the event of a sharp's injury.
- Systems and machinery should be designed and operated so as to reduce the risk of re-infection of linen during the course of the laundering process and, to prevent articles being re-infected after laundering and prior to re issue to the hospital.

Spillage of Contaminated Linen

Wearing gloves, replace the linen in an appropriate bag. Wash the contaminated surface with detergent and water and dry. Wash hands thoroughly after removing gloves.

Antimicrobial Action of Laundering

Antimicrobial activity results from a combination of mechanical, thermal, and chemical processes.
- Dilution and agitation in water removes substantial quantities of microorganisms.
- Soap and detergent have some antimicrobial activity/property.
- Hot water also provides effective means of microbial destruction.

Special Laundry Situations

- Reusable gowns and surgical drapes must be sterilized before use and requires steam autoclaving after laundering.
- Linen used in neonatal ICUs and burn units is also recommended for autoclaving after laundering.

BIOMEDICAL WASTE MANAGEMENT

Definition

Biomedical waste management (BMW) means any waste, which is generated during the laboratory diagnosis, treatment or immunization of human beings or animals or research activities pertaining thereto or in the production or testing of biological or in health camps. The new biomedical waste guideline was published in 2016 with an amendment added in 2018 and 2019. It was implemented with the vision of simplifying categorization of BMWs, while improving the ease of segregation, transportation and disposal methods to decrease environmental pollution.

Salient Features of Biomedical Waste Management (Amendment) Rules, 2018

- Biomedical waste generators including hospitals, nursing homes, clinics, dispensaries, veterinary institutions, animal houses, pathological laboratories, blood banks, healthcare facilities, and clinical establishments will have to phase out chlorinated plastic bags (excluding blood bags) and gloves.
- All healthcare facilities shall make available the annual report on its website within a period of two years from the date of publication of the Biomedical Waste Management (Amendment) Rules, 2018, as per **Figure 10.1**.
- Operators of common biomedical waste treatment and disposal facilities shall establish bar coding and global positioning system for handling of biomedical waste in accordance with guidelines issued by the Central Pollution Control Board.
- The State Pollution Control Boards/Pollution Control Committees have to compile, review and analyze the information received and send this information to the Central Pollution Control Board in a new Form (Form IV A), which seeks detailed information regarding district-wise biomedical waste generation, information on healthcare facilities having captive treatment facilities, information on common biomedical waste treatment and disposal facilities.
- Every occupier, i.e., a person having administrative control over the institution and the premises generating biomedical waste shall pre-treat the laboratory waste, microbiological waste, blood samples, and blood bags through disinfection or sterilization on-site in the manner as prescribed by the World Health Organization (WHO) or guidelines on safe management of wastes from healthcare activities and WHO Blue Book 2014 and then sent to the common biomedical waste treatment facility for final disposal.

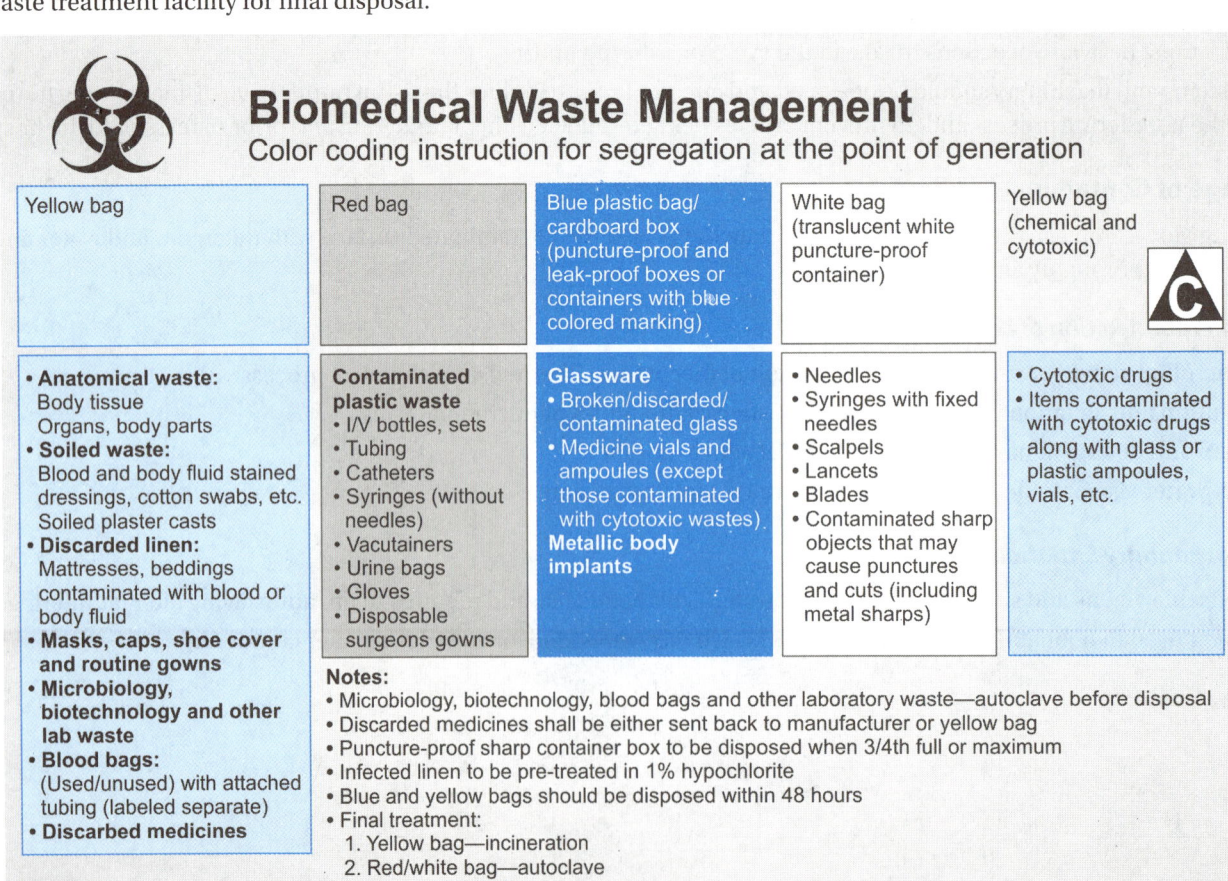

Fig. 10.1: Biomedical waste management. *(For color version, see Plate 7)*

Salient Features of Biomedical Waste Rules

Biomedical Waste Management Rules, categorizes the biomedical waste generated from the healthcare facility into four categories based on the segregation pathway and color code **(Table 10.3)**. Various types of biomedical waste are further assigned to each one of the categories, as detailed below:
1. Yellow category
2. Red category
3. White category
4. Blue category

TABLE 10.3: Color coding and type of container/bags to be used for waste segregation and collection.

Sl. No.	Category	Type of waste	Color and type of container
1.	Yellow category	• Human anatomical • Waste • Animal anatomical waste • Soiled waste • Discarded or expired medicine • Microbiology, biotechnology and other clinical laboratory waste • Chemical waste (yellow) • Chemical liquid waste	Yellow colored non-chlorinated plastic bags **Note:** chemical waste (yellow-e) comprising of unused, residual or date expired liquid chemicals including spent hypo of X-ray, should be stored in yellow container
2.	Red category	Contaminated waste (recyclable)	Red colored non-chlorinated plastic bags (having thickness equal to more than 50 µ) and containers
3.	White category	Waste sharps including metals	White colored translucent, puncture-proof, leak proof, temper-proof containers
4.	Blue category	• Glassware • Metallic body implants	Puncture-proof, leak-proof boxes or containers with blue colored marking

Biomedical Waste Segregation

Biomedical waste generated from a healthcare facility is required to be segregated at the point of generation as per the color coding stipulated under Schedule-I of BMWM Rules, 2016. Following activities to be followed to ensure proper waste segregation:
- Waste must be segregated at the **point of generation** of source and not in later stages. **"Point of Generation"** means the location where wastes initially generate, accumulate and is under the control of doctor/nursing staff, etc., who is providing treatment to the patient and in the process generating biomedical waste.
- Posters/placards for biomedical waste segregation should be provided in all the wards as well as in waste storage area.
- Adequate number of color coded bins/containers and bags should be available at the point of generation of biomedical waste.
- Color coded plastic bags should be in line with the Plastic Waste Management Rules, 2016. Specifications for plastic bags and containers given at Annexure 1.
- Provide Personnel Protective Equipment to the biomedical waste handling staff.

Biomedical Waste Collection

Time of Collection
- Biomedical waste should be collected on daily basis from each ward of the hospital at a fixed interval of time. There can be multiple collections from wards during the day.
- HCF should ensure collection, transportation, treatment and disposal of biomedical waste as per BMWM Rules, and HCF should also ensure disposal of human anatomical waste, animal anatomical waste, soiled waste and biotechnology waste within 48 hours.
- Collection times should be fixed and appropriate to the quantity of waste produced in each area of the healthcare facility.
- Biomedical waste collected by the staff, should be provided with PPEs.

Packaging
- Biomedical waste bags and sharps containers should be filled to no more than three quarters full. Once this level is reached, they should be sealed ready for collection.
- Plastic bags should never be stapled but may be tied or sealed with a plastic tag or tie.
- Replacement bags or containers should be available at each waste-collection location so that full ones can immediately be replaced.
- Color coded waste bags and containers should be printed with the biohazard symbol, labeled with details, such as date, type of waste, waste quantity, senders name and receiver's details as well as bar coded label to allow them to be tracked till final disposal.

Labeling
- All the bags/containers/bins used for collection and storage of biomedical waste, must be labeled with the Symbol of Biohazard or Cytotoxic Hazard as the case may be as per the type of waste in accordance with the BMWM Rules, 2016.
- Biomedical waste bags/containers are required to be provided with bar code labels in accordance with CPCB guidelines for "Guidelines for Barcode System for Effective Management of Biomedical Waste" (**Fig. 10.2**).

Common Biomedical Waste Treatment and Disposal Facility (CBWTF) (Fig. 10.3)

Each healthcare facility should ensure that there is a designated central waste collection room situated within its premises for storage of biomedical waste, till the waste is picked and transported for treatment and disposal at CBWTF. Such room should be under the responsibility of a designated person and should be under lock and key. The following points may be considered for construction of central waste collection room:
- The location of central waste collection room must be away from the public/visitor's access.
- The space allocation for this room must be as per the quantity of waste generated from the hospital.
- The planned space must be sufficient so as to store at least two days generation of waste.
- Central waste collection room must be roofed and manned and should be under lock and key under the responsibility of designated person.
- The entrance of this center must be accessible through a concrete ramp for easy transportation of waste collection trolleys.
- Flooring should be of tiles or any other glazed material with slope so as to ease the cleaning of the area.
- Exhaust fans should be provided in the waste collection room for ventilation.
- It is to be ensured by the healthcare facility that such central storage room is safety inspected for potential fire hazard

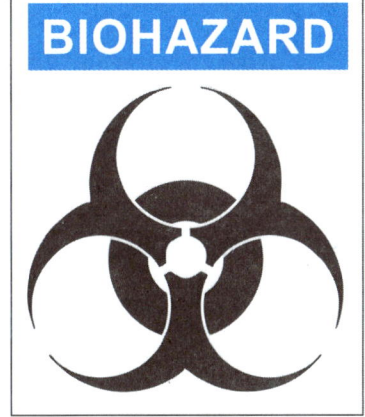
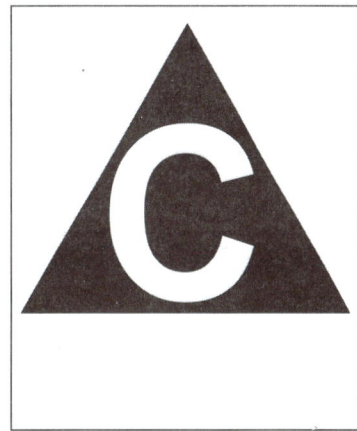

Fig. 10.2: Labels of biomedical waste.

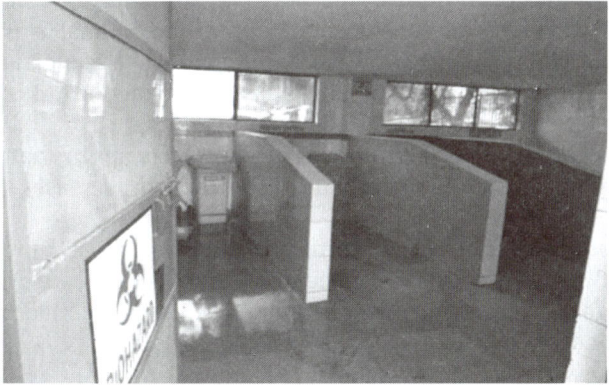

Fig. 10.3: Central waste collection room for biomedical waste.

and based on such inspection preventive measure has to be taken by the healthcare facility, such as installation of fire extinguisher, smoke detector, etc.
- There should also be provision for water supply adjacent to central waste storage area for cleaning and washing of this station and the containers. The drainage from the storage and washing area should be routed to the Effluent Treatment Plant (ETP).
- Sign boards indicating relevant details, such as contact person and the telephone number should be provided.
- The entrance of this station must be labeled with "Entry for Authorized Personal Only" and Logo of Biomedical Waste Hazard.
- It is to be ensured that no general waste is stored in the central waste collection area.

CHAPTER 11

Antimicrobial Stewardship

Chapter Outline

- Antimicrobial Stewardship
  — Purpose
  — Strategic Approaches
- Multidrug Resistant Organisms
  — Infection Control Precautions
- Prevention of MRSA, MDROs in Healthcare Setting

ANTIMICROBIAL STEWARDSHIP

"Antimicrobial stewardship" refers to interventions designed to promote the optimal use of antibiotic agents, including drug choice, dosing, route, and duration of administration. To address antimicrobial resistance, all clinicians must become stewards of antimicrobials by prescribing them appropriately and educating their patients and colleagues on the proper use of this increasingly scarce medical resource.

Antimicrobial stewardship is a coordinated program that promotes the appropriate use of antimicrobials (including antibiotics), improves patient outcomes, reduces microbial resistance, and decreases the spread of infections caused by multidrug-resistant organisms.

Misuse and overuse of antimicrobials is one of the world's most pressing public health problems.

Infectious organisms adapt to the antimicrobials designed to kill them, making the drugs ineffective.

People infected with antimicrobial-resistant organisms are more likely to have longer, more expensive hospital stays, and may be more likely to die as a result of an infection.

Stewardship interventions are listed in three categories below:
1. Broad
2. Pharmacy-driven
3. Infection and syndrome specific.

Purpose of Antimicrobial Stewardship Program

- **Primary goal:** To optimize safe and appropriate use of antibiotics to improve clinical outcomes and minimize adverse effects of antibiotics.
- **Secondary goal:**
  – To reduce healthcare costs without adversely impacting quality of patient care
  – To reduce the incidence of antibiotic induced collateral damage

Strategic Approaches to Antimicrobial Stewardship

- Appropriate antimicrobial therapy.
- Optimizing antimicrobial prophylaxis for operative procedures.

- Developing and implementing an antibiotic policies and standard treatment guidelines (STG).
- Prospective auditing and providing feedback and timely intervention in streamlining the antibiotic prescriptions.
- Formulary restriction/pre-authorization.
- Improving antimicrobial prescribing by educational and administrative means.

CDC's Seven Core Elements of Antimicrobial Stewardship

See **Figure 11.1**.

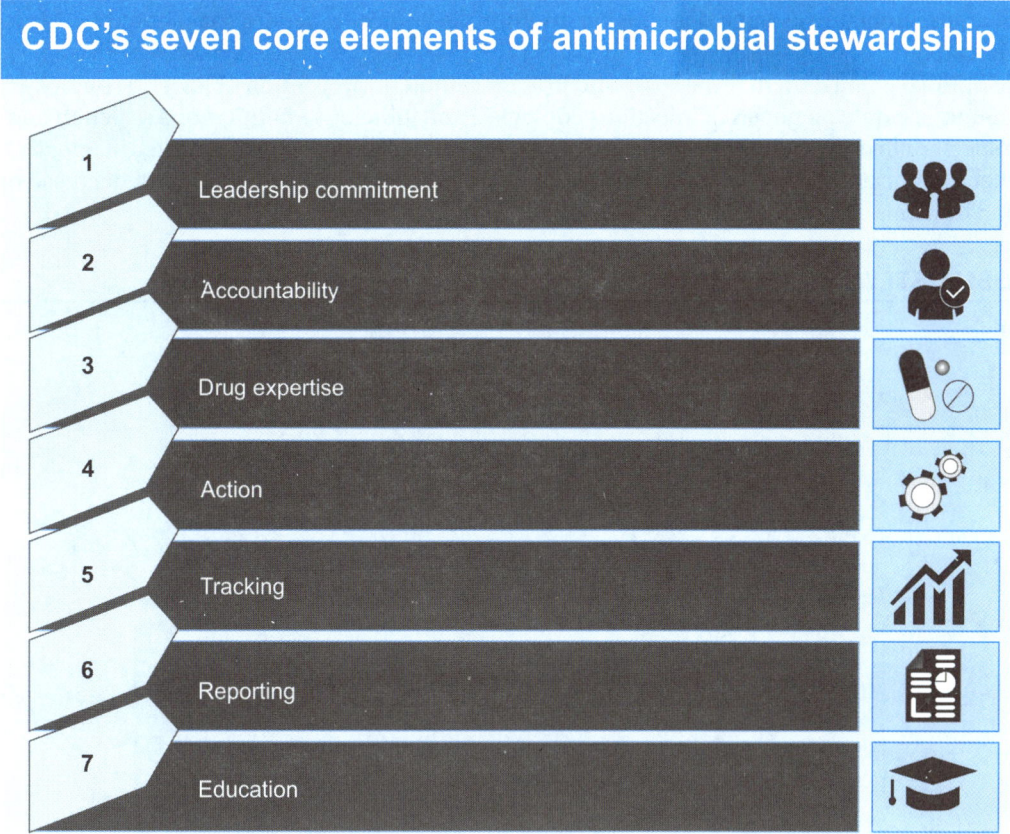

Fig. 11.1: CDC seven core elements of antimicrobial stewardship.

MULTIDRUG RESISTANT ORGANISMS

Recommendations for prevention of transmission of multidrug resistant organisms (MDROs) definition: MDROs are defined as microorganisms, predominantly bacteria, that are resistant to one or more classes of antimicrobial agents, e.g., MRS A, VRE, ESBL producing gram negative bacilli GNB. Organisms, such as *Stenotrophomonas maltophilia*, *Burkholderia cepacia*, and *Ralstonia pickettii* that are intrinsically resistant to the broadest spectrum antimicrobial agents and are also considered as MDRO.

Infection Control Precautions to Prevent Transmission of MDROs

- Fellow standard precautions and contact precautions.
- Use masks according to standard precautions while performing splash generating procedures, (e.g., wound irrigation, oral suctioning, intubation); when caring for patients with open tracheotomies which are potential for projectile secretions; and in circumstances where there is evidence of transmission from heavily colonized sources, (e.g., burn wounds). Masks are not otherwise recommended for prevention of MDRO transmission from patients to healthcare personnel during routine care, (e.g., upon room entry).

PREVENTION OF MRSA, MDROs IN HEALTHCARE SETTING

Methicillin Resistant *Staphylococcus aureus* (MRSA)

Methicillin-resistant *Staphylococcus aureus* (MRSA) is a major *Staphylococcus* infection that is difficult to treat because of resistance to some antibiotics. Staphylococcal infections—including those caused by MRSA—can spread in hospitals, other healthcare facilities, and in the community where you live, work, and go to school.

You can help prevent infections and stop the spread of MRSA/MDROs by:
- Preventing infections by hand hygiene which will reduce the burden of MDROs/MRSA in healthcare settings.
- Prevention of antimicrobial resistance depends on appropriate clinical practices that should be incorporated into all routine patient care.
- These include optimal management of vascular and urinary catheters, prevention of lower respiratory tract infection in intubated patients, accurate diagnosis of infectious etiologies, and judicious antimicrobial selection and utilization.
- Although the specific effect on MDRO infection and colonization rates have not been reported, it is logical that decreasing these and other healthcare-associated infections will in turn reduce antimicrobial use and decrease opportunities for emergence and transmission of MDROs.

ANTIMICROBIAL STEWARDSHIP OCTAGON

See **Figure 11.2**.

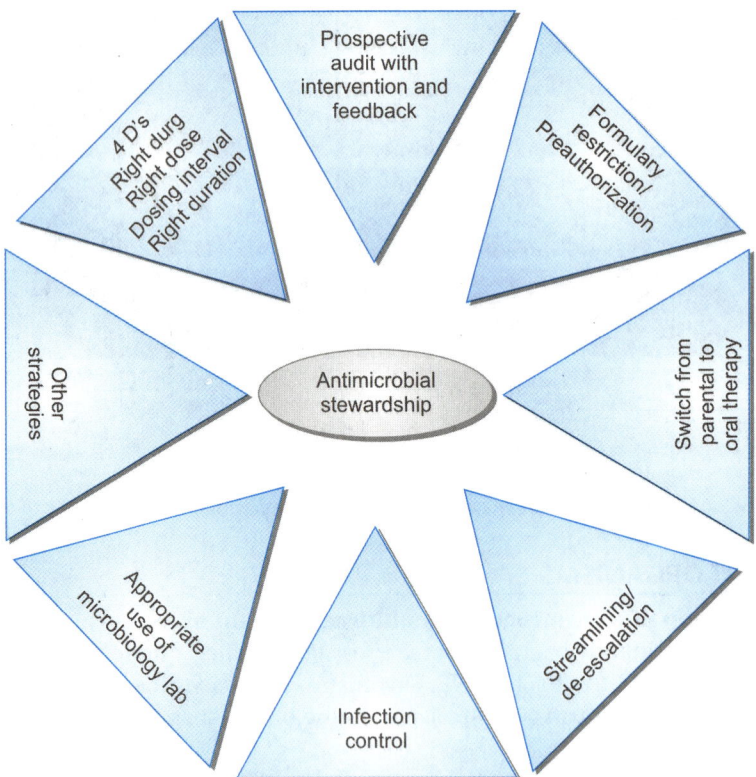

Fig. 11.2: Antimicrobial stewardship (AMS) octagon.

CHAPTER 12

Patient Safety Indicators

Chapter Outline

- Care of Vulnerable Patients
- Prevention of Iatrogenic Injury
- Care of Linens Drains and Tubing
- Restrain Policy and Care: Physical and Chemical
- Blood and Blood Transfusion Policy
- Prevention of IV Complication
- Prevention of Fall
- Prevention of DVT
- Shifting and Transportation of Patients
- Surgical Safety
- Prevention of Communication Errors
- Prevention of Healthcare-associated Infections
- Incidents and Adverse Events

INTRODUCTION

The patient safety indicators (PSIs) provide information on potentially avoidable safety events that represent opportunities for improvement in the delivery of care. More specifically, they focus on potential in hospital complications and adverse events following surgeries, procedures, and childbirth.

It can be used to help hospitals and healthcare organizations to assess, monitor, track, and improve the safety of inpatient care.
- Can be used for comparative public reporting, trending, and pay-for-performance initiatives.
- Can identify potentially avoidable complications that result from a patient's exposure to the healthcare system.
- Include hospital-level indicators to detect potential safety problems that occur during a patient's hospital stay.
- Include area-level indicators for potentially preventable adverse events that occur during a hospital stay to help assess total incidence within a region.

The Agency of Healthcare Research and Quality (AHRQ), quality indicators include four modules:
1. Prevention quality indicators (PQIs)
2. Inpatient quality indicators (IQIs)
3. Patient safety indicators (PSIs)
4. Pediatric quality indicators (PDIs)

CARE OF VULNERABLE PATIENTS

Definition

Those patients who cannot protect or take care of themselves, against exploitation or harm.
- Those patients who are prone to various risks within the hospital, such as fall, injury, neglect, abuse, medical errors and acquiring of infections.
- Vulnerability of a patient can be due to their age, physical or mental condition.
- It is the duty of the hospital staff to identify such patients and provide necessary support so that they are safe in the hospital surroundings.

Patients identified as vulnerable are:
- Old patients >65 years who or as decided by the hospital
- Minor age patients, <12 years or as decided by the hospital
- Patients having physical problems, e.g., limited mobility, blindness, deafness, speech limitations, etc.
- Patients having mental problems, e.g., depression, mental retardation, forgetfulness, etc.
- Patients who are unconscious or in semi-conscious stage
- Those patients who are illiterate and have difficulty in understanding written instructions.

Identifying Vulnerable Patients
- The first and most important step is to correctly identify these patients to whom special attention is required. The senior nurse or the medical officer on duty can be given the responsibility of identifying vulnerable patients in their department.
- They can identify a vulnerable patient through observation, basic details of the patient and by basic assessment of physical/mental limitation.
- After identification a patient ID band of special color or label should be put on their medical file.

Fall Risk Assessment
Fall is one of the most common risks to these patients. Hence, all patients identified as vulnerable, must be assessed for risk of fall. 'Morse fall scale' can be used for this purpose, which gives a risk score. Necessary measures can be taken for a patient with high score to prevent fall.

Morse Fall Scale
The Morse Fall Scale (MFS) is a rapid and simple method of assessing a patient's likelihood of falling. It consists of six variables that are quick and easy to score, and it has been shown to have predictive validity and interrater reliability **(Table 12.1)**.

MFS is used widely in acute care settings, both in the hospital and long-term care inpatient.

Falling History
This is scored as 25, if the patient has fallen during the present hospital admission or if there was an immediate history of physiological falls, such as from seizures or an impaired gait prior to admission. If the patient has not fallen, this is scored 0.

Secondary Diagnosis
This is scored as 15 if more than one medical diagnosis is listed on the patient's chart; if not, score 0.

TABLE 12.1: Morse Fall Scale.

Item	Scale		Scoring
1. History of falling; immediate or within 3 months	No Yes	0 25	
2. Secondary diagnosis	No Yes	0 15	
3. Ambulatory aid bed rest/nurse assist crutches/cane/walker furniture		0 15 30	
4. IV/Heparin lock	No Yes	0 20	
5. Gait/transferring, normal/bedrest/immobile, weak impaired		0 10 20	
6. Mental status, oriented to own ability, forgets limitations		0 15	

Ambulatory Aids

This is scored as 0 if the patient walks without a walking aid (even if assisted by a nurse), uses a wheelchair, or is on a bed rest and does not get out of bed at all. If the patient uses crutches, a cane, or a walker, this item scores 15; if the patient ambulates clutching onto the furniture for support, score this as 30.

Intravenous Therapy

This is scored as 20 if the patient has an intravenous apparatus or a heparin lock inserted; if not, score 0.

Gait

A normal gait is characterized by the patient walking with head erect, arms swinging freely at the side, and striding without hesitant. This gait scores 0. With a weak gait (score as 10), the patient is stooped but is able to lift the head while walking without losing balance. Steps are short and the patient may shuffle. With an impaired gait (score 20), the patient may have difficulty rising from the chair, attempting to get up by pushing on the arms of the chair/or by bouncing, (i.e., by using several attempts to rise). The patient's head is down, and he/she watches the ground. Because the patient's balance is poor, the patient grasps onto the furniture, a support person, or a walking aid for support and cannot walk without this assistance.

Mental Status

When using this scale, mental status is measured by checking the patient's own self-assessment of his/her own ability to ambulate.

Ask the patient, "Are you able to go the bathroom alone or do you need assistance?" If the patient's reply judging his/her own ability is consistent with the ambulatory order, the patient is rated as "normal" and scored 0.

If the patient's response is not consistent with the nursing orders or if the patient's response is unrealistic, then the patient is considered to overestimate his/her own abilities and to be forgetful of limitations and scored as 15.

Scoring and Risk Level

The score is then tallied and recorded on the patient's chart. Risk level and recommended actions, (e.g., no interventions needed, standard fall prevention interventions, and high-risk prevention interventions) are then identified.

Safety of Vulnerable Patient

Following safety practices must be followed for each vulnerable patient:
- Disabled friendly environment should be in the hospital as there can be disable patients
- Vulnerable patients be monitored more frequently for ensuring that they are safe, at-least twice in each shift or as decided for each patient.
- Vulnerable patients should be accompanied by an attendant while going to washroom or any other area.
- The washroom of vulnerable patients use, must have grab bars, anti-skid mats and call alarm system.
- When vulnerable patients are on bed safety railings, they should be put up in place to prevent fall from bed.
- When vulnerable patients are being transported on wheelchairs or stretchers, safety belt should be put up.
- Responsibility shall be given to a senior nurse or a duty doctor to ensure that vulnerable patients are not being neglected or abused.
- Senior nurse or a duty doctor should also ensure that the rights of these patients are being protected.
- The family of vulnerable patients should be explained about various safety precautions needed to be taken with the patient.
- Vulnerable patients who are determined to be at complete bed rest for prolonged periods of time shall receive proper pressure ulcer prevention and care.
- Children shall be admitted to pediatric ward only. In case, hospital does not have any separate pediatric ward, good security arrangement shall be made. Code Pink procedure for prevention of child abduction/missing child shall be in place.
- Elderly patient must be assessed for conditions associated with old age, such as delirium, forget-fullness, impaired vision, etc.
- A double check should be done before administering any medicine or carrying out any clinical intervention on these patients.
- Informed consent should be taken from vulnerable patient as well. In case they cannot provide consent, it must be obtained from their legal guardian.

PREVENTION OF IATROGENIC INJURY

Iatrogenic injury refers to tissue or organ damage that is caused by necessary medical treatment, due to adverse drug interactions or the application of medical devices and has nothing to do with primary disease.

Risk Factors

- **Multiple chronic diseases:** Greater the number of chronic diseases, greater the risk that treatment of one disease will exacerbate others. For example, treatment of arthritis with a nonsteroidal anti-inflammatory drug (NSAID) may exacerbate heart failure, coronary artery disease, or chronic gastritis.
- **Multiple physicians:** Having multiple physicians can result in uncoordinated care and polypharmacy. As a result, a patient's therapeutic regimen is frequently changed without the input of the patient's other physicians, thereby increasing risk of iatrogenic complications.
- **Multiple drugs (polypharmacy) and inappropriate drugs:**
  - Taking multiple drugs concurrently and having multiple chronic diseases markedly increase risk of adverse drug-drug or drug-disease interactions.
  - Specific examples include anticholinergics, such as diphenhydramine, benzodiazepines and other sleep aids, (e.g., zolpidem), opioids, antipsychotics, anticoagulants, and NSAIDs.
  - Iatrogenic complications are more common and often more severe among older adults than among younger patients. These complications include adverse drug effects (e.g., interactions), falls, nosocomial infections, pressure ulcers, delirium, and complications related to surgery. Prevention is often possible.
- **Hospitalization:** Risks due to hospitalization include hospital-acquired infection, polypharmacy, and transfusion reactions. Medical technology may contribute to iatrogenic complications, including sudden death or myocardial infarction after valvular replacement surgery, stroke after carotid endarterectomy, fluid overload after transfusions and infusions, unwanted prolongation of life via artificial life support, and hypoxic encephalopathy after potentially life-prolonging cardiopulmonary resuscitation (CPR).

Prevention of Iatrogenic Injury

- **Care management:** Care managers facilitate communication among healthcare practitioners and ensure that services are provided, and prevent duplication of services. Care managers may be employed by physician groups, health plans, or community or governmental organizations.
- **Geriatric interdisciplinary team:** This team evaluates all of the patient's needs, develops a coordinated care planning, and manages (or, along with the primary care physician, co-manages) care.
- **Pharmacist consultation:** Pharmacist can help prevent potential complications caused by polypharmacy and inappropriate drug use.
- **Acute care for the elderly units:** These units are hospital wards with protocols to ensure that older patients are thoroughly evaluated for potential iatrogenic problems before problems occur and that such problems are identified and appropriately managed.
- **Advance directives:** Patients are encouraged to prepare advance directives, including designation of a proxy to make medical decisions. These documents can help prevent unwanted treatment for critically-ill patients who cannot speak for themselves.

CARE OF LINEN, DRAINS AND TUBINGS

Care of linen: Nursing-in-charge is responsible for inspecting linen for any kind of damage, wear and tear and condemning them when they cannot be used as per the hospital policy. Following points should be considered for care of linen in hospitals.

- Care of linen should be taken to avoid staining. Draw Mackintosh (Rubber sheet) over bed sheets to protect soiling from stain and body fluids.
- Clean linen should be stored above the floor level away from dirt, water and sunlight.
- Soiled (contaminated) linen should not be placed on floor but properly in a designated place.
- Linen such as bed sheets should be changed every day and soiled linen should be sent to laundry
- Linen used for infectious patients should be disinfected with 1% hypochlorite before sending to laundry.
- Fresh stains should be removed using appropriate stain remover.
- All the cycles of laundry must be performed accordingly for effective washing of linen.

Care of Soiled/Contaminated Linen
- Separate laundry trolley must be used for collecting contaminated linen.
- Contaminated linen should be dipped in the bucket containing 1% hypochlorite solution of chlorine for 10 minutes.
- Rinse in water and dry in sunlight.
- Sent for autoclaving which will destroy spores as well.

Care of Blankets
- If washed on daily basis, they will shrink.
- They should be dusted in open place and dried in direct sunlight to disinfect.
- They should be covered with plastic covers to avoid dust.
- They should be kept folded in inventory with naphthalene balls in between.

Care of Drains and Rubber Tubes

Drains
These are often placed in patients to allow for drainage of a site. The most common indication for drains is to evacuate abscesses. They are placed at the end of a surgery to eliminate any fluid if accumulate within the wound. Remove fluid or air from body cavities.
- **Passive drainage:** This allows to help remove excess fluid, without the use of pressure, e.g., Foley catheter
- **Active drains:** They use actual pressure, typically negative pressure, to help remove excess fluid from the body, e.g., Jackson-Pratt (JP) drain or hemovac drain.
- **An open drainage system:** This means that it is open to air, e.g., Penrose drain
- **A closed drain:** This is not open to the environment, here the draining fluid is contained within the system, and the collection bulb or bag is simply emptied from time to time, as an when required.
- **Surgical drains:** These are usually positioned in the operating room or, at the bedside by the physician.
- **Percutaneous drains:** These are placed without surgical intervention.

Rubber Tubes
This includes rectal tube, flatus tube, catheters, Ryles, tube, etc.

Cleaning and Disinfection
- Keep rubber tube upside down under running water.
- Make use of swab sticks to remove any organic matter, if present.
- Run water through the tube to ensure patency of the tube.
- Clean tube with soap and water to remove dirt and grease.
- Hang tube for drying in a shaded place.
- After drying, place same sized tube together.
- Cover the tube with paper lining and store in appropriate place.
- It should be sent for autoclaving if further sterilization is required.

RESTRAIN POLICY AND CARE—PHYSICAL AND CHEMICAL

Restraints
It is defined as 'the intentional restriction of a person's voluntary movement of behavior.'

Nurses are accountable for providing, facilitating, advocating and promoting the best possible patient care and to take action when patient safety and well-being are compromised, including when deciding to apply restraints.

General principles of restraints are:
- Should be selected to reduce client's movement only as much as possible
- Nurse should carefully explain type of restraint and reason for its use.
- Should not interfere with treatment.
- Bony prominences should be padded before applying it.
- Should be changed when they become soiled or damped.
- Should be secured from client's reach.

- Should be attached to bed frame not to slide rails.
- Frequent circulation checks should be performed when extremity is used.

Indications for Restraints
- Displaying behavior that is putting themselves at risk or harm.
- Displaying behavior that is putting others at risk of harm.
- Requiring treatment by a legal order, e.g., Mental Health Act 2007.
- Requiring urgent life-saving treatment.
- Needing to be maintained in secure settings.

There are Three Types of Restraints: Physical, Chemical and Environmental
- **Physical restraints:** Limit a patient's movement.
- **Types of physical restraints are:**
  - *Mummy restraint:* It is used on infants and small children during examinations and treatment of head and neck. It is used to mobilize the arms and legs of child for a brief period of time.
  - *Elbow restraint:* It is used to prevent flexion of the elbow and to hold the elbow in an extended position so that the infant cannot reach the face.
  - *Extremity restraint:* It is used to immobilize one or more extremities. one type of extremity resistant is clove-hitch, restraint which is done with gauze bandage strip (2 inch wide) making figure of eight. The end of the gauze is to be tied up with crib/bed.
  - *Abdominal restraint:* It is used to hold the infant in a supine position on the bed.
  - *Jacket restraint:* It is used to hold up the infant.
  - *Mitten or finger restraint:* It is used for infants to prevent self-injury by hands in case of burns, facial injury or operations of eczema of face or body.
- **Chemical restraints:** A chemical restraint is the intentional use of any medications to subdue, sedate, or restrain an individual. It is any form of psychoactive medication used not to treat illness, but to intentionally inhibit a particular behavior or movement.

  Chemical restraints have been used to restrict the freedom of movement of a patient—usually in acute, emergency, or psychiatric settings. Chemical restraints are often prescribed for what healthcare workers describe as dangerous, uncontrolled, aggressive, or violent behavior.

  Anti-anxiety, antidepressant, and antipsychotic medications are often used to treat the behavioral and psychological symptoms associated with dementia. These medications affect mood, perception, consciousness, cognition, and behavior
- **Environmental restraints:** It is defined as barrier or device that limits the mobility of a patient, e.g., bed rails, person's walker or cane or private quiet room.

Restraint Policy
Restraint may only be used to ensure the immediate physical safety of the patient, staff or others and must be discontinued at the earliest possible time. Alternative and nonphysical interventions are attempted prior to use of restraints.

Patient Rights
When restraints are deemed necessary, such activity will be undertaken in a manner that protects the patient's health and safety and preserves his/her dignity, rights, and well being. Restraints will be used for medical necessity only and not as a means of coercion, discipline, convenience, or retaliation.
- Each patient will be respected as an individual.
- Staff will monitor and meet the patients needs while in restraints.
- Staff will reassess and encourage release from restraints.
- The patient and family will be encouraged to participate in care and receive education as appropriate.
- Provide for safe application and removal of restraint by qualified staff authorized to do so, and whose competencies have been validated.

Organizational Oversight
- Approving the restraint policy/procedure outlining risks, preventive strategies, effective alternatives, criteria for use, education of the patient and family, and the care of the patient in restraints.
- Providing appropriate staffing for safe and effective use of restraint alternative(s) and restraint(s)

- Assuring that staff is trained and competent to minimize the use of restraints and to use restraints safely with consideration of the patient's dignity and well being.
- Including the restraint reduction plan as part of the organization's performance improvement plan
- Refining patient assessment processes to identify earlier the potential risk of dangerous patient behavior and the prevention, when appropriate, of those behaviors.
- Assuring restraints are used in conformity with all prevailing laws, regulations, and accreditation standards.

Restraint Orders

- Restraint(s) is/are used in accordance with the order of a physician or other licensed independent practitioner who is responsible for the care of the patient and is authorized to order restraint or seclusion in accordance with state law.
- Orders for restraints are documented on the Restraint Order Set in the patient's medical record. All orders are time limited, and restraints must be discontinued at the earliest possible time, regardless of the length of time identified in the order.
- **Chemical intervention orders include the following:** Patient name, medication name, dose, route and that it is a STAT or NOW order.

BLOOD AND BLOOD TRANSFUSION POLICY

The policy aims to ensure easily accessible and adequate supply of safe and quality blood and blood components collected/procured from a voluntary non-remunerated regular blood donor in well equipped premises, which is free from transfusion transmitted infections is stored and transported under optimum conditions. Transfusion under supervision of trained personnel for all who need it irrespective of their economic or social status through comprehensive, efficient and a total quality management approach will be ensured under the policy.

Objectives of the Policy

To achieve the above aim, the following objectives are drawn:
- To reiterate firmly, the government commitment to provide safe and adequate quantity of blood, blood components and blood products.
- To make available adequate resources to develop and reorganize the blood transfusion services in the entire country.
- To make latest technology available for operating the blood transfusion services and ensure its functioning in an updated manner.
- To launch extensive awareness programs for donor information, education, motivation, recruitment and retention in order to ensure adequate availability of safe blood.
- To encourage appropriate clinical use of blood and blood products.
- To strengthen the manpower through human resource development.
- To encourage research and development in the field of transfusion medicine and related technology.
- To take adequate regulatory and legislative steps for monitoring and evaluation of blood transfusion services and to take steps to eliminate profiteering in blood banks.

Objective 1

To reiterate firmly, the government commitment to provide safe and adequate quantity of blood, blood components and blood products:
- A national blood transfusion program shall be developed to ensure establishment of non-profit integrated National and State Blood Transfusion Services in the country.
- Trading in blood, i.e., sale and purchase of blood shall be prohibited.
- Transfusion services shall be promoted for making available of safe blood to the people.
- Due to the special requirement of Armed Forces in remote border areas, necessary amendments shall be made in the Drugs & Cosmetics Act/Rules to provide special licenses to small garrison units. These units shall also be responsible for the civilian blood needs of the region.

Objective 2

To make available adequate resources to develop and reorganize the blood transfusion services in the entire country:
- National and State/UT Blood Transfusion Councils shall be supported/strengthened financially by pooling resources from various existing programs and if possible by raising funds from international/bilateral agencies.
- Efforts shall be directed to make the blood transfusion service viable through non-profit recovery system.

Objective 3

To make latest technology available for operating the blood transfusion services and ensure its functioning in an updated manner:
- Minimum standards for testing, processing and storage shall be set and ensured.
- A Quality System Scheme shall be introduced in all blood centers.
- Regular proficiency testing of personnel shall be introduced in all the blood centers.
- An External Quality Assessment Scheme (EQAS) through the referral laboratories approved by the National Blood Transfusion Council shall be introduced to assist participating centers in achieving higher standards and uniformity.
- Efforts shall be made towards indigenization of kits, equipment and consumables used in blood banks.
- Use of automation shall be encouraged to manage higher workload with increased efficiency.
- A mechanism for transfer of technology shall be developed to ensure the availability of state-of-the-art technology from outside India.
- Each blood center shall develop its own Standard Operating Procedures on various aspects of Blood Banking.
- All blood centers shall adhere to bio-safety guidelines as provided in the Ministry of Health and Family Welfare manual 'Hospital Acquired Infections: Guidelines for Control' and disposal of biohazardous waste as per the provisions of the existing Biomedical Wastes (Management and Handling) Rules—1996 under the Environmental Protection Act—1986.

Objective 4

To launch extensive awareness programs for donor information, education, motivation, recruitment and retention in order to ensure adequate availability of safe blood:
- Efforts shall be directed towards recruitment and retention of voluntary, non-remunerated blood donors through education and awareness programs.
- Enrolment of safe donors shall be ensured.
- State/UT Blood Transfusion Councils shall recognize the services of regular voluntary non-remunerated blood donors and donor organizers appropriately.
- National/State/UT Blood Transfusion Councils shall develop and launch an IEC campaign using all channels of communication including mass-media for promotion of voluntary blood donation and generation of awareness regarding dangers of blood from paid donors and procurement of blood from unauthorized blood banks/laboratories.
- National/State/UT blood transfusion councils shall involve other departments/sectors for promoting voluntary blood donations.

Objective 5

To encourage appropriate clinical use of blood and blood products:
- Blood shall be used only when necessary. Blood and blood products shall be transfused only to treat conditions leading to significant morbidity and mortality that cannot be prevented or treated effectively by other means.
- National Guidelines on 'Clinical use of Blood' shall be made available and updated as required from time to time.
- Effective and efficient clinical use of blood shall be promoted in accordance with guidelines.
- Education and training in effective clinical use of blood shall be organized.
- Blood and its components shall be prescribed only by a medical practitioner registered as per the provisions of Medical Council Act—1956.
- Availability of blood components shall be ensured through the network of regional centers, satellite centers and other blood centers by creating adequate number of blood component separation units.
- Appropriate steps shall be taken to increase the availability of plasma fractions as per the need of the country through expanding the capacity of existing center and establishing new centers in the country.
- Adequate facilities for transporting blood and blood products including proper cold-chain maintenance shall be made available to ensure appropriate management of blood supply.
- Guidelines for management of blood supply during natural and man-made disasters shall be made available.

Objective 6

To strengthen the manpower through human resource development:

- In all the existing courses for nurses, technicians and Pharmacists, transfusion medicine shall be incorporated as one of the subjects.
- In-service training programs shall be organized for all categories of personnel working in blood centers as well as drug inspectors and other officers from regulatory agencies.
- Appropriate modules for training of Donor Organizers/Donor Recruitment Officers shall be developed to facilitate regular and uniform training programs to be conducted in all states.
- Short orientation training cum advocacy programs on donor motivation and recruitment shall be organized for community.
- Community-based organizations (CBOs) and NGOs who wish to participate in Voluntary Blood Donor Recruitment Program.
- Inter-country and intra-country exchange for training and experience of personnel associated with blood centers shall be encouraged to improve quality of blood transfusion service.
- States/UTs shall create a separate cadre and opportunities for promotions for suitably trained medical and paramedical personnel working in blood transfusion services.

Objective 7

To encourage Research and Development in the field of transfusion medicine and related technology:

- A corpus of funds shall be made available to NBTC/SBTCs to facilitate research in transfusion medicine and technology related to blood banking.
- A technical resource core group at national level shall be created to coordinate research and development in the country. This group shall be responsible for recommending implementation of new technologies and procedures in coordination with DC.
- Multicentric research initiatives on issues related to blood transfusion shall be encouraged.
- To take appropriate decisions and/or introduction of policy initiatives on the basis of factual information, operational research on various aspects, such as various aspects of transfusion transmissible diseases, knowledge, attitude and practices (KAP) among donors, clinical use of blood, need assessment, etc., shall be promoted.
- Computer-based information and management systems shall be developed which can be used by all the centers regularly to facilitate networking.

Objective 8

To take adequate regulatory and legislative steps for monitoring and evaluation of blood transfusion services and to take steps to eliminate profiteering in blood banks:

- For grant/renewal of blood bank licenses including plan of a blood bank, a committee, comprising of members from State/UT Blood Transfusion Councils including Transfusion Medicine expert, Central and State/UT FDAs shall be constituted which will scrutinize all applications as per the guidelines provided by Drugs Controller General (India).
- Fresh licenses to stand-alone blood banks in private sector shall not be granted. Renewal of such blood banks shall be subjected to thorough scrutiny and shall not be renewed in case of noncompliance of any condition of license.
- A separate blood bank cell shall be created under a senior officer not below the rank of DDC(I) in the office of the DC(I) at the headquarter.
- As a deterrent to paid blood donors who operate in the disguise of replacement donors, institutions who prescribe blood for transfusion shall be made responsible for procurement of blood for their patients through their affiliation with licensed blood centers.
- States/UTs shall enact rules for registration of nursing homes wherein provisions for affiliation with a licensed blood bank for procurement of blood for their patients shall be incorporated.

PREVENTION OF IV COMPLICATIONS

Peripheral intravenous catheters (PIVC) are the most commonly used intravenous device in hospitalized patients. They are primarily used for therapeutic purposes, such as administration of medications, fluids and/or blood products as well as blood sampling.

Definition of Terms

- **Peripheral IV devices:** These are cannula/catheter inserted into a small peripheral vein for therapeutic purposes, such as administration of medications, fluids and/or blood products.
- **Aseptic technique:** It is a part of all procedures which aims to prevent pathogenic microorganisms, in sufficient quantity to cause infection of hands, surfaces and equipment. Therefore, unlike sterile techniques, standard and surgical aseptic techniques are possible and can be achieved in typical hospital and community settings.
- **Decontaminate hands:** Perform hand hygiene in order to protect the patient from organisms which may enter their key sites or devices during a procedure.
- **Key parts:** Part of the device/s that must remain aseptic throughout the clinical procedures. Examples of key parts include—catheter hub, needleless connector, syringe hub, needle, etc.
- **Key sites:** The area on the patient, such as IV insertion site that must be protected from microorganisms.
- **Extravasation:** An extravasation occurs when there is accidental infiltration of a vesicant drug or fluid into the tissue surrounding the venipuncture site.
- **Infiltration:** Occurs when drugs or fluid infiltrates into the tissue surrounding the venipuncture site. This happens when the tip of catheter slips out of the vein, catheter passes through the wall of the vein, or as blood vessel wall stretches which allows fluid to infuse into the surrounding tissue.
- **Phlebitis—a sign of vessel damage:** The cause can be chemical (due to the osmolarity of the solution), mechanical (from trauma at insertion or movement) or infective (microorganisms contaminating the device). Signs include swelling, redness, heat, induration, purulence, a palpable venous cord (hard vein) and pain related to local inflammation of the vein at or near the insertion site.
- **Infusion pump:** Refers to infusions pumps, such as large volume pumps (LVPs)/volumetric pumps, e.g., Alaris Signature Edition (SE), syringe drivers, (e.g., Alaris GH+), Patient Controlled Analgesia/PCA pumps (Alaris PCAM), etc.
- **Double checking:** Refers to the practice of two clinicians [appropriately endorsed enrolled nurses (EN), Registered Nurses (RN), Doctors or Pharmacists] independently checking the medications.

Assessment

Patient and IV site assessments should be done on a regular basis.

PIVC assessment includes:

- **Assessment of PIVC insertion site:** Catheter position, patency/occlusion, limb symmetry, any signs of phlebitis (erythema, tenderness, swelling, pain, etc.), infiltration/extravasation. PIVC are considered as high-risk for pressure injury. PIVC sites should be checked hourly for pressure sore and any signs of infection unless documented.
- **Assessment of PIVC dressing and splints:** Check securement of dressing—if it is intact, clean and dry or if it is loose or if visible ooze was present underneath the dressing. Check splint tapes are not too tight or restrictive.
- **Assessment of IV lines, equipment and IV fluid infusions:**
  - If the patient is receiving continuous IV fluid infusion—observations of the IV site, type of fluid and volume infused, accurate rate of infusion for patient and pressure alarms of infusion pumps are observed hourly and documented in the fluid balance flowsheet.
  - If the patient (inpatient setting) is having intermittent infusion, eight hourly assessments are a minimum. Unstable patients who have signs and symptoms of complications are to be assessed more frequently.

Management

Continuous infusion of IV fluids: Assessment and documentation of findings are to be completed hourly to determine effective delivery of prescribed medications and fluid.

Each bag of fluid is independently double checked, and a signed patient label is put on the bag.

- Check whether the solution is the prescribed one, the rate of infusion, and the amount infused is noted.
- **Document the infused volume:** Hourly on fluid balance flowsheet (it is advised to clear the infusion pump hourly).

- Check the infusion site for any signs of complications and document the assessment findings hourly in fluid balance flowsheet.
- Review the cumulative volume infused and fluid output as required based on patient's clinical condition.
- Pump pressures for each IV line should be documented hourly or when adjusted on the flow sheet.

Table 12.2 depicts the visual infusion phlebitis (VIP) score card.

TABLE 12.2: Visual infusion phlebitis (VIP) score card.

Observation/complication	Score	Management
IV site appears healthy	0	**No sign of phlebitis:** Observe cannula
One of the following is evident: • Slight pain near IV or • Slight redness near IV site	1	**Possible first sign of phlebitis:** Observe cannula
Two of the following are evident: • Slight pain near IV • Erythema • Swelling	2	**Early stage of phlebitis:** Resite cannula
All of the following are evident: • Pain along path of cannula • Erythema • Induration	3	**Medium stage of phlebitis:** • Resite cannula • Consider treatment
All of the following are evident and extensive: • Pain along path of cannula • Erythema • Palpable venous cord	4	**Advanced stage of phlebitis or start of thrombophlebitis:** • Resita cannula • Consider treatment
All of the following are evident and extensive: • Pain along path of cannula • Erythema • Palpable venous cord • Pyrexia	5	**Advanced stage of thrombophlebitis:** • Initiate treatment • Respite cannula

PREVENTION OF FALL

A patient fall is defined as an event that results in a sudden, unplanned fall of a patient to the floor with/without injury.
Falls may be at different levels, i.e., from one level to ground level, e.g., from beds, wheelchairs or down stairs on the same level as a result of slipping, tripping, or stumbling, or from a collision, pushing, or shoving, by or with another person below ground level, i.e., into a hole or other opening in surface.

Not all patient falls are predictable or preventable in acute care hospitals. Some falls are simply the result of individual physiological responses to illness or treatment in care settings in which patient ambulation is essential to recovery.

Types of Fall

1. **Accidental falls:** Occur when patients fall unintentionally because of an environmental hazard or equipment failure (14% of all falls).
2. **Anticipated physiological falls:** Occur in patients with known risk factors for tripping related to the patient's underlying medical condition (78% of all falls).
3. **Unanticipated physiological fall:** Falls which occur in patients who do not have identified risk factors until the fall occurs, e.g., faints, seizures (8% of all falls).

Fall Risk Assessment

IPSG6 (International patient Safety Goals 6), a part of evidence-based fall safety initiative, was developed to prevent patients from falling. For any fall prevention program, the characteristics and activities of patient linked to an increased risk of falling should be the main focus. While there is some form of assessment for risk of falling among patients that is likely to help determine when special prevention interventions are needed, there is currently very little evidence to support the use of fall risk assessment tools.

There is nothing to suggest that the use of a generic assessment tool (identified from the literature) offers greater accuracy than tools developed by institutions based on local patient characteristics.

No interventions have, currently, been proven to be effective in fall prevention in the acute care setting. Expert opinion, however suggests that institutions should have a falls prevention program consisting of multiple interventions aimed at minimizing the individual patient's risk of falling. While the use of multiple fall prevention interventions was the most common approach, results of their effectiveness are contradictory.

How Hospitals can Prevent Patient Falls: The Measures are as Follows (Fig. 12.1):

- Identifying the vulnerable groups
- Assessment of vulnerable patient within 2 hours
- Applying yellow band.
- Applying side railings.
- Applying brakes for all the cots.
- Patient first card at the edge of the cot.
- Education to the relative on fall risk prevention.
- Education of the staff of fall risk assessment.
- Uses of grab bars and call bells.
- Importance of using safety belts on stretcher and wheel chairs.

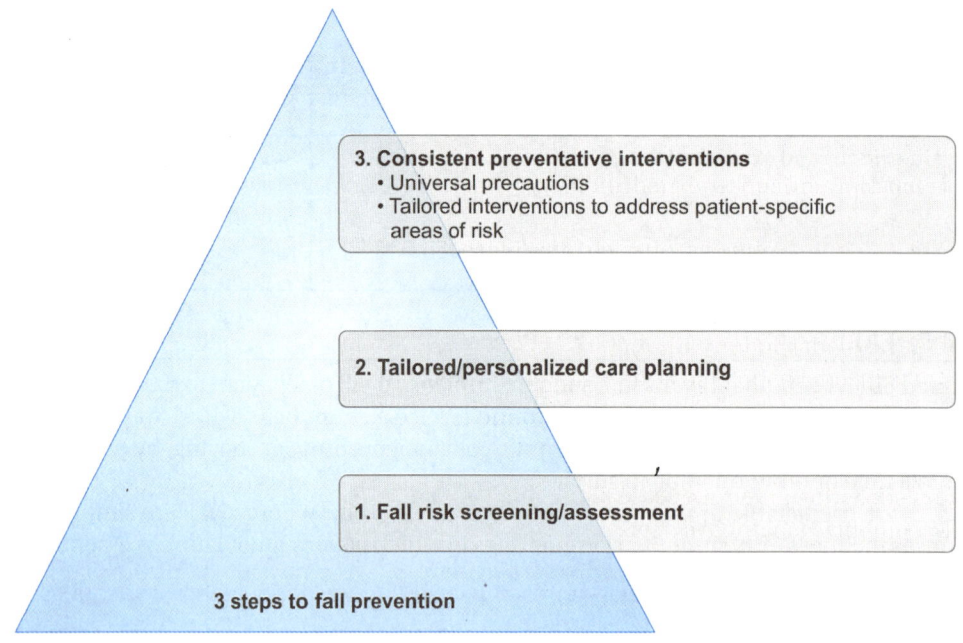

Fig. 12.1: Steps of fall prevention.

PREVENTION OF DVT

Deep vein thrombosis or venous thromboembolism (DVT or VTE), is a term which refers to the formation of blood clots (thrombus) within a deep vein usually in the leg. Infective tissue perfusion related to interruption of venous blood flow can occur, it is an underdiagnosed and serious, yet preventable medical condition that can cause disability and death.

The following are the most common symptoms of DVT that occur in the affected part of the body:
- Swelling
- Pain
- Tenderness
- Redness of the skin

Chapter 12: Patient Safety Indicators **179**

Prevention of DVT (Fig. 12.2)

Move around as soon as possible after having been confined to bed, such as after surgery, illness, or injury:
  – Graduated compression stockings
  – Medication (anticoagulants) to prevent DVT.
- **When sitting for long periods of time, such as when traveling for more than four hours:**
  – Get up and walk around every 1 to 2 hours.
  – Exercise your legs while you are sitting by:
    ◆ Raising and lowering your heels while keeping your toes on the floor
    ◆ Raising and lowering your toes while keeping your heels on the floor
    ◆ Tightening and releasing your leg muscles
- Wear loose-fitting clothes.
- Reduce risk by maintaining a healthy weight, avoiding a sedentary lifestyle, and following your doctor's recommendations based on your individual risk factors.

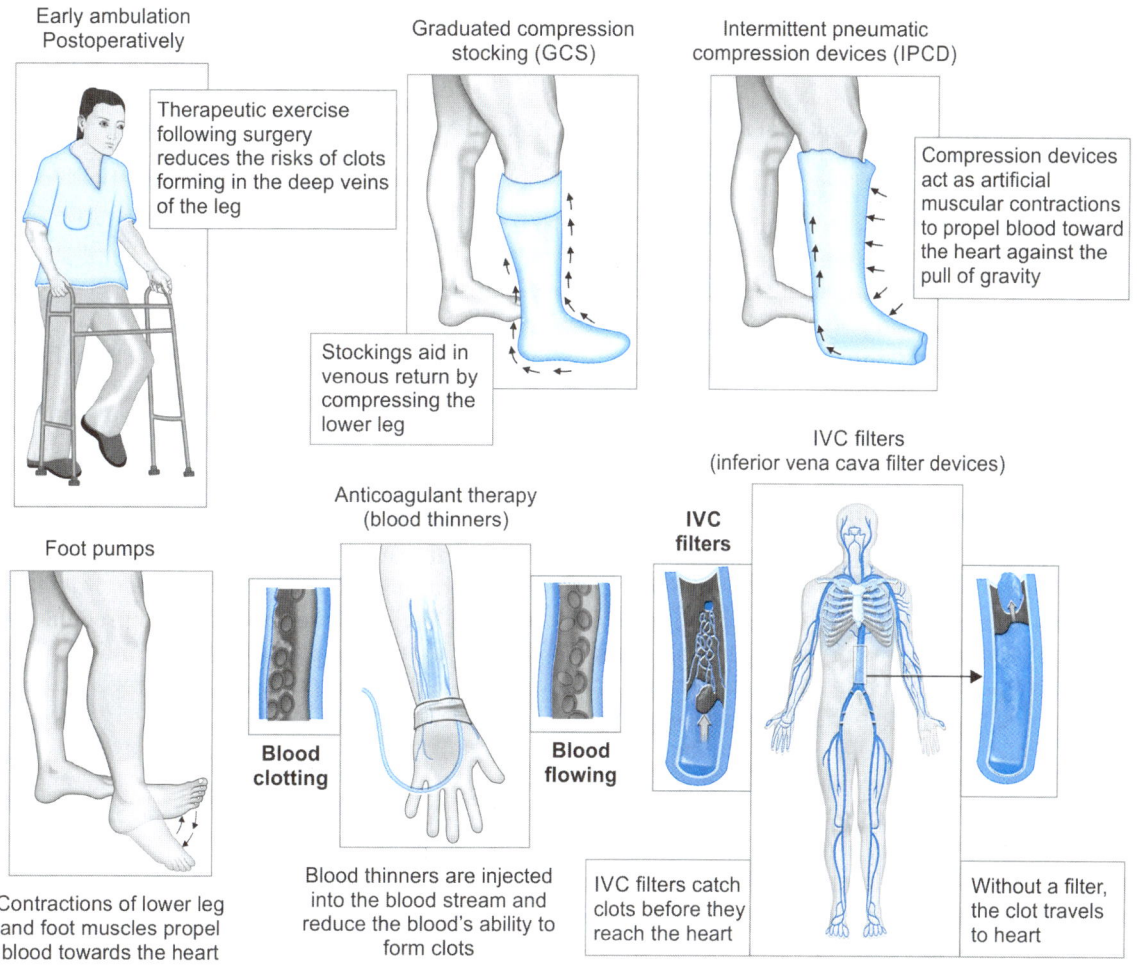

Fig. 12.2: Prevention of deep vein thrombosis.

SHIFTING AND TRANSPORTING OF PATIENTS

Patient care transfer can be defined as moving a patient from one flat surface to another. The most common patient transfers are from a bed to a stretcher and from a bed to a wheelchair.

Patient care transfers are an essential yet often neglected aspect of patient care. Proper transfers are based on the concept that focuses on maintaining continuity of care both during and after the transfer.

Depending on the complexity, patients often receive care in multiple settings during and after hospitalization. While some aspects of patient transport vary depending on the patient's status, intrahospital transports are inevitable, particularly in critically-ill patients. Poorly organized patient transfers can result in increased morbidity and mortality and should be performed with careful attention.

Clinical Significance—Types of Transfer

Transfers from a Bed to a Stretcher

After the pre-transfer checklist is complete, the transfer from a bed to a stretcher may be performed according to the following steps:
1. Identify the number of staff required for the transfer (typically 3–4 providers for a bed-to-stretcher transfer).
2. Explain what the patient can do to help the procedure (hands crossed over the chest, chin tucked, etc.) and obtain necessary supplies.
3. Raise/lower the bed to a safe working height, lock the brakes, lower guard rails, and position the patient closest to the side of the bed where the transfer will take place.
4. Place a sheet on top of the slider board; this is used to transfer the patient onto the stretcher and decrease friction.
5. Roll the patient over to the side opposite to the stretcher and place the slider board underneath the patient, such that the board is between the patient and the bed.
6. Roll the patient back into the supine position, make sure the patient is centered on the slider board and that the feet are in a straight position.
7. Bring the stretcher to the side of the bed near the patient and position the stretcher slightly lower than the bed. Lock the brakes of the stretcher.
8. **Position the healthcare team such that the patient's weight is distributed evenly:**
   – Two on the side of the stretcher, grasping the sheet placed over the slide board
   – One at the head of the bed, grasping the pillow and the sheet.
   – One at the far side of the patient, between the chest and the hips
   – An additional one can be at the foot of the bed.
9. **The leader of the healthcare team will initiate the transfer, counting 1, 2, 3:**
   – The provider on the far side of the bed will push the patient.
   – The two providers on the side of the stretcher will shift their weight from front to back, bringing the patient with them by pulling the sheet.
   – Meanwhile, the providers at the head and foot of the bed will ensure that the patient is secured, lifting the head/shoulders and feet, respectively.

Transfer from a Bed to a Wheelchair

Transferring patients from a bed to a wheelchair requires understanding the needs of the patient. Always communicate with the person being transferred so that assistance is being given at the appropriate time, allowing for coordination of efforts between the assistant and the patient. If the patient can bear weight on both lower extremities and predictably take small steps, a one-person assist may be performed. If these criteria are not met, a two-person transfer or a mechanical lift may be necessary to safely transfer the patient. If transferring a patient from a bed to a wheelchair, first complete the pre-transfer checklist and proceed according to the following steps:
- Apply the patient's footwear before ambulation.
- Raise/lower the bed to a safe working height, lower guard rails, place wheelchair next to the bed at a 45° angle and ensure the brakes are applied. If one side of the patient is weaker, place the wheelchair on the healthier side.
- Place hands on the patient's waist.
- Help the patient shift weight in a rocking motion (front foot to back foot, and so on) until reaching a standing position.
- Once the patient is standing, have them walk a few small steps backward until feeling the wheelchair's back against the legs. Ask the patient to grasp the wheelchair.
- Ensure that the patient is adequately draped and sitting comfortably in the wheelchair.
- Patients may use slide boards for more effortless transfer.
- When the patient transfers back to the bed from the wheelchair, the safest sequence of actions is positioning the chair at a 45° angle to the bed, locking the brakes, raising the footplates, and rotating the leg rests outward. This will allow the patient to stand more easily. Leaning forward or grasping the edge of the bed is likely to cause the wheelchair to tip forward. Assistance can be given to block the person's knees to provide additional support.

Slide Boards Transfer

A sliding transfer board can benefit patients with paraplegia, lower-extremity amputation, and decreased balance or strength at the lower extremities. A patient with quadriplegia would not have the postural support or upper extremity strength to use a

slide transfer board. A patient who can do a stand pivot transfer would not need a slide transfer board. A patient that cannot follow commands will not benefit from a slide transfer board.
- A transfer belt is placed around the patient's hips/buttocks.
- The wheelchair is placed as close to the bed, and brakes are applied. The armrest is removed, and the footrests must be swung away. The patient of the assistant places the sliding transfer board under the patient's buttock/leg. Placing the sliding transfer board under the patient's buttock/leg will prevent the patient from falling off the board. Fingers should not be under the board to avoid pinching the fingers.
- The assistant places one knee between the patient's knees and the other knee near the wheelchair's front, close to the other surface.
- The assistant holds the transfer belt and slowly slides the patient across the board.

Log-rolling Procedure
- The purpose of the log-rolling procedure is to move a patient without flexing the spinal column. The entire body is transferred as a single object.
- If a neck injury is a concern, a firm neck support should be in place, and in-line traction should be maintained with multiple assistants while performing the procedure.
- The patient should not ambulate until proper examination and radiographs are obtained.
- Keep the patient's arms on the side of the body at all times. Some recommend that the patient's arms be crossed over the chest.
- A pillow can be placed between the legs for support while turning.

SURGICAL SAFETY

WHO Second Global Patient Safety Challenge is "Safe Surgery Saves Lives". Safe Surgery Saves Lives set about to improve the safety of surgical care around the world by defining a core set of safety standards that could be applied in all WHO Member States.

Surgical Safety Checklist
See **Figure 12.3**.

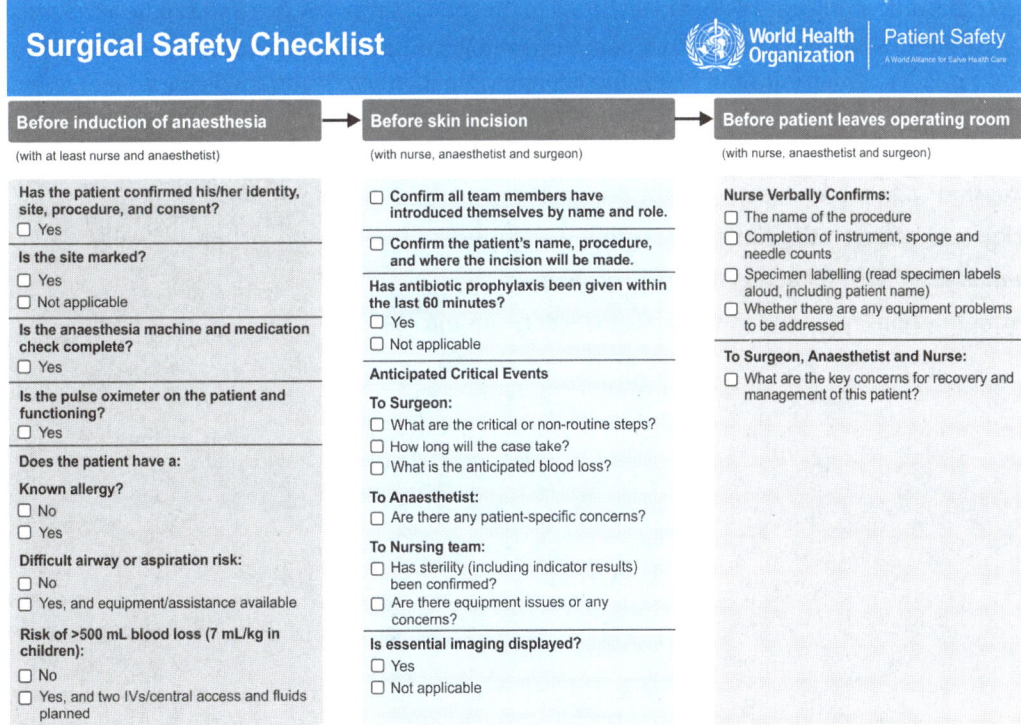

Fig. 12.3: Surgical safety checklist.

PREVENTION OF COMMUNICATION ERRORS

Communication is the process of exchanger of information, through ideas, thoughts and feelings between two are more individuals through a common system of signs, symbols or behavior.

Levels of Communication

Communication Level

1. Intrapersonal communication or self talk
2. Interpersonal communication
3. Group communication
4. Organizational communication

Forms of Communication

1. Verbal communication
2. **Nonverbal communication: also known as body language:**
   – Physical appearance
   – Facial expression
   – Posture and gait
   – Eye contact
   – Body movement and gestures
   – Touch
   – Tone of voice
   – Symbols
   – Signals

The following communication strategies were included in the toolkit interventions and can be accessed.

Situational briefing guide SBAR: A standardized communication format, the SBAR, was utilized as a situational briefing guide for staff and provider communication regarding changes in patient status or needs for nonemergent events, related issues, or for events on the unit, in the lab, or within the healthcare team.

SBAR stands for:

- **Describe Situation:** Where is going on with the patient?
- **Provide Background:** What is the clinical background or context?
- **Provide Client assessment:** What do I think the problem is?
- **Make Recommendation:** What do I think needs to be done for the patient?

Barriers of Communication

See **Table 12.3**.

TABLE 12.3: Barriers of communication.

Barriers	Description	Methods to overcome
Physiological barrier	• Poor retention due to memory problems • Lack of intention • Discomfort due to illness • Poor sensory perception • Hearing problems • Poor listening skills • Information overload • Gender physiological differences	• Sender and recipient must keep each other's retention and recollection abilities in mind • Sender and recipient should pay complete attention when information is being shared • Sender and recipient should ensure each other's comfort before starting communication • Intactness of communication between sender and recipient must be ensured • While communicating limitations of hearing abilities must be kept in mind • Sender and recipient should ensure active listening between each other • Overload of information must be avoided • Difference in communication on account of gender must be kept in mind while communication
Environmental barriers	• Loud background noise • Poor lighting • Uncomfortable settings • Unhygienic surroundings and bad odor • Very hot or cold room distance	• Good lightening must be ensured • Comfortable sitting arrangements must be ensured • Proper hygienic and odor free environment should be ensured • Optimal temperature should be maintained • Distance should be maintained proper
Psychological barriers	• Misperception and misunderstanding • Disrupt and unhappy emotions • Emotional disturbance, e.g., anger, jealously and suspicion • Prejudice, resentment and antagonism • Psychotic or neurotic illness • Worry and emotional disturbance • Fear, anxiety and confused thinking	• Carry out communication in happy and trustworthy way • Sender and recipient should not harbor negative emotions, e.g., anger, jealously and suspicion • Feelings of prejudice, resentment and antagonism must be avoided by sender and recipient • During communication, sender and recipient must be free from fear, anxiety and confusion
Social barriers	• Difference in social norms, values and behavior • Social taboos • Social status	• Difference in social norms, values and behavior should be considered while communication • Social beliefs should be kept in mind while communicating
Cultural barriers	• Ethics, religious and cultural differences • Cultural traditions, values and behavior	• Cultural differences must be given due consideration while communicating • Cultural traditions, values and behavior must be kept in mind during communication
Semantic barriers	• Language barrier, language jargons • Faulty language translations • Individual differences in expression and perception • Past experience of individual • Failure to listen	• Sender and recipient must use same language when communicating • Individual differences in expression and perception should be kept in mind during communication
Organizational barrier	• Organizational policy, rules and regulations • Technical failure • Time pressure • Complexity of organizational structure due to hierarchy • Size of organization	• Organizational policy, rules and regulations must be pro-communication • Organizational structure should be simple • Organization must be technically strong in communication • Large organizations must be divided into smaller subsets to promote effective communication
Communication process-related barriers	• Unclear and conflicting message • Inappropriate channels • Lack of poor feedback	• Appropriate channel must be used • Stereotypical approach should be avoided • Message should be clear and non-conflicting • Proper feedback must be ensured by recipients

DOCUMENTATION

Documentation is the written or electronic legal record of all pertinent interactions with the patient—assessing, diagnosis, planning, implementing, and evaluating.

Documentation is necessary for:
- Communication between healthcare providers
- Meeting legislative requirements: Documentation is a valuable method of demonstrating that you have applied nursing knowledge, skill and judgment within a nurse-client relationship.
- Quality improvement requires clear, complete and accurate nursing documentation, which facilitates quality improvement initiatives and risk management analysis for clients, staff and organizations.
- Documentation is used to evaluate quality of services and appropriateness of care through chart audits and performance reviews
- Helps in clinical research
- Support decision analysis
- Legal proof of healthcare provided, the client record is a legal document and can be used as evidence in a court of law or in a professional conduct proceeding.

Patient Record

It is a compilation of a patient's health information (PHI).

It is mainly the responsibility of nurse to maintain patient record, as this is the only permanent legal document that witness's to the nurses interactions with patient.

Guidelines for Effective Documentation

Content
- Information should be entered in a complete, concise, current and accurate way.
- This should be made sure properly that this document reflects ones nursing process/professional responsibilities.
- Patient's findings (observations of behavior) should be recorded instead of one's own interpretation of these findings.
- Avoid using such words which can be interpreted differently (dual meaning words) by different persons, such as good, average, sufficient, etc.
- All the precautions and preventive measures used should be recorded.
- Document is a legal record. Adhere to professional standards and institutional policy for documentation.
- Avoid copying and pasting notes in EHRs as data can be outdated or inaccurate, check that thing.
- Document the nursing response to questionable medical orders or treatment or failure to treatment. Note the date and time the healthcare provider was notified of the concern and the exact healthcare provider response. If all this occurs on phone, appoint a second nurse to listen the conservation and co-sign the note. If nursing administrator was notified document this event also.
- Document should have legal protection to nurse, other caregivers, the healthcare facility and the patient.

Timing
- Document in a timely manner
- If one forgets, record it as soon as possible, follow procedure for late entries
- In each entry indicate date and time, when the entry was written and time of observation and interventions. This is crucial when case is being reconstructed for legal purposes.
- Document nursing intervention as closely as possible to their execution.
- Write progress notes on admission, transfer to another unit, discharge, when procedure is performed, before procedure and post-procedure, upon communication with healthcare provider regarding patients health and for any change in patients status.

Format
- Check to make sure you have the correct chart before writing.
- Record on proper forms and formats or screens as per institutional policy
- Use correct grammar and spelling, use standard terminology.
- Follow computer documentation guidelines when recording on digital screen.
- Put date and time at each entry.
- Record nursing interventions chronologically in consecutive lines.

Accountability
- Sign from first entry to last entry wherever staff notes are written.
- Do not sign note notes, if describing interventions not performed by you.
- Recognize that patient record is permanent. Follow facility policy pertaining to the color of ink and type of pen or ink to be used.
- Ensure that patient record is complete before sending it to medical records.
- Anything omitted in care, must be recorded as what was omitted, why it was omitted and who omitted it.

Confidentiality
- Information contained in patient health record should be kept private.
- Staff should be familiar with hospital policy about who has access to patient records other than the immediate care giver team, and process used to obtain access.
- Students using patient's records for educational reasons are bound professionally and ethically to keep in strict confidence all the information they learn from patient record.

PREVENTION OF HEALTHCARE ASSOCIATED INFECTIONS

Prevention of HAI is an important practice as it not only reduces the economical burden of the patient but also saves the patient's life from life-threatening infections. This can be studied under two categories:
1. Standard precautions
2. Transmission based precautions.

Standard Precautions

- Standard precautions apply to: (1) blood; (2) all body fluids, secretions, and excretions except sweat, regardless of whether or not they contain visible blood; (3) non-intact skin; and (4) mucous membranes.
- Standard precautions are designed to reduce the risk of transmission of microorganisms from both recognized and unrecognized sources of infection in hospitals. Every person is potentially infected or colonized with an organism that could be transmitted in the healthcare setting.

Key Components

- Hand hygiene and hand hygiene moments
- Personal protective equipment
- Respiratory hygiene
- Patient placement
- Patient-care equipment and instruments/devices
- Care of environment
- Care of textiles/laundry
- Safe injection practices
- Handling needles and sharps

Transmission-based Precautions (TBP)

These are the set of infection control practices which should be followed above and over the standard precautions. Precautions are needed to prevent infection transmission.

They should be followed while giving care to the patients infected with infectious agents having specific mode of transmission, such as contact, droplet and airborne.

They are of three types **(Flowchart 12.1):**

Flowchart 12.1: Transmission-based precautions.

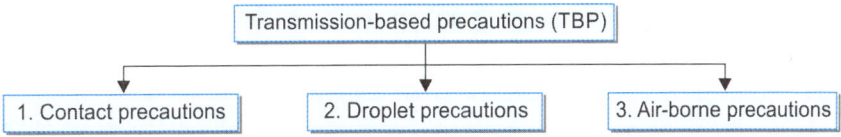

1. Contact Precautions

These should be followed when there is a suspected or definitive evidence of infectious agents that can be transmitted by direct or indirect contact while giving patient care **(Table 12.4)**.

TABLE 12.4: Direct, indirect transmission and agents transmitted via contact transmission.

Direct transmission	Indirect transmission
• It occurs when infectious agents are transferred from one person to another directly • **Examples:** Direct transmission via contaminated hands, direct contamination with blood and body fluids of infectious person, etc.	• Here the infectious agents transferred through intermediate contaminated objects • **Example:** Infected clothes, infected patient care devices, infected environmental surfaces, etc.
Agents transmitted via contact transmission: • Methicillin-resistant *Staphylococcus aureus* (MRSA) • Carbapenem-resistant Enterobacteriaceae (CRE) • Vancomycin-resistant *Enterococcus* (VRE) • Multi-drug resistant (MDR) non-fermenting gram negative bacilli, such as *Acinetobacter, pseudomonas*, etc. • Adenovirus, gonococcus, Chlamydia (gents of conjunctivitis) • Group A *Streptococcus* (GAS), *Staphylococcus*, scabies, rotavirus, cholera, etc.	

Infection Control Measures

- Strict adherence to **hand hygiene**
- **Proper use of PPE** and also the PPE must be removed before leaving the patient care areas and proper disposal of those used PPEs.
- **Use disposable or dedicated patient-care equipment** (e.g., blood pressure cuffs). If common use of equipment for multiple patients is unavoidable, clean and disinfect such equipment before use on another patient.
- **Ensure appropriate patient placement** in a single patient isolation room with bathroom facility available. If isolation room is not available then **cohorting** is recommended, which can be carried in many ways, such as:
  - Patient with same infection can be placed in similar room or in same corner of the ward, or
  - Spatial separation of minimum 3 feet between the beds with privacy curtains
- **Transfer of the patients** should be limited and should be moved only for medically necessary purpose.
- **Proper disinfection** of the room and the equipments in the room on regular basis should be done.

2. Droplet Precautions

These precautions are to prevent the spread of infectious agents that are transmitted via respiratory droplets. Respiratory droplets are large particles (>5 μm in size) generated while coughing, sneezing or taking. Transmission via these droplets require distance of <3 feet usually, but infection can occur greater then this distance also as seen in the COVID-19 cases **(Box 12.1)**.

> **BOX 12.1:** Droplet precautions are indicated for the patients with following infective agents.
>
> Droplet precautions are indicated for the patients with following infective agents:
> - Diphtheria, pharyngeal
> - *Haemophilus influenzae* type B (epiglottis, pneumonia, meningitis)
> - *Neisseria meningitis*—meningitis, pneumonia, sepsis
> - Pertussis (whooping cough)
> - Pharyngitis
> - GAS disease
> - Influenza virus, seasonal
> - EBOLA, corona virus mumps, measles, rubella, adenovirus, Lassa virus, parvovirus B19, etc.

Infection Control Measures

In addition to standard precautions following infection control measures should be applied:
- Strict adherence to **hand hygiene**
- **Proper use of PPE** (gloves, face shield/goggles, surgical mask) and also the PPE must be removed before leaving the patient care areas and proper disposal of those used PPEs. For certain disease, such as influenza seasonal, COVID-19, etc., HCWs should wear N95 respirators during aerosol generating procedures.

- **Respiratory hygiene and cough etiquette:** The individuals with respiratory symptoms should follow the following measures:
  - Direct coughing or sneezing on hands or rubbing of the nose should be strictly avoided.
  - Covering of mouth and nose with tissue when sneezing or coughing, after which the tissue should be disposed of in proper bin.
  - In case, there is no tissue available coughing or sneezing should be done into the inner elbow, turning away from other patients.
  - Hand hygiene should be performed after having contact with respiratory secretions.
  - Contaminated hands should be kept away from eyes and mucous membranes.
- In outpatient settings, patients with respiratory symptoms should be segregated, poster on respiratory hygiene should be displayed.
- Patient education should be done in waiting areas on respiratory hygiene for this purpose nursing and paramedical staff can be engaged.
- Persons with respiratory symptoms should always maintain a distance of 1 meter (**social distancing**).
- **Ensure appropriate patient placement** in a single room if possible if not cohorting, spatial separation of >3 feet's and drawing the curtains between patient beds should be done.
- **Transfer of the patients** should be limited and should be moved only for medically necessary purpose with the precautions that patient should wear a surgical mask while being transferred and follow Respiratory hygiene and cough etiquettes. also, the HCWs transferring the patient should wear PPE properly.
- **Proper disinfection** of the room and the equipments in the room on regular basis should be done with appropriate disinfectant.

Air-borne Precautions

In addition to standard precautions, airborne precautions are supposed to prevent the infectious agents that are transmitted via respiratory aerosols. Aerosols are small particles (<5 μm in size) generated by infectious person while coughing, sneezing or taking. These are also generated while performing certain aerosol generating procedures, (e.g., intubation). These smaller particles remain suspended in the air for long period of time and may get dispersed to distant places with air current **(Box 12.2)**.

> **BOX 12.2:** Agents causing aerosol transmitted disease (ATD).
>
> - *Mycobacterium tuberculosis*
> - Chickenpox and zoster
> - SARS-CoV
> - Smallpox
> - *Bacillus anthracis* spores
> - *Aspergillus* spp.
> - COVID-19
> - Influenza

Infection Control Measures

In addition to standard precautions following infection control measures should be applied:
1. Strict Adherence to hand hygiene
2. **Proper use of PPE:** (Gloves, face-shield, gown respirator) HCWs must should wear N95 respirators during aerosol generating procedures **(AGP)**. There should be proper fit checking and fit testing of PPE.
3. **Ensure appropriate patient placement:** Patient should be placed in airborne infection isolation room (AIIR), components of which are:
   - Adequate ventilation through mechanical ventilation (negative pressure room) and air exchanges 10–12/hr
   - Ultraviolet germicidal irradiation (UVGI)
   - Air leaving the room should be directly to outside or through HEPA filters (high efficiency particulate air)
4. Transfer of the patients should be done only when it is absolutely necessary with following measures: Patient should wear a surgical mask while being transferred and follow respiratory hygiene and cough etiquettes. Also, the HCWs transferring the patient should wear PPE properly.
5. Entry of visitors and staff should be restricted, or they should wear proper PPE for entering the room.

INCIDENTS AND ADVERSE EVENTS

Capturing of Incidents

Incident reporting is an essential responsibility of healthcare organizations to improve patient safety and quality care today. Incident and event reporting helps to identify areas of quality improvement in healthcare.

Benefits of Healthcare Incident Reporting

- **Incident reporting improves quality and safety:** The number one benefit of healthcare incident reporting is improving quality of care and patient safety. Healthcare organizations focus on improving patient safety and care quality by consistently evaluating and improving their clinical processes and other patient-related operations.
- **Reduces risk of reoccurrence**: One of the most powerful benefits of incident reporting in healthcare is reducing the risk of reoccurrence. When healthcare providers can easily capture, analyze, and share data, they can proactively act on potentially harmful situations to minimize further escalation.
- **Facilitates a learning culture:** The majority of clinicians and healthcare staff want to learn and readily accept instruction on improving. That is true whether an incident involves them, a coworker in their department, or a staff member in another part of the organization.
- **Analytics:** Accurate data is essential for increasing patient safety. Utilizing customized dashboards with drill-through analytics tools allow healthcare teams to drill down into data across multiple departments and turn vast amounts of data into actionable decisions.
- **Improves employee engagement:** It encourages and engages employees to participate in the safety of their workplace and patients. Using a healthcare incident reporting system that recognizes employees for noticing and reporting patient safety risks, such as good catches and near misses, helps improve employee engagement through healthcare incident reporting.

ROOT CAUSE ANALYSIS

A root cause analysis is done in the healthcare industry to give professionals a systematic and precise view of their existing problems in detail so that they can improve the overall quality and safety of the services they provide.

Seven Powerful Problem-solving Root Cause Analysis Tools

1. The Ishikawa Fishbone Diagram (IFD)
2. Pareto Chart
3. 5 Whys
4. Failure Mode and Effects Analysis (FMEA)
5. Scatter Diagram
6. Affinity Diagram
7. Fault Tree Analysis (FTA)

Also called the **Ishikawa diagram, a fishbone diagram** is a useful tool in conducting root cause analysis (**Fig. 12.4**):

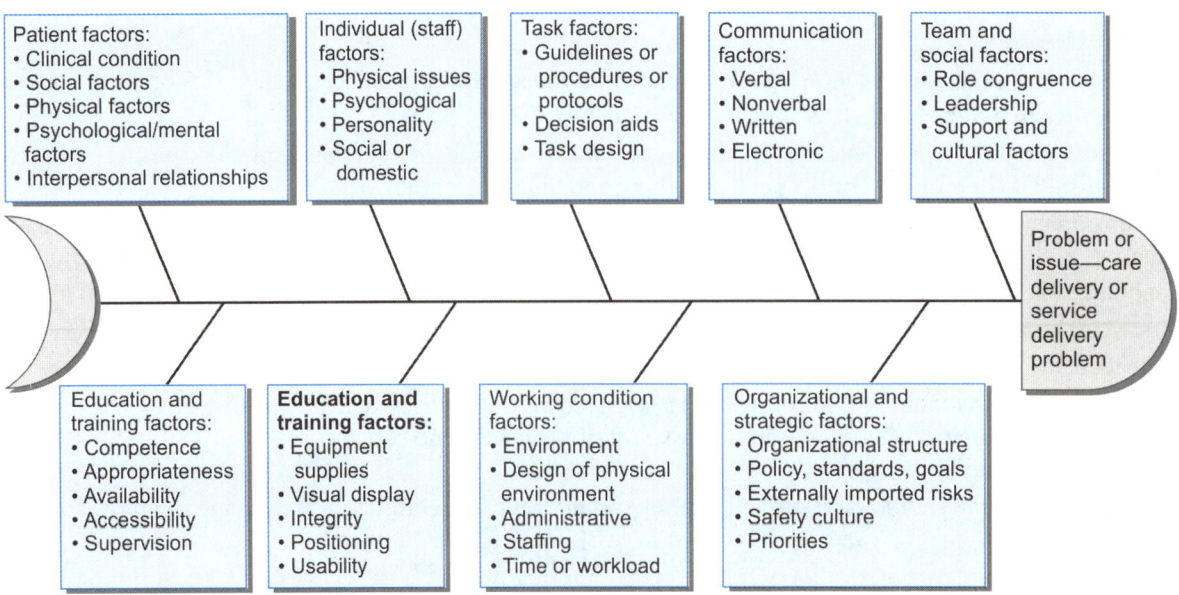

Fig. 12.4: Ishikawa diagram.

Corrective and Preventive Action (CAPA)

Definition

CAPA is the acronym for **Corrective Action and Preventive Action** (CAPA). It is a system that all medical devices companies need to have in place to identify all quality-related issues, investigate the root cause, and implement corrective actions and preventive actions to ensure that such problems do not arise again.

Corrective and Preventive Action (CAPA) program can be a powerful tool for improving product quality, streamlining production and ensuring regulatory compliance.

Examples of CAPA-related deficiencies reported include deviation of reports containing insufficient information to describe the investigations conducted or demonstrate the evidence supporting the proposed root cause **(Flowchart 12.2)**.

Seven Steps for Effective CAPA Analysis

1. Identify the potential or actual problem
2. Evaluate the potential impact and risk level
3. Develop an investigation procedure
4. Analyze the problem using available information.
5. Create an action plan using the analysis.
6. Implement and document action plan tasks
7. Verify completion and effectiveness of actions

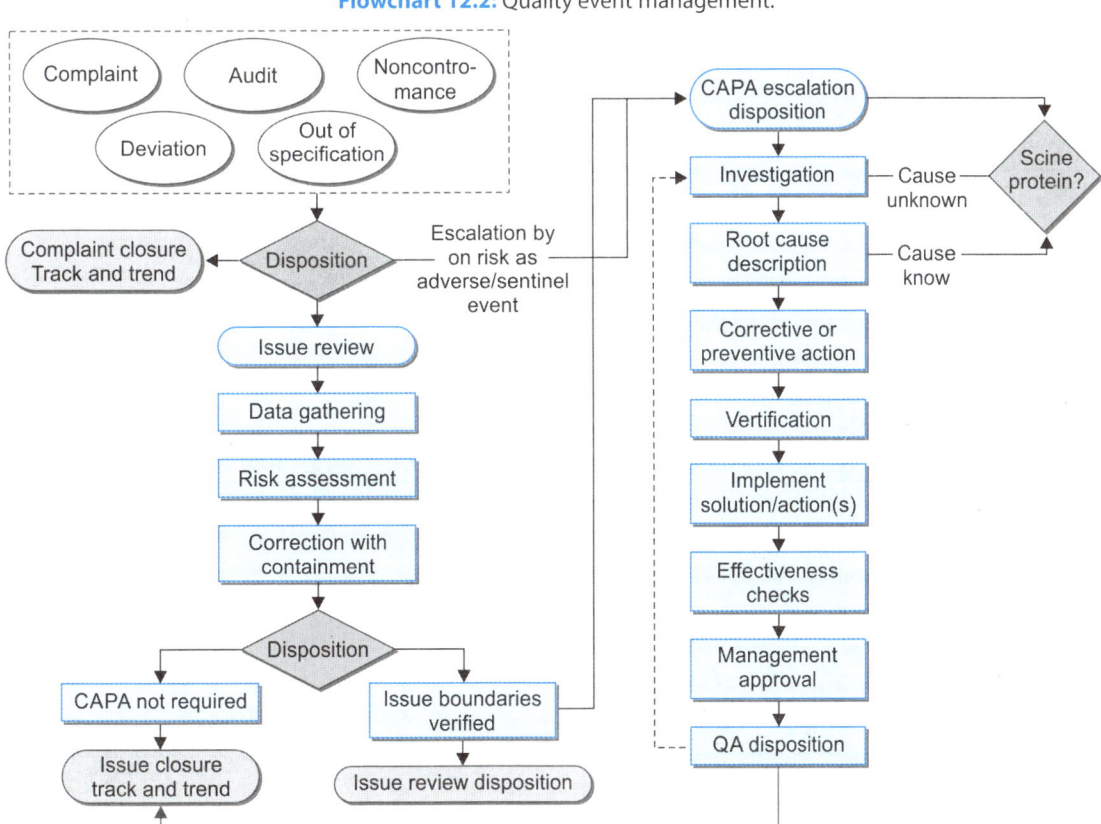

Flowchart 12.2: Quality event management.

CHAPTER 13

International Patient Safety Goals

Chapter Outline

- International Patient Safety Goals
- Hospital National Patient Safety Goals

INTRODUCTION

International Patient Safety Goals (IPSGs) help accredited organizations address specific areas of concern in some of the most problematic areas of patient safety.

Objectives

- To promote specific improvements in patient safety.
- Represent proactive strategies to reduce the risk of medical error.
- Provide clear priorities and solutions improving patient safety.

INTERNATIONAL PATIENT SAFETY GOALS AS PER JCI STANDARDS 5TH EDITION (FIG. 13.1)

Goal 1: Identify patients correctly
Goal 2: Improve effective communication
Goal 3: Improve the safety of high-alert medications
Goal 4: Ensure safe surgery
Goal 5: Reduce the risk of healthcare-associated infections
Goal 6: Reduce the risk of patient harm resulting from falls

HOSPITAL NATIONAL PATIENT SAFETY GOALS

Goal 1: Identify Patients Correctly

- Ask for two identifiers including the "Full Name" and "Medical Record Number."
- Verify patient identification before all invasive and diagnostic procedures.
- Patient identification wristbands for inpatients.
- "Time out" before starting all surgical and invasive procedures (preventing wrong site, wrong procedure, wrong patient surgery)
- Not use the identifications: Patient's *room number and location*

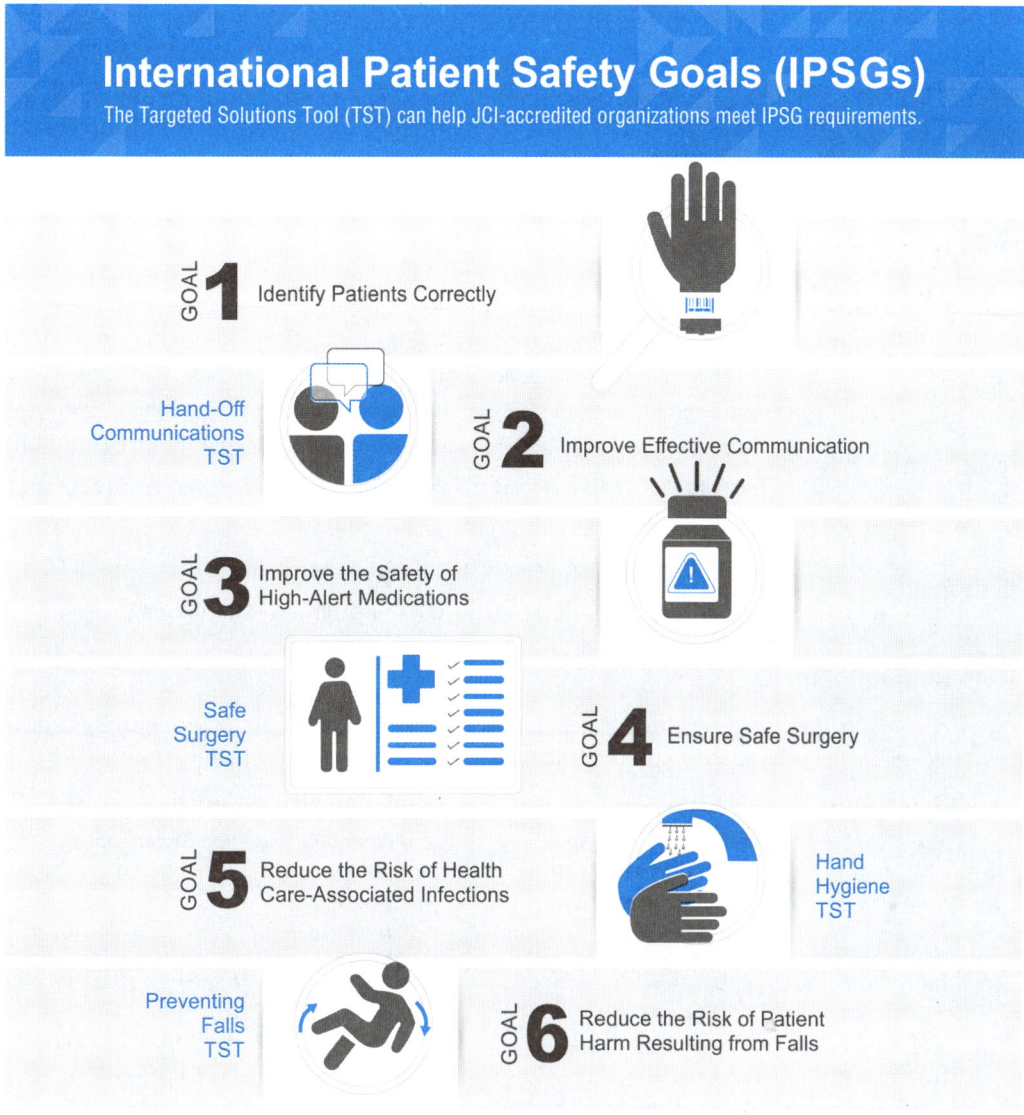

Fig. 13.1: The Joint Commission International (JCI): International Patient Safety Goals IPSG.
[*Source:* The Joint Commission International (JCI): International Patient Safety Goals IPSG 5th edition].

Goal 2: Improve Effective Communication

Standard 2: Verbal/telephone order
- Hospital develops and implements a process to improve the effectiveness of verbal and telephonic conversation among caregivers.
- Effective communication is timely, accurate and complete, unambiguous and understood by the recipient, reduce errors and results in improved patient safety.

Standard IPSG 2.1: Hospital develops and implements a process for reporting critical results of diagnostic tests. Hospital develops and implements a process for handover communication. Adapted **SBAR tool** is used in hospitals which states as **(Fig. 13.2)**:
  – **S**—Describe the **Situation**
  – **B**—Provide **Background**
  – **A**—Provide **Assessment**
  – **R**—Make **Recommendation**

Adapted SBAR Tool

S — Describe SITUATION

My name is.........and I work.........(your service)

I need to talk to you about:
- ❏ an urgent safety issue regarding.........(name of client)
- ❏ a quality of care issue regarding.........(name of client)

I need about.......(minutes) to talk to you, if not now, when can we talk?

I need you to know about:
- ❏ changes to a patient status
- ❏ changes to treatment plan, procedures or protocols
- ❏ environmental/organizational issues related to patient care

B — Provide BACKGROUND

Are you aware of ....(specific problem)

The patient is ...(age) and has a diagnosis of...(diagnosis) as well as ....(diagnosis)

He/She was admitted on.......(date) and is scheduled for discharge on........(date)

His/Her treatment plans related to this issue to date include........(treatment)

He/She is being monitored by ....(specialist) and has appointments for........(procedures)

This patient/family/staff is requesting that........(requests)

A — Provide client ASSESSMENT

I think the key underlying problem/concern is........(describe)

The key changes since the last assessment related to the specific concern are:

Person Level Changes
- ❏ Vital Signs/GI/Cardio-Respiratory
- ❏ Neurological
- ❏ Musculoskeletal/Skin
- ❏ Pain
- ❏ Medications
- ❏ Psychosocial/Spiritual
- ❏ Sleep
- ❏ Cognitive/Mental Status/Behavioral
- ❏ Nutrition/Hydration

Activity/Participation/Functional Changes
- ❏ ADL
- ❏ Transfers
- ❏ Home/Community Safety

Environmental Changes
- ❏ Organizational/Unit Protocols/Processes
- ❏ Discharge Destination
- ❏ Social/Family Supports

R — Make RECOMMENDATION

Based on this assessment, I request that:
- ❏ We discontinue/continue with........
- ❏ We prepare for discharge OR extend discharge date
- ❏ You approve recommended changes to treatment plan/goals including ....
- ❏ You reassess the patient's........
- ❏ The following tests/assessments be completed by........
- ❏ The patient be transferred out to......../be moved to........
- ❏ You inform other team members/family/patients about change in plans
- ❏ I recommend that we modify team protocols in the following ways...............

To be clean, we have agreed to.......Are you ok with this plan?
- ❏ I would like to hear back from you by........
- ❏ I will be in contact with you about this issue by........

Fig. 13.2: Adapted SBAR model.

Goal 3: Improve the Safety of High-Alert Medications (Box 13.1)
- **IPSG 3:** Hospital develops and implements a process to improve the safety of high-alert medications.
- **IPSG 3.1:** Hospital develops and implements a process to manage the safe use of concentrated electrolytes.

> **BOX 13.1:** High-alert medications.
>
> **The top five high-alert medications:**
> 1. Insulin
> 2. Opiates and narcotics
> 3. Injectable potassium chloride or phosphate
> 4. Injectable anticoagulant
> 5. Sodium chloride solution above 0.9%

Goal 4: Ensure Correct Site, Correct Procedure, Correct Patient Surgery

Essential procedures found in Universal Protocol are:
- Marking the surgical site as depicted in **(Fig. 13.3)**.
- A preoperative verification process.
- A time out that is held immediately after the procedure.

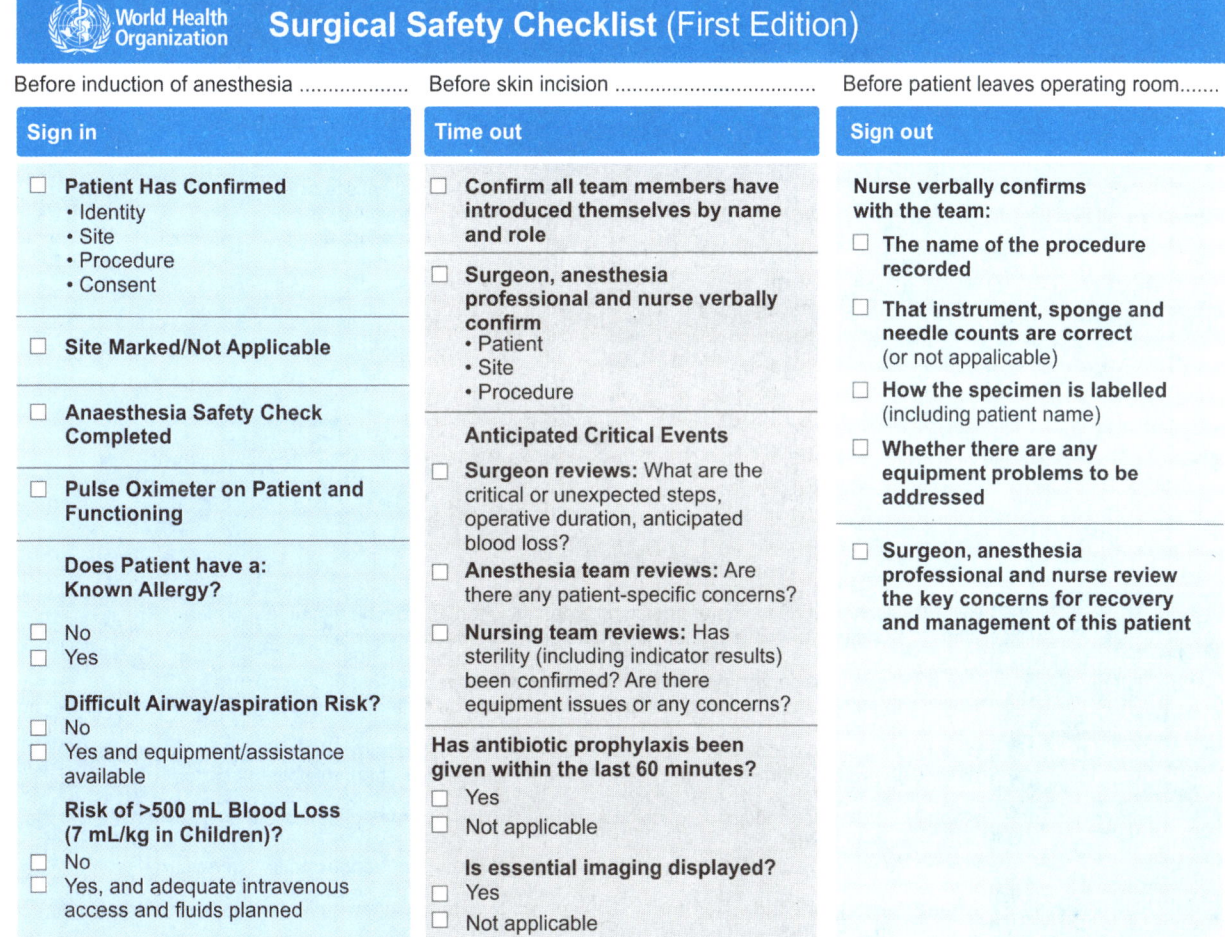

Fig. 13.3: Surgical checklist as per WHO.

(*Source:* WHO Guidelines on Surgical Safety Checklist 1st edition).

Goal 5: Reduce the Risk of Healthcare-associated Infections

- Infection prevention and control
- Prevention of catheter-associated urinary tract infections (CAUTI), central line-associated infections (CLABSI), ventilator-associated pneumonias (VAP), surgical site infections (SSI).
- CDC bundle care and hand hygiene are shown in **Figure 13.4**.

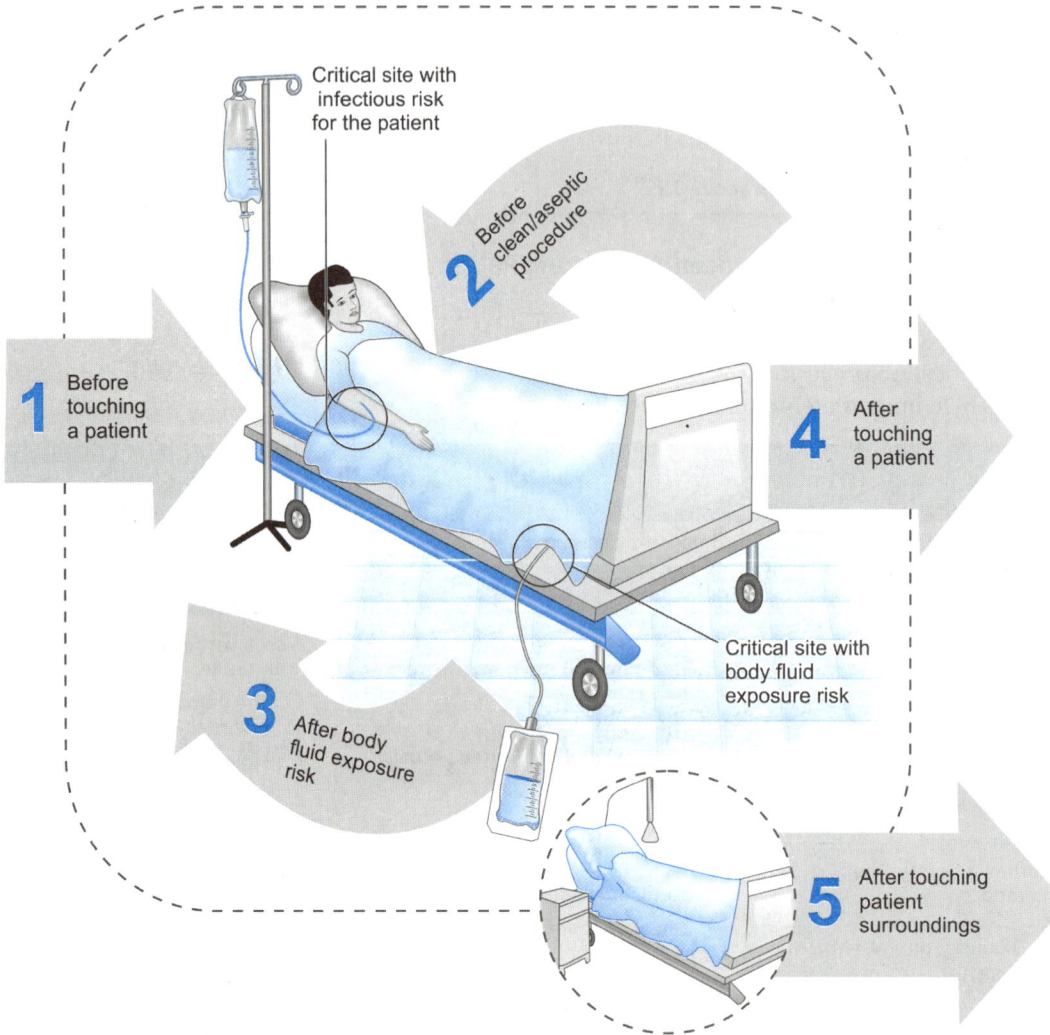

1 Before touching a patient	**When?**	Clean your hands before touching a patient when approaching him/her.
	Why?	To protect the patient against harmful germs carried on your hands.
2 Before clean/aseptic procedure	**When?**	Clean your hands immediately before performing a clean/aseptic procedure
	Why?	To protect the patient against harmful germs, including the patient's own, from entering his/her body.
3 After body fluid exposure risk	**When?**	Clean your hands immediately after an exposure risk to body fluids (and after glove removal)
	Why?	To protect yourself and the healthcare environment from harmful patient germs.
4 After touching a patient	**When?**	Clean your hands after touching a patient and her/his immediate surroundings, when leaving the patient's side.
	Why?	To protect yourself and the healthcare environment from harmful patient germs.
5 After touching patient surroundings	**When?**	Clean your hands after touching any object or furniture in the patient's immediate surrounding. When leaving—even if the patient has not been touched.
	Why?	To protect yourself and the healthcare environment from harmful patient germs.

Fig. 13.4: Five moments of hand hygiene.

[*Source:* WHO Guidelines on Hand hygiene in Health Care: A summary (2009)].

Goal 6: Reduce the Risk of Patient Harm Resulting from Falls
- Evaluate patient's risk for falls.
- Take action to reduce the risk of falling and to reduce the risk of injury for fall to occur.
- Evaluation includes fall history, medication and alcohol consumption review, gait and balance screening, walking aids used by the patients.

Preventing patient's fall by:
- Training to patient and patient's relatives.
- Not leaving bed without any help.
- Nurse call and frequently used objects are placed near the patient.
- Bed height is fixed at the lowest level.
- All side rails in the up position.
- Instruct the patient to wear non-skid footwear.
- Unused equipment to be removed from the room.
- Proper lighting.

CHAPTER 14

Safety Protocol

Chapter Outline

- 5'S (Sort, Set in Order, Shine, Standardize, Sustain)
- Radiation Safety
- Laser Safety
- **Fire Safety:** Types, Classification, Fire Alarms, Firefighting Equipments
- **HAZMAT Safety:** Types of Spills, Spillage Management, MSDS
- **Environmental Safety:** Risk Assessment Aspect Impact Analysis, Maintenance of Temperature and Humidity
- Emergency Codes in Hospitals
- Role of Nurse in Times of Disaster Management

5'S (SORT, SET IN ORDER, SHINE, STANDARDIZE, SUSTAIN)

Application of 5S (Sort, Set, Shine, Standardize and Sustain) for improvement of working environment.
- Continuous quality improvement (CQI) or KAIZEN activities for evidence-based participatory problem solving at the workplace for continuous quality improvement; and
- Total quality management (TQM) as an approach to make maximal use of capacity of the entire organization.

Five S (5S) is the principle directed to improve work environment and is derived from the Japanese words Seiri, Seiton, Seiso, Seiketsu, and Shitsuke. In English, the 5S means Sort, Set, Shine, Standardize, and Sustain **(Table 14.1)**.
- It is also helpful in improving the quality, efficiency and safety. 5S is, therefore, the key activity in the way to Continous Quality Improvement and to achieve Total Quality Management.
- 5S is applied to make a breakthrough to improve work environment and motivation of staff working in the hospital.
- 5S includes a set of actions that needs to be conducted systematically with full participation of staff serving the hospital.
- 5S activities should be practiced in a real participatory manner to improve the quality of both work environment and service components delivered to the clients.
- 5S is a sequence of activities to make the work environment convenient and comfortable.
- **5S can be divided into two steps:** Achievement of initial 3S (Sort, Set and Shine) and subsequent practices of remaining 2S (Standardize and Sustain).

TABLE 14.1: Showing 5S's.

Principles	Meaning
Sort	Identify and remove unwanted/unused items from the workplace; and reduce clutter (removal/organization)
Set	Organize everything needed in proper order for easy operation (orderliness)
Shine	Maintain high standard of cleanness (cleanness)
Standardize	Set up the above 3S as norms in every section of the workplace (standardize)
Sustain	Train and maintain discipline of the personnel engaged (self-discipline)

A. Sort

Sort means separation (sorting) and removing/discarding unwanted and unnecessary items from the workplace. Without "Sorting," it is not possible to have the next step of putting things in an appropriate order (setting) in the workplace. There are several steps to implement sorting.

1. **Identification and segregation of unwanted items:** The "Sort" activity starts with identification of unwanted items in the workplace. During the sorting stage, lots of unwanted items can be identified at different sections. Color codes should be used to mark the unwanted items, which are identified during the sorting process and routine work. Green, yellow or red color tags (labels) with explanation of the problems may be used for easy identification of the unwanted items in the store.
2. **Sorting from indoor to outdoor:** Sorting may start from any section (or any part) of the hospital. It may be good to start sorting from inside the hospital building.
3. Initiation of "Reduce, Reuse, Recycle Concept" with "Sort" activities
4. **Improvement of waste management system:** The first step
5. Organize "Big sorting day"

B. Set

"Set" is the second step of 5S and is mainly a process to put orderliness in every workplace for better work efficiency. It requires team work for achieving a specific target. The process should start once all the clutters and unnecessary items are removed from the workplace during the sorting stage.

The stepwise activities for this stage are (Table 14.2):

A. Select target places for setting.
B. Expansion to other sections
C. Use of visualized information

TABLE 14.2: Tools used to enhance "Set" activity.

• Red tag	• Zones
• Alignment	• Symbols
• X-axis, Y-axis	• Street lines
• Theory	• Name boards
• Numbering	• Directions
• Alphabetical order	• Safety signs
• Ascending order	• Checklists
• Left to right order	• Instructions sheets
• Top to bottom order	• Color code

C. Shine

- **Everyone should participate:** "Shine" is the participatory activity for maintaining cleanliness at every workplace regardless of the category and location. All staff in the hospital are allocated a specific territory as his/her working area. Regardless of the category, rank and gender of the staff, everyone is expected to join in the "Shine" activity and control the work environment on cleanliness.
- **Periodical implementation of cleaning:** Periodical implementation of "Shine" is important.

D. Standardize

Make 3S as a part of routine work. The "Standardize" stage of 5S is for development of standards for the initial 3S activities, i.e., sort, set and shine. The other objective of this step is to make "Sort", "Set", and "Shine" as part of all staff's routine work in all the sections of the hospital.

E. Sustain

Train and maintain discipline of the personnel engaged (self-discipline).

RADIATION SAFETY

To minimize exposure, you need to take five routine precautions:
1. **Recognize radiation sources:** Radiation sources are marked by the international radiation hazard symbol—a purple trefoil on a bright yellow background. When you see this sign **(Fig. 14.1)**:
    – Make sure you are aware of the source of the hazard.
    – Take appropriate precautions to reduce exposure and avoid contamination.
    – Do not handle material labeled as radioactive unless you are trained and authorized to do so.
2. **Reduce your exposure time:** The key to reducing your exposure time is planning. Make sure in advance that you have everything you need so that you can complete necessary procedures near a radiation source as quickly as possible.
3. **Increase your distance from radiation:** Radiation levels vary inversely with the square of the distance from their source—that is, levels decrease sharply with distance. The farther away you place yourself, the less radiation you are exposed to.
4. **Shield yourself from radiation:** Shielding will also reduce the level of radiation. Shielding is very effective with X-rays. Wear a lead apron, where provided. If your hands may be in the X-ray beam, wear lead gloves unless doing so would compromise patient care. Use lead shields when available. In diagnostic nuclear medicine and radionuclide therapy, a lead apron is not effective. An appropriate bedside shield is effective in some situations (such as brachytherapy), and should be used wherever provided.
5. **Avoid radioactive contamination:** If possible, try to avoid radioactive contamination by taking the precautions you would use with infectious agents:
    – Wear gloves, a gown, and shoe covers if indicated.
    – Avoid contact with objects or areas that may be contaminated.
    – Do not eat, drink, or smoke in areas where radioactive materials are in use.
    – Do not apply cosmetics or groom your hair while in the area.
    – Wash your hands while leaving the area.
    – Read and follow all signs and instructions.
    – Do not handle radioactive materials unless you are trained and authorized to do so.

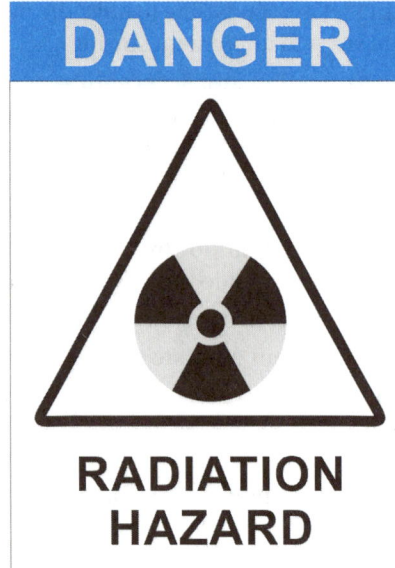

Fig. 14.1: Radiation hazard symbol.

LASER SAFETY

Lasers that are capable of producing hazardous diffuse reflections within the Nominal Ocular Hazard Area (NOHA), may cause skin injuries and could also constitute a fire hazard. Their use requires extreme caution **(Fig. 14.2)**.

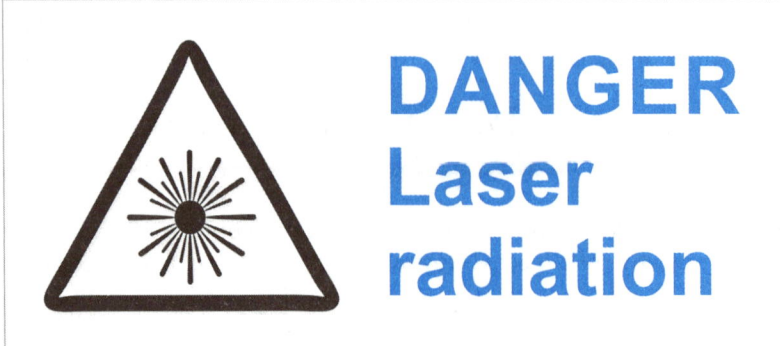

Fig. 14.2: Hazardous laser radiation symbol.

Objectives
- To ensure staff is appropriately trained in the safe use of lasers.
- To minimize the health risks from lasers to patients and personnel.
- To ensure efficient and effective use of laser equipment.

Implementation
- Provision of training to staff commensurate with the degree of potential laser hazards.
- Appointment of a Laser Safety Officer whose primary function is to implement and monitor laser safety policy in healthcare settings and reports via theatre manager to the Quality and Risk Committee.
- Appointment of Deputy Laser Safety Officers (DLSO's) who will carry out the day-to-day aspects of laser safety. There will be a DLSO assigned to each case where a laser is in use.
- Appropriate signage at entrance to theatre alerting to the use of a laser.
- All departments using laser equipment must maintain documentation relating to the provision of safety and control measures.
- Completion of a laser checklist.
- Completion of a logbook.
- Completion of education program every two years inclusive of:
  - Laser education package
  - Laser safety questionnaire
  - Skills validation checklist
- Preventive maintenance of the laser and accessories including:
  - Appropriate checking prior to being put into service.
  - Calibration of the output power, energy and temporal characteristics.
  - Copies of all instruction manuals stored for easy access.
  - A schedule for recommended testing, maintenance, safety checks and calibration.

Five laser safety measures to follow are:
1. Wear laser safety glasses
2. Utilize proper storage
3. Follow standards and regulations
4. Work with trained personnels
5. Use warning signs

FIRE SAFETY
Any healthcare facility should have fire safety system in place. Classification of fire is listed in **Table 14.3**.

TABLE 14.3: Classes of fire.

Class A	Ordinary solid combustibles such as paper, wood, cloth and some plastics.
Class B	Flammable liquids such as alcohol, ether, oil, gasoline and grease, which are best extinguished by smothering.
Class C	Electrical equipment, appliances and wiring in which the use or a nonconductive extinguishing agent prevents injury from electrical shock. Do not use water.
Class D	Certain flammable metallic substances such as sodium and potassium. These materials are normally not found in the medical center.
Class F	Fires that involve cooking oils and fats, such as vegetable oil, sunflower oil, olive oil, maize oil, lard, or butter (typically those used for deep-fat fryers).

Basic principles of fire safety are (Fig. 14.3):
- **Rescue:** Rescue anyone in immediate danger of fire
- **Alarm:** Pull the nearest fire alarm and call fire response
- **Contain:** Contain the fire by closing all doors in fire area
- **Extinguish:** Extinguish small fires. If not, leave area and close the door

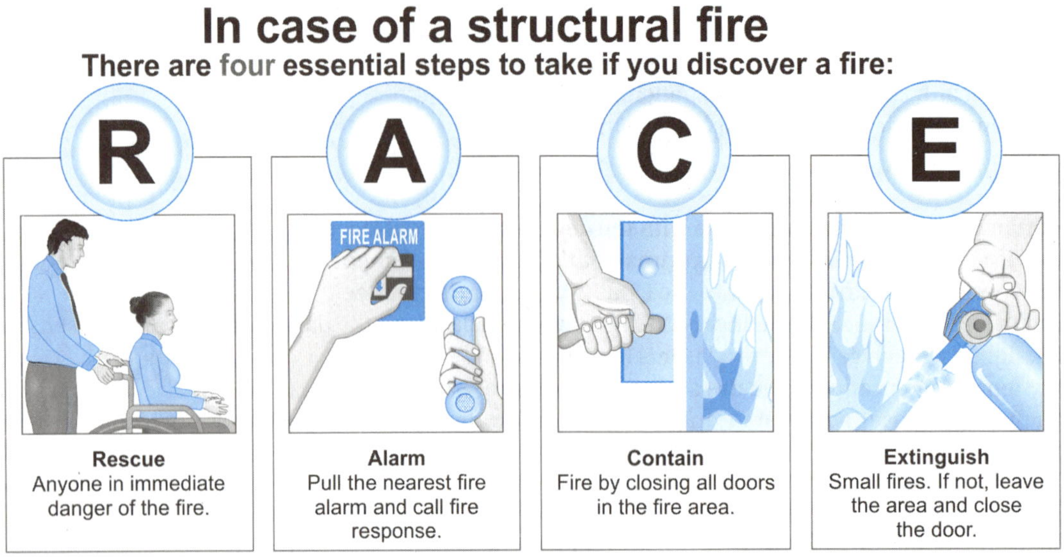

In case of a structural fire
There are **four** essential steps to take if you discover a fire:

R — **Rescue** Anyone in immediate danger of the fire.

A — **Alarm** Pull the nearest fire alarm and call fire response.

C — **Contain** Fire by closing all doors in the fire area.

E — **Extinguish** Small fires. If not, leave the area and close the door.

Fig. 14.3: Principles of fire safety.

To use a fire extinguisher, follow the acronym PASS (Fig. 14.4):
- **Pull:** Pull the pin on the extinguisher.
- **Aim:** Aim the nozzle at the base of the fire
- **Squeeze:** Squeeze the trigger to release the product
- **Sweep:** Sweep the nozzle from side to side (slowly)

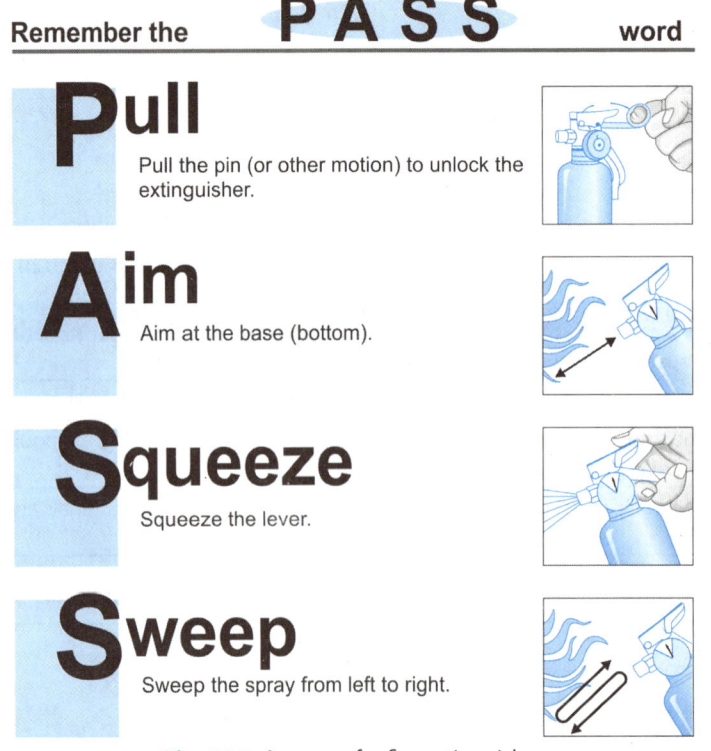

Remember the **PASS** word

Pull — Pull the pin (or other motion) to unlock the extinguisher.

Aim — Aim at the base (bottom).

Squeeze — Squeeze the lever.

Sweep — Sweep the spray from left to right.

Fig. 14.4: Acronym for fire extinguisher.

Types of Fire Fighting Equipments

See **Table 14.4.**

TABLE 14.4: Types of fire fighting equipments (Figs. 14.5 to 14.9).

Type	Uses	Warning
1. **Water extinguishers (type A):** There are two main types water extinguishers	• Water extinguishers are only suitable for class A fires, which means they can fight fires that involve wood, cardboard, paper, plastics, fabric and textiles, and other solid material • Do not use on Class B or C fires; may cause fire spread or electrical shock.	Do not use water extinguishers on burning fat and oil fires and electrical appliances.
i. Standard water extinguishers	• These will be solid red and will have the word 'WATER' or 'AQUA SPRAY' printed across them in a signal red band, often with a white border. • They dispense water at a high pressure to extinguish flames.	
ii. Dry water mist extinguisher	• These types of fire extinguishers will be solid red and will usually have the words 'WATER MIST' printed within a white rectangle. • Dry water mist extinguishers are unique as it can combat almost all types of fires, including class F fires that are usually difficult to attack.	
2. **Powder extinguishers:** There are three types of powder extinguisher	Dry chemical effective on all classes of fires	
i. ABC powder	• These types of extinguishers will say 'POWDER' in white text over a blue rectangle, and underneath the rectangle will be written 'ABC POWDER'. • As their name suggests, these are designed to **combat class A, B, and C fires**—those involving solids, liquids, and gases. • The powder acts as a thermal blast that cools the flames so burning cannot continue. • Due to their non-conductive nature, they are also suitable for fighting electrical fires.	Do not use on domestic chip or fat pan fires **(class F).**
ii. M28 powder and L2 powder extinguishers	M28 and L2 are unique extinguishers in that they are designed for tackling **Class D fires**—those involving combustible metals including powder, which are often produced in engineering factories. Metals includes lithium, magnesium, sodium, or aluminum.	Do not use on any other fire type, especially live electrical fires.
3. **Foam extinguishers**	**They are suitable for fighting class A and B fires.** Foam extinguishers are identifiable by the word 'FOAM' printed within a cream rectangle on their bodies. They are primarily water based but contain a foaming agent, which has rapid flame knock-down and a blanketing effect.	These should not be used on any other fire classes, especially electrical fires or chip or fat pan fires.
4. **Carbon dioxide (CO_2) extinguishers:** Type BC:	• These types of extinguishers can be identified by the text 'CARBON DIOXIDE' or 'CO_2' printed in white on a black rectangle. • Carbon dioxide to used for combating class B and electrical fires. • They are particularly useful for offices and workshops where electrical fires may occur.	They must not be used on hot cooking oil and fat (class F) fires. The strong jet from the extinguisher would push the burning oils or fats and spread the fire to surrounding areas.
5. **Wet chemical extinguishers:** Type K:	• These types of fire extinguishers are identifiable by the words 'WET CHEMICALS' printed across a yellow rectangle. • They are designed for combating fires that involve class F fires. • Used in kitchens on grease fires	Wet chemical extinguishers are usually not recommended for class B fires—those involving liquids.

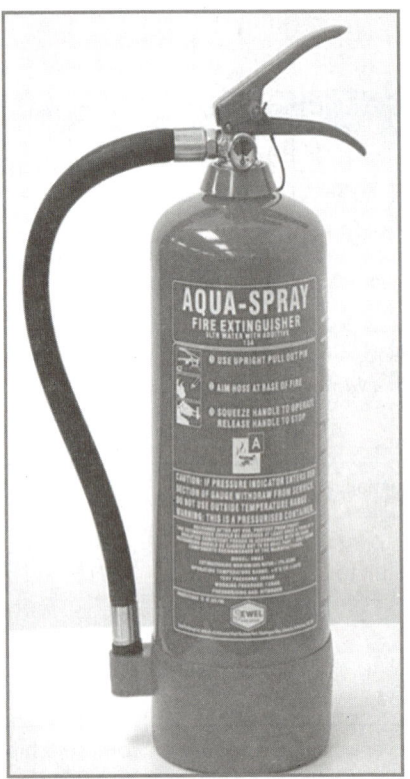

Fig. 14.5: Basic fire extinguisher.

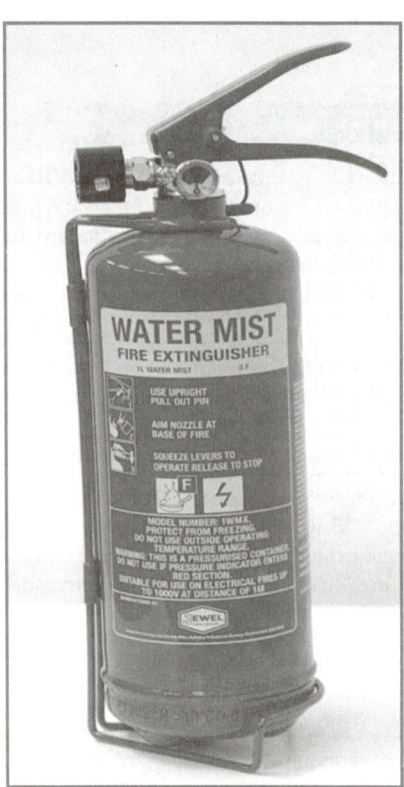

Fig. 14.6: Water mist fire extinguisher.

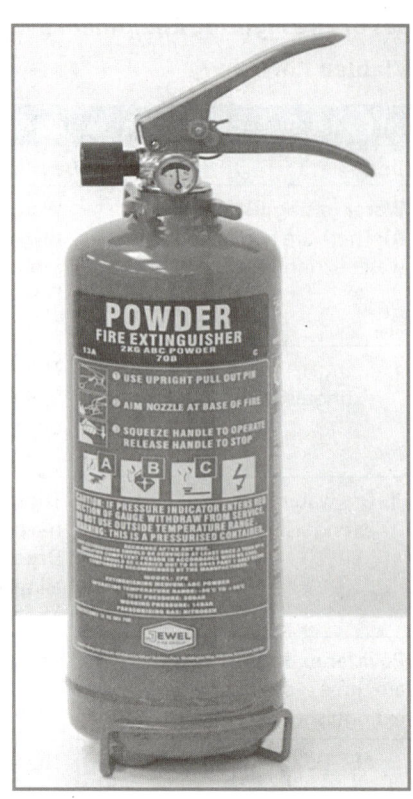

Fig. 14.7: Powder fire extinguisher.

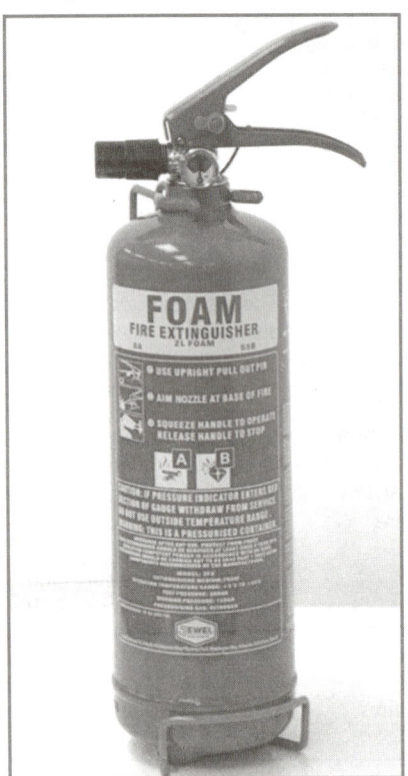

Fig. 14.8: Foam fire extinguisher.

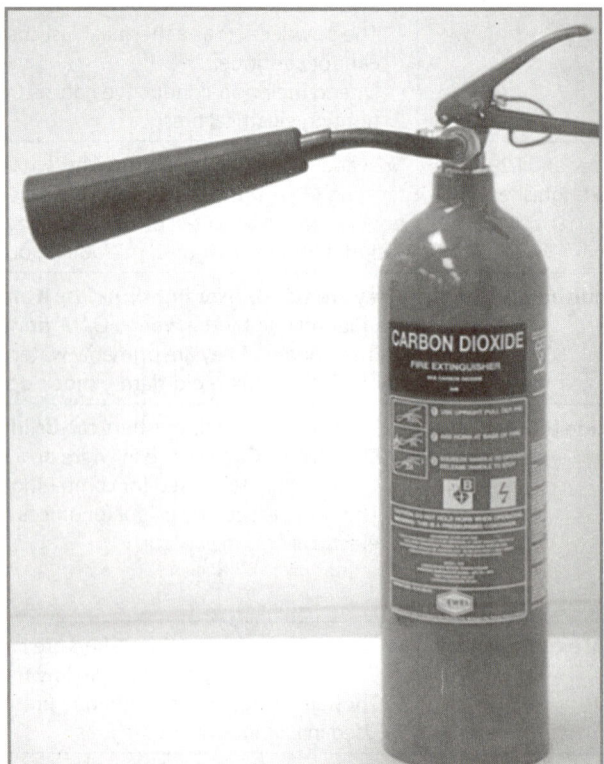

Fig. 14.9: CO_2 fire extinguisher.

Fire Safety Signs

See **Table 14.5**.

TABLE 14.5: Fire safety signs (for emergency exits).

Sign	Description
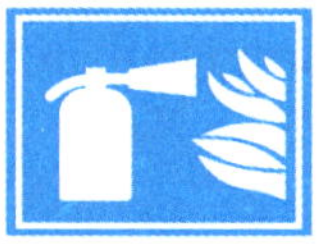	**Fire extinguisher sign:** Displayed next to all fire extinguishers to easily identify the location of the nearest extinguisher
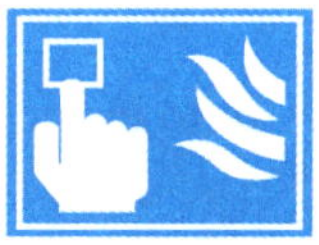	**Fire alarm call point sign:** Located at all fire alarms
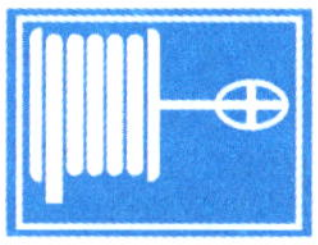	**Fire hose reel sign:** Located at all fire hose points
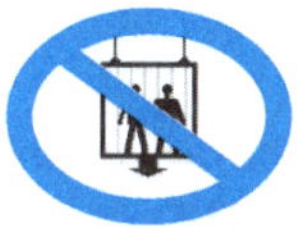	**In case of fire, do not use the lift sign:** Displayed at all lifts alongside the 'USE STAIRS' sign to indicate safe escape route
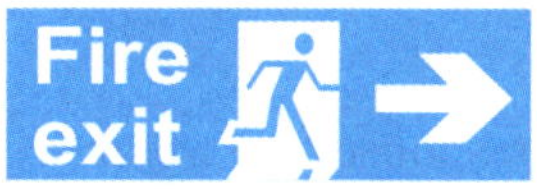	**Fire exit sign:** Displayed along all designated fire escape routes (with arrows) and above all emergency exits (without arrows)
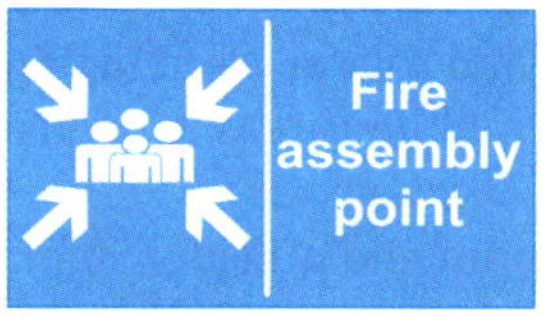	**Fire assembly point:** A pictogram or written sign displayed at the outside point of assembly where people must gather after evacuation.
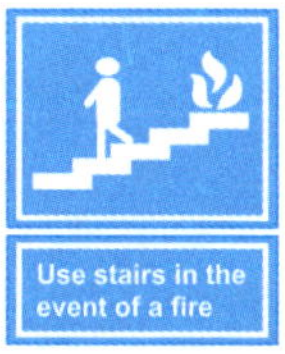	**In case of fire, use stairs sign:** An information sign displayed next to lifts and at the top of staircases so people know not to use the lift for safety reasons
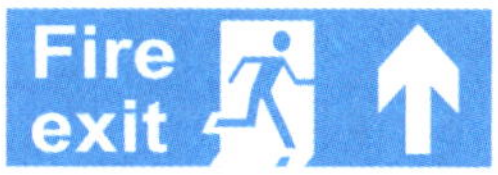	Progress forward from here (indicating direction of travel)
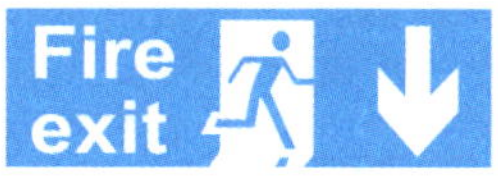	Progress down from here (indicating direction of level)
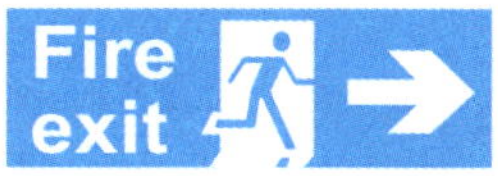	Progress to the right from here (indicating direction of travel)
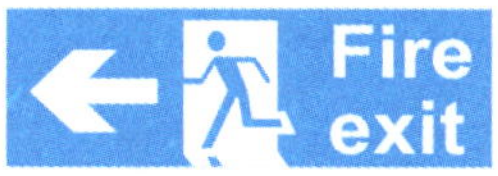	Progress to the left from here (indicating direction of travel)
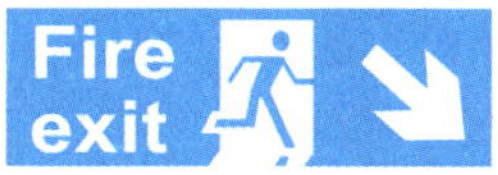	• Progress down to the left (indicate change of level) • Progress forward and across to the left from here when suspended within an open area
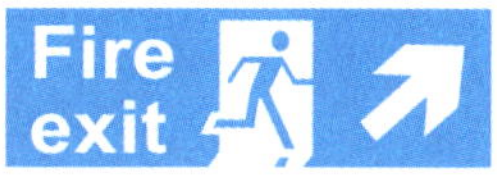	• Progress up to the right (indicate change of level) • Progress forward and across to the right from here when suspended within an open area

Fire Alarms and Fire Fighting Systems

The fire alarm system is designed to give an early warning when there is a smoke or fire condition in building. According to the **National Fire Protection Association (NFPA) 101 Life Safety Code:**

"All healthcare facilities shall be designed, constructed, maintained, and operated to minimize the possibility of a fire emergency requiring the evacuation of occupants. Because the safety of healthcare occupants cannot be ensured adequately by dependence on the evacuation of the building, their protection from fire must be provided by appropriate arrangement of facilities, adequate staffing, and development of operating and maintenance procedures."

If Case of a Fire or Smoke Condition

- Do not panic.
- If the fire is in a room or small area, confine the spread of the smoke and fire by closing the room doors prior to leaving the building, but only if it is safe to do so.
- Evacuate the building to the outside and warn others of the fire on the way out.
- Once you have reached a safe area, call on emergency number.
- Never re-enter the building.
- Seek out the first arriving personnel, police officer, fire fighter, and give them the specific location of the fire or smoke.
- If you know someone is still inside, try to give the fire fighters the last known location where you saw them.

Types of Fire Alarms

1. **Fire alarm panels:** One panel is placed in every protected building. Fire brigade panels are located near all entrances and in all nurses stations. Loop powered panels communicate and are powered through the detection loop **(Fig. 14.10)**.
2. **Standard detectors (Fig. 14.11):**
   – This smoke, heat and multisensors covers most needs for fire detection.
   – Smart technology offers longer life, better protection against unwanted alarms, and shorter response time to fires.
3. **Flame detectors:** Flame detector is ideal for the protection of facades usually in storage area **(Fig. 14.12)**.
4. **Aspirating smoke alarms:** Smoke alarms that are properly installed and maintained, play a vital role in reducing fire deaths and injuries. High-sensitivity smoke detection is designed for use in particularly clean or polluted areas in need of extra protection **(Fig. 14.13)**.
   – A closed door may slow the spread of smoke, heat and fire. Install smoke alarms in every room and outside. Smoke alarms should be interconnected. When one sounds, they all sound.

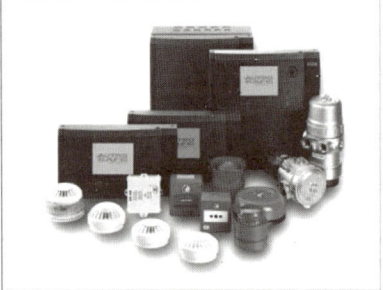

Fig. 14.10: Fire alarm panels.

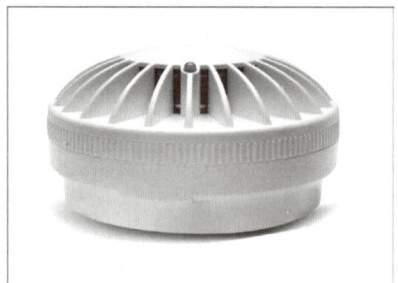

Fig. 14.11: Standard detectors.

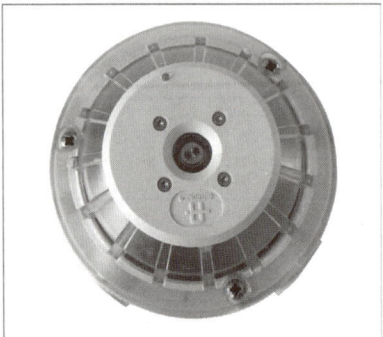

Fig. 14.12: Flame detectors.

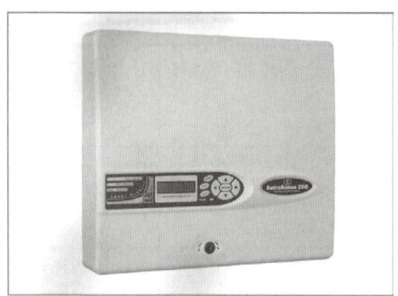

Fig. 14.13: Smoke alarms.

HAZARDOUS (HAZMAT) MATERIALS SAFETY

HAZMAT is an abbreviation for "hazardous materials"—substances in quantities or forms that may pose a reasonable risk to health, property, or the environment. HAZMATs include substances which are toxic chemicals, fuels, nuclear waste products, and biological, chemical, and radiological agents. HAZMATs may be released as liquids, solids, gases, or a combination or form of all three, including dust, fumes, gas, vapor, mist, and smoke.

Spill Management

In hospital settings spillage of blood, body fluids or chemicals can occur at any time due to broken or faulty equipment or human error. Any such spill poses risk to the staff, visitors and patients. Therefore, it is essential to manage this spill in order to prevent its hazardous effects. Hospital should have the desired spill management kit, standard operating procedures (SOPs) and a well trained staff to manage the spill.

Prevention of Spill

Spillage of any fluid can be easily prevented by properly following standard precautions while handling the fluids like blood or other body fluids and via proper way of collection and transportation.

Spill Management of Blood and Other Body Fluids

If spillage comes in contact with skin, mucous membranes, eyes or open wounds: The first step is to irrigate the area continuously. Management will depend on the size of spillage. Types of spills and its management are depicted in **Tables 14.6 and 14.7** respectively.

TABLE 14.6: Types of spills management of blood and other body fluids.

Spot	Small ≤10 cm	Spill management for spill >10 cm
• Select appropriate PPE • Wipe spot quickly with a damp cloth, tissue or paper towel • Discard contaminated materials in 1% sodium hypochlorite • Perform hand hygiene	• Select appropriate PPE • Wipe spot quickly with a absorbent material, soaked with 1% hypochlorite • Place contaminated absorbent material into impervious container or plastic bag for disposal • Mop the area with cloth soaked in 1% sodium hypochlorite and allow to dry	

Spill management of blood and other body fluids (large spill >10 cm)		
Blood and blood stained body fluids	**Pus/sputum/feces/vomits**	
	Is visible blood present or not	
	Yes	**No**
• Prepare all items required to manage the spill and don PPE • If spillage is large place disposable paper towels over spill to absorb and contain it • Cover the spill with an absorbent pad poured with 10% hypochlorite or chlorine granules and wait for 5 minutes (or 1% hypochlorite for 15–20 minutes) • Discard these absorbent paper towel into yellow bag • Use disposable paper to clear the area and discard these into appropriate bin.	Manage as for blood Note: • Where organic matter is present (e.g., feces) first absorb the spillage using absorbent towel and then clean with detergent and water before applying disinfectant ↓ • Wash area using fresh paper towel, general purpose detergent and water, rinse and dry then wipe over with a concentration of 1000 ppm available chlorine and dry ↓ • Ensure non-disposable items used, e.g., buckets etc., are cleaned, dried and stored properly • Discard disposable used items immediately into appropriate waste bin including disposable PPE worn and perform hand hygiene	• Remove with disposable paper towel and discard quickly in appropriate waste bin ↓ • Wash area using fresh paper towel, general purpose detergent and water, rinse and dry

TABLE 14.7: Components of spill kit (Fig. 14.14).

Blood and body fluid spill kit	*Chemical spill kit*
This should include the following items: • **PPE:** Gloves, apron, mask, shoe cover and face shield eye protector • Absorbent material like newspaper, disposable towel, etc. • Waste collection bag • Scoop and scarper • Disposable forceps • Bucket and mops of spill should be different from the one routinely used • Signage board or no entry	**This should include the following items:** • **PPE:** Chemical resistant safety gloves, e.g., nitrile gloves, safety goggles', apron, footwear, shoe cover, dust mask or respirator. • Absorbent pads and rolls such as "HAZMAT" absorbent. • Chemical neutralizer for various chemicals **Clean up material for spill:** • Brooms, plastic dustpan, plastic tongs or scoops. • Chemical resistant bin with close fitted lid. • Heavy duty plastic bags for wrapping contaminated PPE.

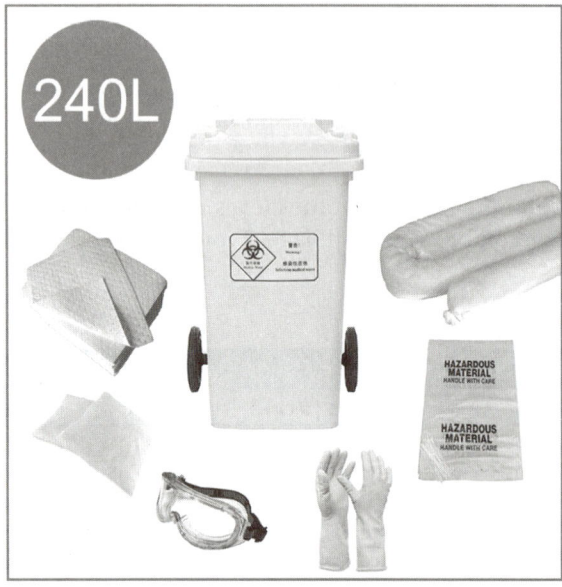

Fig. 14.14: Spill kit.

Mercury (Hg) spill kit

This should include the following items:
- 4–5 zip lock type bags (4–5 µm in thickness)
- Waste bags of 2–6 mm thickness, plastic container with lid
- Nitrile or latex gloves, paper towels, cardboard strips
- Syringe without needle or eye dropper
- Face mask with 0.3 µm HEPA, designed particularly for mercury management

Vapor suppressing agents:
- Powdered sulfur or zinc or copper
- Commercial absorbent pads or vapor upper suppressant containing sodium thiosulfate, copper sulfate, calcium chloride, potassium iodide and propylene glycol solution

Materials for decontamination:
- Vinegar, hydrogen peroxide and cotton swabs for final cleaning using sulfur powder
- 10% sodium thiosulfate solution or a mixture of sodium thiosulfate and EDTA

Small Volume of Spill (Few Drops)
- Wear appropriate PPE.
- If sharps are involved pick up by using forceps and discard into a sharp box.
- **Disinfection:**
  - Wipe spot quickly with a absorbent material, soaked with 1% hypochlorite (1% dilution containing minimum 10,000 ppm chlorine).
  - Discard the absorbent material as infected waste, wipe the area with a cloth mop moistened with 1% hypochlorite solution and allow drying naturally. All contaminated items used in the clean-up should be placed in a biohazardous bag for disposal.

Large Volumes (>10 mL) of Spills
- Confine contaminated area.
- Wear gloves and other PPE appropriate to the task.
- **Disinfection:**
  – Cover the spill with appropriate absorbent material to prevent from spreading.
  – Flood the spill with 10% hypochlorite solution. While flooding the spill with 10% hypochlorite solution it is to be ensured that both the spill and absorbent material is thoroughly wet.
  – Wait for five minutes.
  – Remove and discard the paper as infected waste.
- **Redisinfection:**
  – Wipe the area with paper moistened with 10% hypochlorite again and a cloth mop and allow drying naturally.
  – All contaminated items used in the clean-up should be placed in a biohazardous bag for disposal.

HAZMAT Placards

HAZMAT is a term used to describe incidents involving hazardous materials or specialized teams who deal with these incidents. Hazardous materials are defined as substances that have the potential to harm a person or the environment upon contact. These can be gases, liquids, or solids and include radioactive and chemical materials.

Table 14.8 represent the different hazardous classes and their divisions (class numbers are located at the bottom of the sign and division numbers are in the middle).

TABLE 14.8: Different hazardous classes and their divisions (Fig. 14.15).

Class 1: Explosives • Products with the potential to create a mass explosion • Products with the potential to create a projectile hazard • Products with the potential to create a fire or minor blast • Products with no significant risk of creating a blast • Products considered very insensitive that are used as blasting agents • Products considered extremely insensitive with no risk to create a mass explosion	**Class 4:** Flammable materials • Flammable solids • Spontaneously combustible • Dangerous when wet
	Class 7: Radioactive
Class 2: Gases • Flammable gases • Nonflammable gases • Toxic gases	**Class 5:** Oxidizer and organic peroxide • Oxidizing substances • Organic peroxides
	Class 8: Corrosive
Class 3: Flammable and combustible liquids	**Class 6:** Poisons • Toxic substances • Infectious substances
	Class 9: Miscellaneous

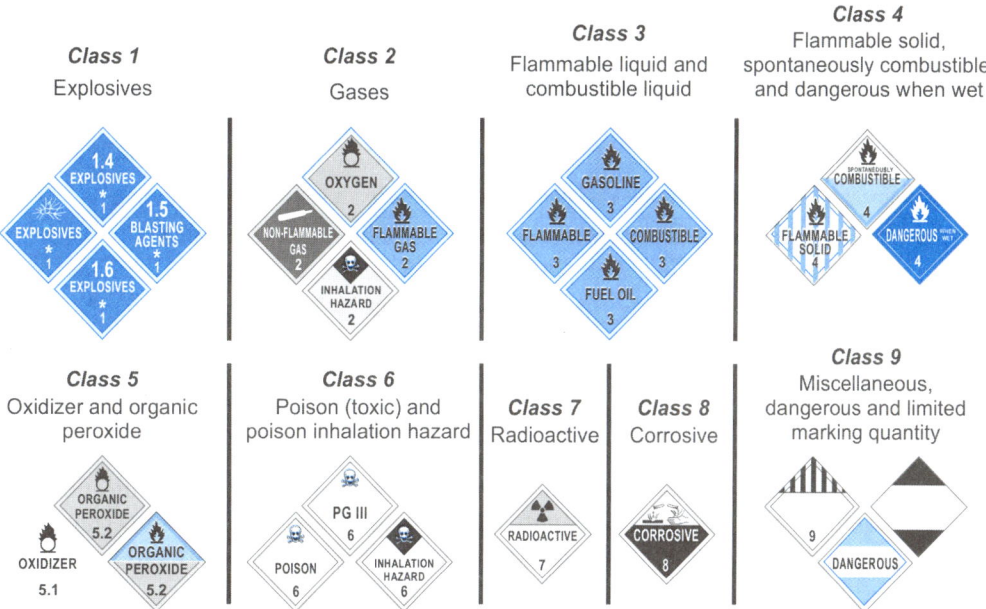

Fig. 14.15: Different hazardous classes and their divisions.

Material Safety Data Sheet (MSDS)

Material safety data sheet (MSDS) is a data sheet which contains the health and safety information about products, substances or chemicals which may be hazardous. It is made for both workers and emergency personnel **(Fig. 14.16)**.

An MSDS usually follows two formats:
1. Occupational Safety and Health Administration (OSHA) format
2. American National Standards Institute (ANSI) format

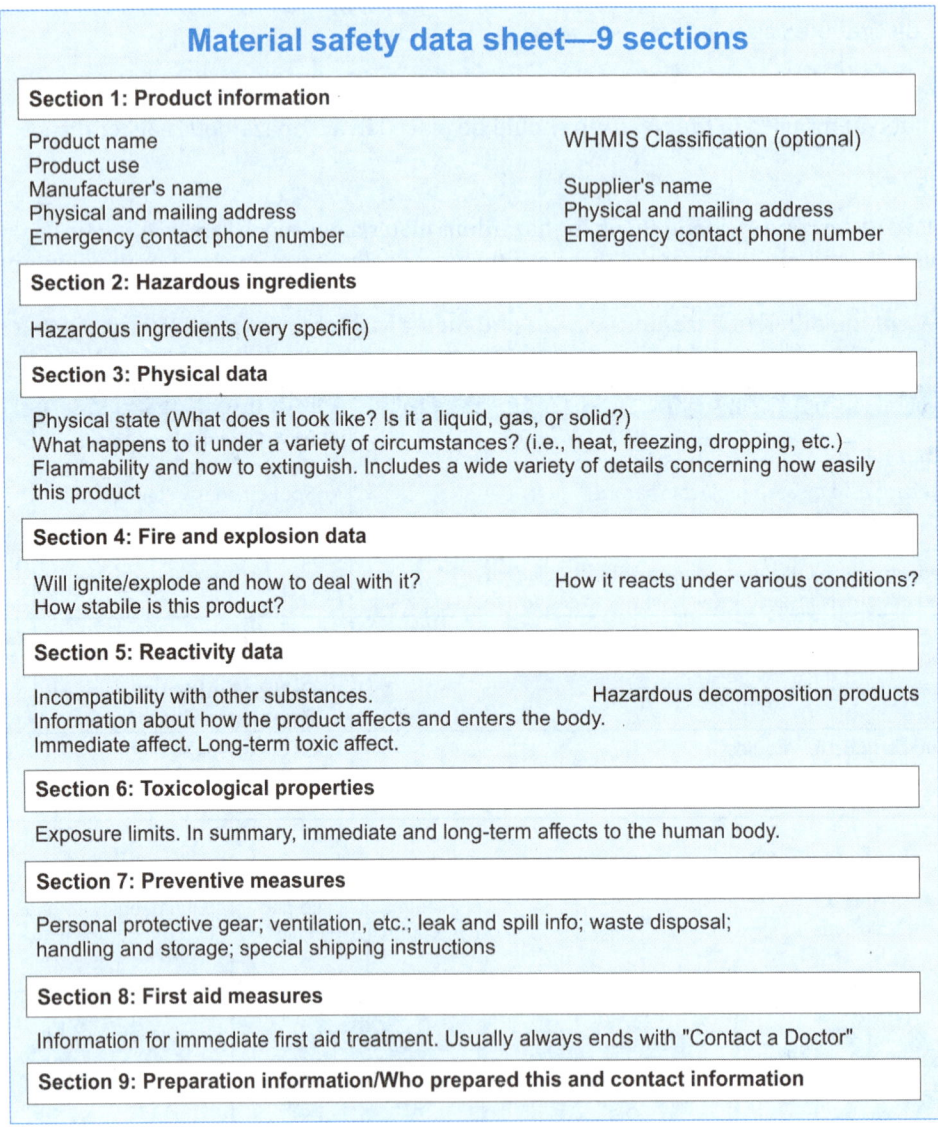

Fig. 14.16: Material safety data sheet.

ENVIRONMENTAL SAFTEY

Risk Assessment

It is a term used to describe the overall process or method where a person works. It is a thorough look at workplace to identify those things, situations, processes, etc., that may cause harm, particularly to people. After identification is made, analyze and evaluate how likely and severe the risk is, is done. When this determination is made, decision is taken that what measures should be in place to effectively eliminate or control the harm from happening **(Flowchart 14.1)**.

Flowchart 14.1: Plan a risk assessment.

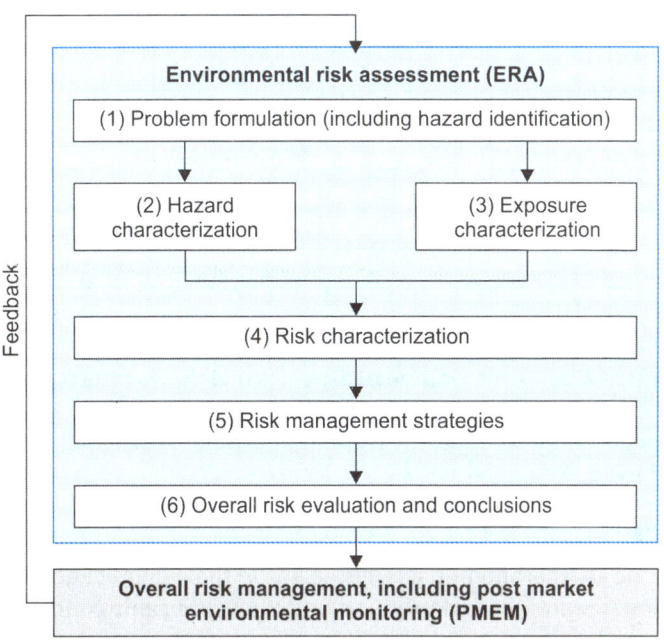

- **Hazard identification:** Identify hazards and risk factors having the potential to cause harm.
- **Risk analysis, and risk evaluation:** Analyze and evaluate the risk associated with that hazard
- **Risk control:** Determine appropriate ways to eliminate the hazard, or control the risk when the hazard cannot be eliminated.
- **Risk evaluation:** The process of comparing an estimated risk against given risk criteria to determine the significance of the risk.
- **Risk control:** Actions implementing risk evaluation decisions.

Ranking Risks

It is the way to help or determine which risk is the most serious one and which risk is to be controlled first. For simple or less complex situations, an assessment can literally be a discussion or brainstorming session based on knowledge and experience. In some cases, checklists or a probability matrix can be helpful. For more complex situations, a team of knowledgeable personnel who are familiar with the work is usually necessary **(Fig. 14.17)**.

Description	Color code
Immediately dangerous	
High risk	
Medium risk	
Low risk	
Very low risk	

Fig. 14.17: Ranking risk factors.

Environmental Aspects and Impacts Analysis

Environmental Aspects

An environmental aspect is anything resulting from the organization's activities, products or services that has the potential to cause an environmental impact, even if it is presently controlled, or prevent such impact. The fact that the potential exists (if something goes wrong, for instance) makes it an environmental aspect:
- Negative environmental aspects include emissions to the air or water, discharge of oil to the land or water, generation of hazardous waste, generation of solid waste, community impact, and the generation of dust and noise.
- Positive environmental aspects include recycling of used materials such as steel, aluminum, copper, glass bottles and paper, removal of pollutants from the air or water, and restoring land by removing decontaminated soil.

Environmental Impact

An environmental impact is any change to the environment, whether adverse or beneficial, wholly or partially resulting from the organization's activities, products or services. Essentially, the environmental impact is the result of the environmental aspect.

For example, suppose a company is discharging wastewater to a nearby stream. A potential environmental impact of that activity is pollution to the water. Few more examples are shown in **Table 14.9**.

TABLE 14.9: Examples of environmental aspects and impacts.

Environmental aspects	Environmental impacts
Storage of fuel	Spills and leaks
Delivery of cement to ready mixed concrete production facility	Air emission, noise
Delivery of concrete	Air emission, noise
Truck washout	Process water, track out and housekeeping
Electricity use	Air pollution and global warming
Use of recyclable paper	Conservation of natural resources

Direct and indirect environmental aspects
- **Direct environmental aspects:** A direct environmental aspect is one that is directly attributable to an activity or process and can therefore be controlled.
- **Indirect environmental aspects:** They are typically those that arise before an activity (known as upstream aspects) or after the activity (known as downstream aspects).

Aspects and Impacts Analysis

A suggested approach to determine aspects and impacts, according to their significance, includes the following five steps:
1. Identifying activities, component processes and products under all applicable conditions.
2. Determining their environmental aspects.
3. Determining the impacts of these aspects.
4. Assessing the significance of these impacts.
5. Ranking the impacts according to their significance

EMERGENCY CODES IN HOSPITALS

A hospital emergency, outbreak or an emerging new virus can occur without warning. At any given time hospitals must be prepared to respond to all emergencies that may arise within hospital facilities or the community at large. In order to ensure that healthcare systems has a coordinated effective emergency response, it is imperative that hospital emergency plans and emergency codes are regularly implemented, tested and maintained **(Fig. 14.18)**.

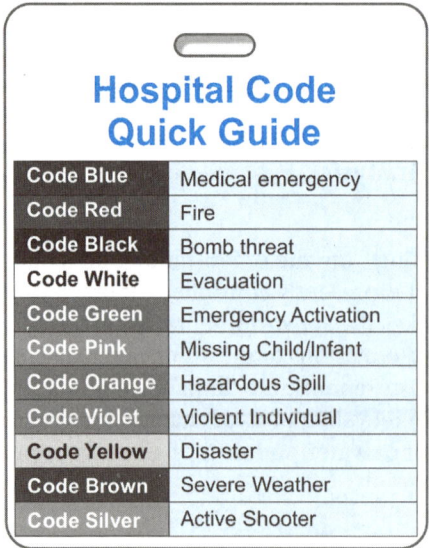

Fig. 14.18: Emergency codes in hospitals.

DISASTER MANAGEMENT CYCLE (FIG. 14.19)

The disaster management cycle is a series of steps that organizations and individuals use to prepare, contain and mitigate unexpected events. These can include natural disasters, unexpected damage to property or events that otherwise endanger the lives of others.

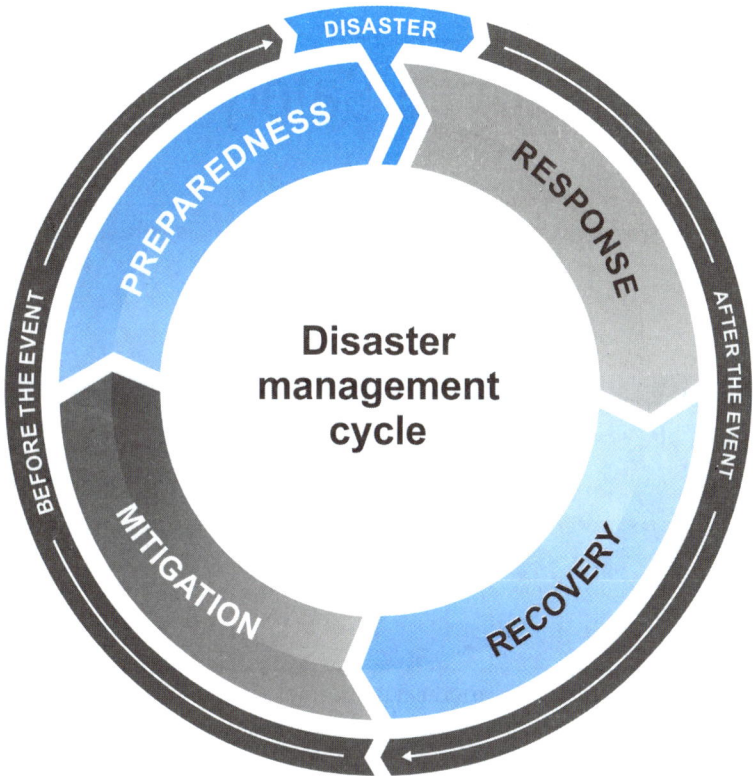

Fig. 14.19: Disaster management cycle.

ROLE OF NURSES IN TIMES OF DISASTER MANAGEMENT

"Disaster preparedness, including risk assessment and multidisciplinary management strategies at all system levels, is critical to the delivery of effective responses to the short, medium, and long-term health needs of a disaster-stricken population."

Major Roles of Nurse During Disaster Management

- Determine magnitude of the event. Define and understand the health needs of the affected groups
- Prepare the priorities and objectives. Identify actual and potential public health problems at the earliest.
- Estimate resources needed to respond to the needs identified
- Collaborate with other professional disciplines and governmental and non-governmental agencies.
- Maintain a proper chain of command. Maintain better communication.
- Emotional support to the individuals/family.
- Assist in providing safe drinking water.
- Assist in activities in daily living in case patient got injured.
- Administration of vaccination. Administration of medications.
- Distributing of relief materials if such a condition occurs.
- Rapport development. Gathering the information about diseases, incidents, etc.
- Reporting the details. Maintain records and reports.
- Collaborate with government and non-government organizations.
- Self-care/protection with required precautions.
- Keen observer for any diseases which starts to spread.
- Special care to infants/pregnant women.
- Health education to the needy.
- Identify psychologically affected and counsel them properly.

CHAPTER 15

Employee Safety Indicators

Chapter Outline

- Vaccination
- Annual Health Check
- Occupational Health Ordinance
- Needle Stick Injury Prevention

VACCINATION

Healthcare workers (physicians, nurses, emergency medical personnel, dental professionals, students, medical and nursing students, laboratory personnel's, pharmacists, hospital volunteers, and administrative staff) are at risk for exposure to serious, and sometimes deadly diseases. Appropriate vaccines can reduce the risk from diseases **(Table 15.1)**.

TABLE 15.1: Recommended vaccines for healthcare personnel.

Vaccine	Dosage

Hepatitis B	• 3-dose series of Recombivax HB or Engerix-B
	  – Dose 0 now
	  – Dose 1 at 1 month
	  – Dose 2nd at 6 months.
	                                       Or
	• 2-dose series of hepatitis-B, with the doses separated by at least 4 weeks.
	• Post-vaccination protective titer: Anti-HBs titer of ≥10 μ/mL

COVID-19	Two vaccines were granted emergency use authorization by the Central Drugs Standard Control Organization (CDSCO) in India: 1. Covishield® (AstraZeneca's vaccine manufactured by Serum Institute of India) 2. Covaxin® (manufactured by Bharat Biotech Limited). Sputnik-V has been granted EUA in the month of April 2021. The time interval between two doses of the Covishield vaccine has been extended from four-eight weeks to 12–16 weeks. The second dose of Covaxin can be taken four to six weeks after the first.
Flu (influenza)	1 dose of influenza vaccine annually
MMR (Measles, Mumps, and Rubella)	2 doses of MMR (1 dose now and the 2nd dose at least 28 days later).

Contd...

Contd...

Vaccine	Dosage
Varicella (chickenpox)	If one have not had chickenpox (varicella): 2 doses of varicella vaccine, 4 weeks apart
Tdap (Tetanus, Diphtheria, Pertussis)	One-time dose of Tdap. Get either a Td booster shot every 10 years thereafter, single dose IM deltoid region
Meningococcal polysaccharide vaccine	Microbiologists who are routinely exposed to *Neisseria meningitidis* should get meningococcal conjugate vaccine and serogroup B meningococcal vaccine. Single dose IM Booster shot every 5 years thereafter.
Typhoid vaccine	**Typhoid vaccine is recommended for:** • Travelers to parts of the world where typhoid is common • People in close contact with a typhoid carrier • Laboratory workers who work with *Salmonella typhi* bacteria **Inactivated typhoid vaccine:** • Is administered as an injection (shot). • Given to people who are 2 years or above. • One dose is recommended at least 2 weeks before travel. • Repeated doses are recommended every 2 years for people who remain at risk. **Live typhoid vaccine:** • Administered orally (by mouth). • Given to people who are 6 years or above. • One capsule is taken every other day, for a total of 4 capsules. • The last dose should be taken at least 1 week before travel. • Each capsule should be swallowed whole (not chewed) about an hour before meals with cold or lukewarm water. • A booster vaccine is needed every 5 years for people who remain at risk. • Important: live typhoid vaccine capsules must be stored in a refrigerator (not frozen).
Hepatitis A	Persons working with HAV research laboratories 2 dose schedule 0 and 6–12 months.

Post-vaccination Screening

- Post-vaccination screening (anti-HBs levels for assessing seroconversion at 1–2 months after last dose) is recommended for all healthcare workers with direct patient contact like doctors, nurses OT staff, laboratory staff, Blood Bank staff, dialysis staff.
- Ideally the levels for anti-Hbs (positive) levels is 10 or more than 10 IU/mL, which means patient has developed antibodies.
- If the test is negative (i.e., <10 IU/mL), repeat the 3 dose series and follow with anti-HBs screening, 1–2 months after the last dose.
- If repeat screening is negative, person should be tested for HBsAg to determine their HBV infection status.
  - Person who tests negative for HBsAg is considered vaccine non-responder and susceptible to HBV infection. They should be counseled about precautions to prevent HBV infection and the need to obtain hepatitis B immune globulin (HBIG) prophylaxis for any known or likely exposure to HBsAg-positive blood or blood or body fluids from a person whose HBsAg status is unknown.

Screening of Food Handlers

- All staff, to be recruited directly or on contract basis, as food handler in the Food and Beverages (F & B) department shall be screened for ova/cyst and carriage of pathogenic bacteria in their stool samples and allowed to join if the result is negative. Screening may be done in the hospital laboratory or a report from a list of laboratories approved by the hospital.
- In case of positive test results, the tests are to be repeated after the person undergoes appropriate therapy, the subsequent test result should be negative.
- Hepatitis A vaccine and typhoid vaccine are recommended for all food handlers.

Maintenance of Vaccination Record

The HR Department shall keep a copy of all records related to vaccination, serology and screening in the personal files of staff. The infection control nurse will have an oversight on the vaccination status of the employees.

Vaccination Schedule Completion

- List of persons eligible for second or third dose of vaccination of Hepatitis B shall be generated by HR department on a weekly basis.
- List will be sent to the Infection Control Nurse, Chief of Nursing, Head Admin and Medical Superintendent.
- Information will be sent to all persons on the list by email or notice.

Emergency Vaccination

Employees may need extra vaccination at the time of joining or within the course of their work due to unexpected circumstances like influenza outbreaks, etc. In such cases, recommendation made by the Hospital Infection Control Committee/Officer shall be considered and appropriate steps taken. COVID-19 vaccination drive started wherein all the healthcare workers were vaccinated as per National Guidelines.

ANNUAL HEALTH CHECK

Regular check-ups can help find potential health issues before they become a problem. Early detection provides the best chance for getting the right treatment quickly, avoiding any complications in future. Good health begins with prevention and that all starts with the individual. The aim of annual health check up help find, prevent or lessen the effect of disease **(Table 15.2)**.

The benefits of regular health checkups are as following:

- Reduces the risk of getting sick
- Detects potentially life-threatening health conditions or diseases early
- Increases chances for treatment and cure
- Limits the risk of complications by closely monitoring existing conditions
- Increases life span and improve health
- Reduces healthcare costs over time by avoiding costly medical services

TABLE 15.2: Health checks to be done at different life stages.

In 20s and 30s	• Blood pressure • Cholesterol and glucose levels • BMI, waist and hip measurements • Dental check • Eye examination • Immunizations • Testes self-checks (men) • Breast self-checks (women) • Sexually transmitted infections (STI) screenings • Pap smear every two years (women)
In 40s	• Type 2 diabetes risk assessment • Cardiovascular risk assessment • Sono-mammography (women)
In 50s and 60s	• Osteoporosis risk assessment • Bowel cancer screening (also called FOBT—fecal occult blood test) • Visual acuity and hearing impairment tests

OCCUPATIONAL HEALTH ORDINANCE

The Occupational Safety and Health Administration (OSHA) were established by the Williams-Steiger Occupational Safety and Health Act (OSH Act) of 1970, in 1971. It was to ensure that every working man and woman in the nation is employed under safe and healthful working conditions.

The OSH Act of 1970 also established a research institute called the National Institute of Occupational Safety and Health (NIOSH). Since 1973, NIOSH has been part of Centers for Disease Control (CDC). The purpose of NIOSH is to gather data documenting incidences of occupational exposure, injury, illness and death in the United States.

Purposes of Ordinance

The purposes of this ordinance are as follows:
- To ensure the safety and health of employees when they are at work
- To prescribe measures that will contribute to making the workplaces of employees safer and healthier for them
- To improve the safety and health standards applicable to certain hazardous processes, plant and substances used or kept in workplaces
- Generally to improve the safety and health aspects of working environments of employees

OSHA Record-Keeping Requirements

OSHA requires all companies subject to its workplace standards to abide by a variety of occupational regulations. All employers covered by the OSH Act are required to keep four kinds of records:
1. Records regarding enforcement of OSHA standards
2. Research records
3. Job-related injury, illness, and death records
4. Job hazard records

PREVENTION OF NEEDLE STICK INJURY

Precautions During Handling Needle

The following precautions should be taken during handling needles to prevent occupational exposures:
- **Standard precautions:** These must be followed such as hand hygiene and appropriate use of PPE while handling blood or body fluids.
- **Work surfaces:** It must be disinfected with 0.5% sodium hypochlorite solution
- **HBV vaccination**: HCWs must be immunized against HBV and protective titer must be documented.
- **Spill management:** Spill of blood and other body fluids must be properly cleaned, and surface to be 0.5% sodium hypochlorite solution.
- **Disposable needles** should be used. Needles should be never reused.
- **Never recap needles:** If unavoidable, single hand scoop technique may be followed.
- **Disposal after use:** Needles must be disposed into the sharp box immediately after use. Needles/sharps should not be left on trolleys and bedside tables.
- **Engineering control measures:** Various devices are specially designed with safety features to prevent NSI such as retractable lancets, safety lock syringes with a protective sheath and needleless IV system.

POST-EXPOSURE PROPHYLAXIS

- **First aid:** It has to be started as early as possible. Dos and Don'ts of first aid management shown in **Table 15.3**.
- **Report to the designated nodal center:** Every hospital must have a nodal center for management of NSI. In most hospitals HICC office acts as a nodal center, others hospitals may designate staff clinic or causality for the purpose **(Fig. 15.1)**.

TABLE 15.3: First aid management of exposed site.

Do's	Don'ts
• Earlier the first aid lesser is the chances of transmission BBV • For the splash injury: Irrigate thoroughly the site vigorously with water at least for 5 minutes. • Spit out immediately if gone into mouth and rinse the mouth several times. • If wearing contact lenses, leave them in place while irrigating. once the eye is cleaned, remove the contact lens and clean them in a normal manner	• Do not panic • Do not place finger into the mouth reflexively • Do not squeeze blood from wound • Do not use antiseptic and detergents.

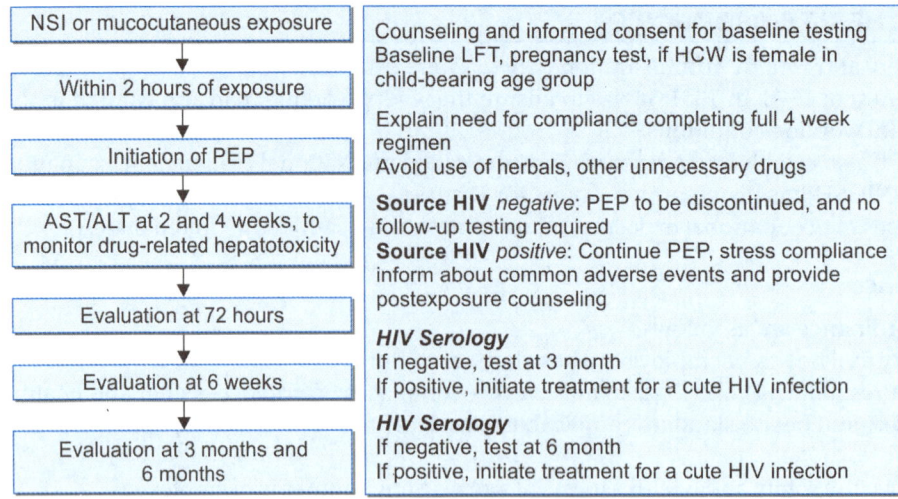

Fig. 15.1: Depicting necessary steps after needle stick injury.

- **Testing for BBVs:** The following tests are done for both source and HCW. Test method should be rapid and result should be available within 1–2 hours.
    - Anti-HIV antibody detection
    - HBsAg detection
    - Anti-HCV antibody detection
    - Anti-HBV antibody (done if previously vaccinated for HBV and titer not tested).
- **Take first dose of PEP for HIV:**
    - It should b taken as early as possible. Effect is minimum if taken <2 hours, effect is nil if taken after 72 hours.
    - **NACO recommendations:** The first dose regimen comprises of fixed dose combination of five tablets; given on the first day of exposure.
        - Tenofovir 300 mg + Lamivudine 300 mg, one tablet once daily
        - Lopinavir 200 mg + Ritonavir 50 mg two tablets twice daily.
    - If the HIV negative status of the source is documented in patients case report then first dose of PPE is not required.
    - If test report is not available then administrate the first dose regimen immediately without waiting for laboratory result.

Pathogen	Infection risk after needlestick*	Post-exposure prophylaxis (PEP) What to do?	When to Act?
Human immunodeficiency virus (HIV)	0.3%	A four-seek course of a combination of either two or three antiretroviral drugs determined on a case-by-case basis	As quickly as possible, preferably within hours
Hepatitis B virus (HBV)	Approximately 0% with PEP; 6% without PEP	HBIG alone or in combination with vaccine (if not previously vaccinated)	Preferably within 24 hours, no later than 7 days
Hepatitis C virus (HCV)	1.8%	No recommendation	N/A

- **Decision on post-exposure prophylaxis (PEP):** For HIV and HBV is taken based on guidelines (NACO for HIV and CDC for HBV).
- **Informed consent and counseling:** Almost every person feels anxious after exposure. Person should be counselled and provided with psychological support.
    - They should be informed about the risk and benefits of PEP medications.
    - PEP is not mandatory, if the exposed person refuses to take PEP, it should be documented. However, he should be made to understand about the risk of acquiring infection if PEP is not taken.
- **Documentation and recording of exposure:**
    - Structural performa should be used to collect detailed information related to exposure as date, time, and place of exposure, duration of exposure, source status, volume and type of specimen involved
    - *Consent form:* For prophylactic treatment the exposed form must sign a consent form. If the individual it should be documented.

- **Follow-up:** Testing of HCWs for BBVs should be done if the source status is positive/unknown
  - *HIV testing follow up is done:* At 6 weeks, 3 months and 6 months after exposure.
  - HBV and HCV follow up testing is done at 6 months after exposure.
- **Precautions during the follow-up period:** If the source status is positive/unknown the following precaution should be adopted by the HCW during the follow up period, especially the first 6–12 weeks.
  - Refraining from blood, semen, organ donation.
  - Abstinence from sexual intercourse or use of latex condom.
  - Women should not breastfeed their infants
  - The exposed person is advised to seek medical evaluation for any febrile illness that occurs within 12 weeks of exposure. Tables 15.4 to 15.6 show the PEP after exposure to HIV, HBV, Influenza and MMR.

TABLE 15.4: NACO guidelines for PEP for HIV (2018).		
Exposure code	**HIV source code**	**PEP recommendation**
1, 2 or 3	Negative	PEP not warranted
1	1	PEP not warranted
1	2	PEP recommended
2	1	Duration: 28 days Regimen (TL): Single daily dose of: • Tenofovir 300 mg + • Lamivudine 300 mg
2	2	
3	1 or 2	
2/3	Unknown (in area of high prevalence)	
Source	Blood, body fluids or other potentially infectious material like CSF, synovial, pleural, pericardial, amniotic fluid pus, etc., or any instrument contaminated with these substances.	

Exposure code:
1. **EC1 (mild exposure):** Mucous membrane or non intact skin exposure with small volumes or less duration, e.g.
  – Superficial wound with a plain or low caliber needle, or
  – Contact with eyes or mucous membranes, subcutaneous injections following small bore needle
2. **EC1 (moderate exposure)**
  – Mucous membrane or non-intact skin exposure with large volumes for several minutes or more duration or
  – Percutaneous superficial exposure with solid needle or superficial scratch.
3. **EC3 (severe exposure):** Percutaneous exposure with:
  – Large volume transfer
  – By hollow needle, wide bore needle, deep puncture
  – Visible blood on device
  – Needle used in patient artery or vein		

Regimens for PEP		
Primary regime for adults	*Alternate regimen for adults includes*	*Primary regime for children's*
TL: Single daily dose of Tenofovir 300 mg + Lamivudine 300 mg For pregnant women its same	**TLE:** Single daily dose of Tenofovir 300 mg + Lamivudine 300 mg + Efavirenz 600 mg **LR:** Lopinavir 200 mg + Ritonavir 50 mg two tablets daily	Zidovudine (preferred) OR Abacavir + Lamivudine + Lopinavir/Ritonavir
Side effects and compliance of PEP **Common side effects:** Nausea, diarrhea, muscular pain, headaches and fatigue, rash, fever, jaundice or abdominal or flank pain, anxiety, nightmares, psychosis, depression. Anemia, leukopenia, thrombocytopenia as side effect of zidovudine.		

TABLE 15.5: Post-exposure prophylaxis (PEP) for HBV exposure.

HCWs status	Post exposure testing		Post exposure prophylaxis		Post vaccination serological testing
	Source patient (HBsAg)	HCW testing (Anti-HBsAg)	Hepatitis B Immunoglobulin (HBIG)[0]	Vaccination	
Documented responders[1] after complete series >3 doses	No action needed				
Documented non-responders[2] after 6 doses	Positive/unknown	--------------[3]	HBIG × 2 doses, separated by 1 month	---	No
	Negative	No action needed			
Response unknown after 3 doses	Positive/unknown	<10 mIU/mL[3]	HBIG × 1 doses	Initiate revaccination with second series	Yes
	Negative	<10 mIU/mL	None		
	Any result	≥10 mIU/mL	No action needed		
Unvaccinated/incompletely vaccinated or vaccine refusers	Positive/unknown	--------------[3]	HBIG × 1 doses	Complete the vaccination	Yes
	Negative	--------------	None	Complete the vaccination	Yes

0 = administrated intramuscularly as soon a possible after exposure, if administrated >7 days effectiveness is unknown. Dosage is 0.06 mL/kg (or 10–12 IU/kg)

1 = a responder is a person with anti-HBs ≥10 mIU/mL after >3 doses of HB vaccine

2 = HCWs with anti-HBs <10 mIU/mL after >6 doses of HB vaccine

3 = HBsAg testing: HCWs with anti-HBs <10 mIU/mL, or who are vaccinated or incompletely vaccinated and sustain and expose to a source patient who is HBsAg positive or unknown, should undergo baseline testing for HBV infection (HBsAg) as soon as possible after exposure and follow up testing approximately 6 months later.

Anti-HBs antibody testing: Should be performed after 1–2 months of last dose of HB vaccine series and 4–6 months after administration of HBIG, using quantitative methods.

TABLE 15.6: Post-exposure prophylaxis (PEP) for measles influenza, pertussis and meningococcal meningitis.

	Vaccine status or type of exposure	*Recommendations*
Measles	HCEs without evidence of immunity	• First dose of MMR should given • Exclude from work from day 5 after first exposure till day 21 after the last exposure regardless of they receive Ig or not.
	If received one dose of vaccine	They may remain at work and should receive the same dose
	If received two dose of vaccine	Can continue to work with infection control measures (e.g., N95 mask)
Influenza	Close contacts, not protected	On exposure with symptomatic patients with laboratory conformed seasonal influenza A, B or H1N1 infection from 1 day before onset of symptoms until 24 hours after resolution of fever; **Chemoprophylaxis:** This is given for 7 days or during outbreaks for a minimum of 2 weeks and up to 1 week of last exposure • Oseltamivir 75 mg orally once daily • Zanamivir 10 mg (2 inhalations) once daily.
Pertussis	Close exposure defined as within 3 feet of a symptomatic patient (within 21 days of symptom onset) or coming in contact with their respiratory secretions.	Azithromycin PO, 500 mg on day 1, followed by 250 mg daily for 4 days.
Meningococcal meningitis	Close contacts, within 3 feet or contact with respiratory secretions	PEP should be taken within 24 hours of exposure if possible. • Ceftriaxone 250 mg IM single dose • Rifampicin 600 mg PO BD for 2 days • Ciprofloxacin 500 mg PO single dose.

Index

A

Absidia 84
Acid-fast bacilli 4
Acid-fast staining 30, 70
Active immunization 196
Acute pyogenic meningitis 47
Adenoviruses 73
    aerobes facultative 20
    aerobes obligate 20
Acquired active immunity 96
Albert's staining 29
Alcohols 144
Aldehydes 144
Alkaline peptone water 63
Amastigote 90
Amoebiasis 86
Anaerobes 86
Anaerobic culture methods 36, 37, 86
Ancylostoma duodenale 88
Anthrax 53
Antibodies 98
Antigen 97
Antigen-antibody reactions 97
    agglutination reaction 101
    precipitation reactions 100
Antibiotic stewardship 164
Antiretroviral drugs 80
Arboviruses 74
Ascaris lumbricoides 87
Aspergillosis 83
Aspergillus
    flavus 83, 84
    niger 83, 84
Aspergillus fumigatus 84
Atopy 94
Atypical mycobacteria 69
Australia antigen 76
Autoclave 143

B

Babes-Ernst granules 29
Bacillus antigen 53
Bacillus cereus 54
Bacteria 12
    capsule 14
    cell division 18
    cell wall 11
    cytoplasmic membrane 13
    fimbriae 16
    flagella 14
    morphology 10
    nutrition 18
    slime layer 14
    spore 17
    viable count 18
Bacterial growth curve 19
BCG vaccine 63, 108
Biomedical waste 161
Biomedical waste management 160
Biomedical waste treatment 162
Blastomyces dermatitidis 82
Blood agar 33
Blood and blood transfusion policy 174
Blood stream infections (BSI) 113
Botulism 57
Brain heart infusion agar 36

C

CAMP reaction 36
Candida albicans 82
Candidiasis 82, 83
CAPA 189
Cary-Blair medium 63
Casteneda medium 36
Catalase test 21
Catheter associated urinary tract infection (CAUTI) 115
Cell wall 11
    gram-negative 12
    gram-positive 12
Cetrimide agar 65
CLABSI 113, 114
Classical filariasis 92
Clostridium 54
Clostridium botulinum 57
Clostridium perfringens 54, 55
Clostridium tetani 55, 56
CMV 73
Coagulase negative staphylococci (CONS) 41
Coagulase test 22
Coccidioidomycosis 36
Collection of specimens 147
Complement fixation test 103
Cooked meat broth 36
Coombs' test 102
Corynebacterium diphtheriae 50
Counterimmunoelectrophoresis 101
COVID-19 vaccine 213
CPIS score 118
Cryptococcus neoformans 83
Cutaneous larva migrans 87
Cysticercus bovis 87
Cysticercus cellulosae 87
Cytomegalovirus
    laboratory diagnosis 73

D

Dane particle 76
Dengue virus 74
Dermatophytes 81
Diarrheal diseases 59, 74
Differential media 33
Dimorphic fungus 82
Disc diffusion method 34
Disinfection 142
DNA viruses 73
Donning and doffing 131, 132
Dysentery 156

E

Edward Jenner 5
Elek's gel precipitation test 52
ELISA 105
Emergency code 211
Enriched media 33, 36
Enrichment media 36
Entamoeba histolytica 85, 86
Enterobacteriaceae 58
Enterococcus faecalis 45
Enterohemorrhagic *E. coli* 59
Enteroinvasive *E. coli* 59
Enteropathogenic *E. coli* 59
Enterotoxigenic *E. coli* 59
Epidermophyton 81
Epstein-Barr virus 74
Escherichia coli 59
ETO—ethylene oxide 145
Eukaryotes 9
Extensively drug resistant tuberculosis 68

F

Filariasis 92
Filariform larva 88
Fire alarm 205
Fire extinguisher 201, 202
Fire safety 199
Food poisoning 40, 54, 57

G

Gas gangrene 54
Generation time 18
Giardia lamblia 86
Gonorrhea 49
Gram staining 28
Group B streptococci 44
Group D streptococci 44
GTTA 63

H

Hand hygiene 128, 129, 137, 141
Hand hygiene moments 194
HAV 175
HAZMAT 205
HBcAg 76
HBeAg 76
HBIG 77
HBsAg 76
HBV 76
HCV 77
HDV 77
Healthcare associated infection 111
    prevention 185
Hemagglutination test 101
Hepatitis A virus 75
Hepatitis B virus 76
Hepatitis C virus 77
Hepatitis E virus 77
Herpes zoster 72
Herpesviruses 72
Histoplasma capsulatum 82
Histoplasmosis 82
HIV 78
Hospital acquired infection 111
Human immunodeficiency virus 78

I

Iatrogenic injury 170
Immunity 94
Immunization 107
Immunofluorescence 103
Immunoglobulin classes 98, 99
India ink preparation 83
Indole test 22
Infection control committee 123
Infection control team 124, 125
Infectious hepatitis 75, 76
Innate immunity 95

Inspissation 143
Intestinal amoebiasis 86
IPSG 190
Ishikawa Fishbrne diagram 188
Isolation precautions 127

K

Killed vaccines 106
Klebsiella pneumoniae 60
Koch's phenomenon 5, 68
KOH mount 31

L

Laser safety 198
Leishmania donovani 90
Lepromin test 69
Live attenuated vaccines 106
Louis Pasteur 4
Lowenstein-Jensen medium 34
LPCB mount 31

M

MacConkey's agar 33
Malaria 91
Mantoux test 68
McIntosh and Filde's anaerobic jar 37
MDR TB 68
MDRO 165
Meningitis 47, 152
Meningococcus 47
Metachromatic granules 50
Micrococci 41
Microfilaria 92
Microsporon 81
Midstream urine specimen 59
MMR 108
Morse Fall scale 168
MR test 24
MSDS 208
Mucor 84
Multidrug resistance tuberculosis 68
Mycetoma 81
Mycobacterium leprae 69
Mycobacterium tuberculosis 66

N

Needle stick injury 215
Neisseria 47
Neisseria meningitidis 47
Non-tuberculous mycobacteria 69
NTEP 68
Nutrient agar 33

O

Occult filariasis 92
Occupation health ordinance 215

OF test 26
Oral polio vaccine 107
Orthomyxovirus 74
Oxidase test 21

P

Paracoccidioidomycosis 82
PASS 200
Pasteurization 143
Paul-Bunnell test 74
PEP 80, 46, 47, 218
Personal protective equipment (PPE) 129
Petroff's method 67
Photochromogens 69
Plasmodium 91
Pneumococcus 45
Polioviruses 74
PPA test 27
Precipitation reaction 100
Prokaryotes 9
Promastigote 90
Proteus 60
Pseudomonas aeruginosa 65
Pulmonary tuberculosis 67
PUO 151

Q

Quantitative buffy coat test 92
Quellung reaction 46

R

Rabies virus 74
RACE 200
Radiation safety 198
Radioimmunoassay 104
Rapid growers 69
Restraints 171, 172
Rhinosporidiosis 82
Rhizopus 84
Rickettsia 72
Ridley and Jopling's classification 69
RNA viruses 74
Robert Koch 4
Robertsoncooked meat media 36
Root case analysis 188
Rotaviruses 74

S

Salmonella 61
Salmonella typhi 61,62
SBAR 182, 192
Scotochromogens 69
Serum hepatitis 75
Shigella 60
Significant bacteria 60
Sore throat 45, 154
Spaulding's principle 146

Staphylococcus aureus 39, 40
Staphylococcus epidermidis 41
Staphylococcus saprophyticus 41
Sterilization 142
Streptococcus 42
Streptococcus pneumoniae 45
Streptococcus pyogenes 42
Superficial mycoses 81
Surgical safety 181, 193
Surgical site infection rate 122
Surgical site infections (SSIs) 119
Surveillance 123

T

Taenia saginata 87
Taenia solium 87
TCBS agar 34, 64
Tetanus 56
Thayer-Martin medium 33, 47
Trichophyton 81
Triple sugar iron test (TSI) 23
Trypanosoma 90
TSST 40

U

Universal immunization program 107
Urease test 23
Urine analysis 154
UTI 59

V

Viral transport medium (VTM) 35
VP test 25

Vibrios 63
Vaccines 106
VAE 116
Vaccination 212
Vaginal swab 155
Vulnerable patients 168
Vacutainers 148, 149

W

Western blot test 80
Widal test 62
Wilson and Blair media 34
Wuchereria bancrofti 92

Z

Ziehl-Neelsen staining 30
Zoonosis 71